PENGUIN BOOKS
THE FAMILY FITNESS HANDBOOK

Bob Glover is president of Robert H. Glover and Associates, Inc., a fitness and marketing consulting firm. He developed and serves as the national director for the Post Raisin Bran Family Fitness Program. Glover started coaching youth sports at the age of thirteen and has thirty years' experience working in the area of youth fitness with such organizations as the U.S. Army Special Services, Little League and Babe Ruth League Baseball, and the YMCA. He directed a model family fitness program at the Rome (NY) Family Y that served thousands of youngsters of all ages and their parents, and now enjoys coaching "Sports Club" for his son and his son's grade-school friends. He founded and directs the New York Road Runners Club's youth fitness program, which serves thousands of youngsters. Additionally, he serves as director of adult educational programs for the twenty-five-thousand–member organization and coaches three thousand members per year in his classes for beginning and competitive runners. He also co-founded the Achilles Track Club (for disabled youth and adult athletes) and founded and coaches the elite women's racing team Atalanta, which has won many national titles in both the open and masters categories. An all-around athlete who has played, officiated, and coached in all major sports, he gained his most satisfaction as a long-distance runner. A high-school county champion at two miles and a three-time gold medalist at the Hue Sports Festival during the Vietnam War, he competed for thirty years at distances ranging from a quarter-mile to fifty miles. Glover consults with many major corporations and athletic clubs, is a member of the board of advisors for the American Running & Fitness Association, a member of the American Alliance for Health, Physical Education, Recreation and Dance, and is a columnist for *Runner's World* magazine. He is author of six books, with combined sales approaching the one million mark, including his first book, *The Runner's Handbook*, which was an immediate best-seller. Glover lives in New York City with his wife, Virginia, and their son, Christopher, born in 1981, who was an honorary co-author of this book by being a role model.

Jack Shepherd is author of eight books, including the national best-seller *The Adams Chronicles*, and, with Bob Glover, *The Runner's Handbook*. He graduated from Haverford College and Columbia University, earning his Ph.D. at Boston University. As a foreign-policy specialist, he has worked for the Carnegie Endowment for International Peace in Washington, D.C. His articles have appeared in *Newsweek, Harper's,* the *Atlantic, Vermont Life, Saturday Review,* the *New York Times Magazine, Reader's Digest,* and other periodicals. He and his wife, Kathy, live in Norwich, Vermont, where they both run, cross-country ski, canoe, and hike in the Green and White mountains. Their two children, born in 1964 and 1967, are active young adults who go rock climbing, kayaking along the Alaskan coastline, cross-country skiing, and mountain climbing. Their son Caleb was captain of his New Hampshire high-school lacrosse team in both his junior and senior years and tri-captain of the Haverford College lacrosse team. Their daughter Kristen works for the Washington Wilderness Coalition, lobbies for environmental protection, and hikes in the Olympic and Cascade mountains.

Also by Bob Glover

The Runner's Handbook: The Classic Fitness Guide
for Beginning and Intermediate Runners
by Bob Glover and Jack Shepherd (1978, 1985)

The Runner's Handbook Training Diary
by Bob Glover and Jack Shepherd (1978, 1989)

The New Competitive Runner's Handbook
by Bob Glover and Pete Schuder (1983, 1988)

The Injured Runner's Training Handbook
by Bob Glover and Dr. Murray Weisenfeld (1985)

Bob Glover
and Jack Shepherd

The Family Fitness Handbook

PENGUIN BOOKS

PENGUIN BOOKS
Published by the Penguin Group
Viking Penguin, a division of Penguin Books USA Inc.,
40 West 23rd Street, New York, New York 10010, U.S.A.
Penguin Books Ltd, 27 Wrights Lane,
London W8 5TZ, England
Penguin Books Australia Ltd, Ringwood,
Victoria, Australia
Penguin Books Canada Ltd, 2801 John Street,
Markham, Ontario, Canada L3R 1B4
Penguin Books (N.Z.) Ltd, 182-190 Wairau Road,
Auckland 10, New Zealand

Penguin Books Ltd, Registered Offices:
Harmondsworth, Middlesex, England

First published in Penguin Books 1989
Published simultaneously in Canada

10 9 8 7 6 5 4 3 2 1

Grateful acknowledgment is made for permission to
reprint the following:
Excerpts from *The Aerobics Program for Total Well Being* by
Kenneth H. Cooper, M.D., M.P.H. Copyright © 1982 by
Kenneth H. Cooper. Reprinted by permission of Bantam Books, a
division of Bantam Doubleday Dell Publishing Group, Inc.
Excerpts from "The Shape of the Nation: A Survey of State
Physical Education Requirements" and "The Bill of Rights for
Young Athletes." Used by permission of the American Alliance for
Health, Physical Education, Recreation, and Dance.
"Code of Ethics" from *Parenting Your Superstar*
by Robert J. Rotella and Linda K. Bunker.
Reprinted by permission of Leisure Press, Champaign, Illinois.

LIBRARY OF CONGRESS CATALOGING IN PUBLICATION DATA
Glover, Bob.
The family fitness handbook.
1. Physical fitness.   2. Physical fitness for
children.   I. Shepherd, Jack.   II. Title.
GV481.G56 1989   613.7'042   88–29004
ISBN 0 14 046.863 3 (pbk.)

Printed in the United States of America
Set in Meridien
Designed by Victoria Hartman

Dedication

Mike Wiley

On Friday the 13th of March 1987, luck ran out on a happy-go-lucky guy named Mike Wiley. Mike, who was always helping others, had stopped to aid a stranded motorist. He was hit by a speeding car and killed. The previous May, his eight-year-old son, my buddy Sam Wiley, had been struck by lightning while playing basketball with his dad, and killed. Only a few weeks earlier, my son and I had played ball with them on the same field. Oh, how Mike and I had rejoiced at re-living our youth through our young sons!

Mike Wiley was my roommate when I started my fitness career in Rome, New York. He was my volleyball mentor, basketball teammate, running partner, and partying buddy. Most of all, he was my best friend and greatest inspiration. It was Mike who challenged me, with a bet after an all-night party, to run my first marathon. That experience, the 1973 Kansas Relays Marathon, changed my life and led me down the road to a successful career as a running/fitness coach. And it was Mike who, by his example, also challenged me to commit myself to a career of helping others.

As much as I remember Mike Wiley as an athlete and friend, it was his love for his family that I most admired. Mike and his sons shared more than simple father-son love. They were best friends and confidants. I loved Mike and Sam in such a special way: they were mirror images of my son, Christopher, and me. The two sudden unexpected deaths of Mike and Sam stole my best friend and his son from me, but they gave something back. To Brenda Wiley and Mike's other son, Jay, I promise that Mike's friendship and spirit will forever push me to help others. That promise lies at the heart of this book: to give the gift of health and fitness to parents and their kids who love each other the way Mike and Sam did.

Elan Benjamin

We would also like to dedicate this book to the memory of Christopher's classmate Elan Benjamin, who loved sports and was good at telling jokes.

Acknowledgments

A book of this length is always the work of more people than the author alone. This book on family fitness must start with my thanks to my own family.

My parents, Corinne and H. Ross Glover of Dansville, New York, played sports with me as a child and encouraged me in fitness activities throughout my lifetime. My mother always managed to find the time to cheer her sons on in our sports activities and set an early example of good nutritional habits for lifetime gifts. I fondly recall my father playing catch with me and my brothers in the backyard for hours, his volunteering to coach our Little League Baseball team, and his efforts to get a Babe Ruth League started so we could play as thirteen-to-fifteen-year-olds and then an American Legion Baseball League so we could play as sixteen-to-eighteen-year-olds.

My brother Don contributed in ways he probably doesn't recall. We rode bikes together, played catch, and took up each sport in season. He made it all the way from the Dansville Little League state finalist team to pitch his high-school team to its only Section V state baseball championship. Now, certainly in part because of our upbringing, Don and I are encouraging our own children to be physically active. His four boys—Matthew, Mark, Michael, and Daniel Glover—are all sports players and fitness enthusiasts.

On my team, Virginia has continued our parents' good nutritional habits for our son, Christopher (and for me), and she serves as a daily role model for him by running, biking, skating, and taking aerobics classes.

In truth, one of the most important people in the development of this book was our son, Christopher Glover. Thank you, buddy, for all the fun we had exercising together, which became the inspiration for this book, and for testing and helping to invent the games and fitness activities we've put in here.

In turn, Christopher wants to thank his friends in the Sports Club we started whose enthusiasm has been infectious. They include: Bradley Bayer, Adam Cohen, Chris Hamilton, Taylor Harris, Hunter Knight, Liam Millhiser, Kayle Morrison, Tim Sacks, Owen Strock, and Ryan Young. Chris also wants to thank the sports partners he has had since he was two years old: Alan Flamenhaft, Jason McKenney, and Justin Pront. Last, but never least, is his sports friend and fellow runner David Pena.

Christopher's cousins Katharine and Jennifer Thomas joined our family as subjects for the cover of this book, and we appreciate their help.

Dozens of men and women have influenced my attitudes about sports and fitness—too many to name them all. You know who you are, and I thank you for your contributions to my development as a fit person and a fitness specialist. Some, however, deserve special mention.

Robert Elia, executive director of the Enterprise, Alabama, YMCA, was my first employer when I returned from the Vietnam War. He guided me into "People Work." George Goyer hired me as fitness director of the ambitious, new Rome (New York) Family Y, despite my lack of experience (I did not lack enthusiasm). He taught me the basics of family fitness programming. The late Bill Coughlin, then athletic director at Rome Free Academy, served as my Sports-Fitness Committee chairman and provided expertise and friendship that proved invaluable.

Alexander Melleby has been my role model as a fitness leader and was perhaps the finest physical education instructor in the long history of the YMCA's service. Al hired and trained me to be his fitness director at one of the largest and most active Y's in the United States, the West Side YMCA in New York City. His professional training and friendship have shaped me and are deeply appreciated.

Much of the fitness philosophy in my work and writing is based on the teaching and research of Dr. Hans Kraus, the co-developer with Al Melleby of the Y's "Way to a Healthy Back" program. Dr. Kraus, who served as fitness advisor to Presidents Eisenhower and Kennedy, has also been my unofficial grandfather. Now in his eighties, he still practices what he preaches by leading an active life. His help with my career and the research and development of this book, and his wise words in the foreword, are greatly appreciated.

Two organizations and one school helped significantly with this book. The New York Road Runners Club, directed by president Fred Lebow, enthusiastically embraced my idea of promoting youth fitness through running. As a result, the pre-school and youth running programs I developed for the NYRRC served as the basis for those sections of this book, and a source of fitness and fun for Christopher.

The American Alliance for Health, Physical Education, Recreation and Dance has developed surveys and programs to promote fitness and health for our children and their schools. The AAHPERD's leadership is making a major impact on our nationwide youth fitness problem. They deserve our support. Thanks, therefore, to Lisa Clough, director of media services for AAHPERD, for her help in researching this book.

I also must thank the Allen-Stevenson School in New York City—Christopher's school—which served as the model for the physical education discussed in Chapter 8. Special appreciation goes to Headmaster Desmond Cole, Deputy Head Jessie-Lea Hayes, and Physical Education Director Patrick Lappin for working closely with me in developing a model school fitness program.

Bruce Grieve, group brand manager for General Foods U.S.A., Breakfast Food Division, and his associates made a commitment to combating the problem of declining youth fitness by sponsoring the Post Raisin Bran Family Fitness Program under my direction and in coordination with the publication of this book. Their insight and enthusiasm are greatly appreciated.

Finally, Jack Shepherd should be thanked—I *think*—for starting me on all this writing. He took my Beginner Runner class at the West Side Y in 1975, and has been running ever since. He suggested that we collaborate on *The Runner's Handbook,* and when it reached the *New York Times* national best-seller list, I was hooked on writing and Shepherd was hooked on running. He's even finished two New York City marathons—which he swears are easier than writing books. I agree. I certainly appreciate, as you undoubtedly will also, his clear and enthusiastic writing style. More than that, I value his friendship.

Contents

Dedication   vii
Acknowledgments   ix
Foreword   xxv
Introduction   xxvii

PART ONE: THE UNFITNESS REVOLUTION

Chapter 1 ▪ The Epidemic of Unfitness   3
   The Unfitness Revolution
   Fitness History
   Today's Parents vs. Their Kids
   Causes of Unfitness
         Lifestyle
         Parents
         Schools
         Community
   The Challenge

Chapter 2 ▪ The Benefits of Fitness   18
   What Is Physical Fitness?
   Health-Related Fitness
         Cardio-respiratory Endurance
         Body Composition
         Flexibility
         Muscular Strength and Endurance
   The Benefits
         Physical Benefits
         Psychological Benefits
         Intellectual Benefits

Fitness Activities and Competitive Sports
Benefits of Team Sports

PART TWO: CHILD/PARENT/FAMILY

Chapter 3 ▪ The Role of the Parent and Family   33
Where to Start
The Parental Role Model
    The Exerciser's Triangle
Family Involvement
    The Aerobic Family
Family Exercise
    The Three F's: Fun, Fellowship, and Fitness
    Learn to Play Like a Child
    Tips for Family Exercise
Parental Responsibilities
    Education
    Nutrition
    Start Early
    Eliminate Shortcuts
    Control TV Watching
    Think Long Term
Encourage Your Child
    Give Your Kids a Place to Play
    Don't Hold Them Back Too Much
    Encourage, Don't Compare
    Establish Incentive Goals and Rewards
Encourage a Variety of Activities
    Playgrounds and Parks
    Give Your Kids Active Toys
    Encourage After-School Activities
    Balance Lifetime Sports with Competitive Sports

Chapter 4 ▪ Family Fitness Evaluation Tests   57
Test #1: Kraus-Weber
Test #2: Flexibility
Test #3: Muscular Strength and Endurance
Test #4: Aerobic Tests

PART THREE: CHILD/TEACHER/SCHOOL

Chapter 5 ▪ Physical Education in the School   81
Tools for Parents

Chapter 6 ▪ The Square Deal: The Four Critical Cornerstones of a Quality Physical Education Program   89
Appropriate, Year-round, Quality Physical Activity
Fitness Testing and Reporting
Wellness Education in the Classroom and Lunchroom
Parental Involvement

Chapter 7 ▪ A Parent's Guide to Evaluating Your Child's School Physical Education Program   97
Administration
Physical Activity
Fitness Testing and Reporting
Wellness Education in the Classroom and Lunchroom
Parental Involvement

Chapter 8 ▪ A Model School Physical Education Program   103
The Allen-Stevenson Model
  School Philosophy
  The Four Cornerstones of Physical Education
Fitness and Sports Activities
  Quality of Activity
  Aerobic Activity
  The Fitness Class
  Walking
  Running
  Activity Sessions
Fitness Testing
Wellness Education in the Classroom and Lunchroom
Parental Involvement

Chapter 9 ▪ Other Innovative School Programs   118
Southside Elementary School, Johnson City, Tennessee
South Huntington School District, Huntington Station, New York
Leal Elementary School, Urbana, Illinois
Black Elementary School, Sterling Heights, Michigan
P.S. 118, Queens, New York

South Bronx High School, Bronx, New York
P.S. 20, Brooklyn, New York
The Horizon School, Phoenix, Arizona
Elkton Elementary School, Elkton, Virginia
Beverly Hills School District, Beverly Hills, California

PART FOUR: GETTING FIT

Chapter 10 • Getting Fit: Exercise Principles 131
    Exercise Principles
        Principle 1: Overload—The FIT Training Method
        Principle 2: Progressive Stress—Train, Don't Strain
        Principle 3: Recovery—The Hard-Easy Method
        Principle 4: Regularity
        Principle 5: Specificity
        Principle 6: Variation
        Principle 7: Adaptability
        Principle 8: Being Patient
        Principle 9: Moderation
        Principle 10: Share the Flowers
    The 1-2-3 Method
        1. The Warm-up
        2. Peak Work
        3. The Cool-down
    A Sample Total Fitness Workout

Chapter 11 • Getting Fit: Flexibility and Muscular Strength and Endurance 140
    Flexibility
    Guidelines for Flexibility Exercises
    A Relaxation and Stretching Program for the Family
    Muscular Strength and Endurance
    A Strength Training Program for the Family
    Weight Training
        Youths to Age Sixteen
        Adolescents and Adults
    Sample Weight Training Routine

Chapter 12 • Getting Fit: Cardio-respiratory Endurance 154
    Aerobic Exercise
    Aerobic Exercise for Kids
    What Kinds of Aerobic Exercise?

Three Key Variables to Aerobic Training
    Frequency
    Time
    Intensity

Chapter 13 ▪ Imaginative Fitness Workouts 166
The Warm-up
    Relaxation Exercises
    Stretching Exercises
    Strengthening Exercises
    Cardio-respiratory Warm-up
Safari Aerobics
Fitness Freeze Aerobics
The Cool-down

Chapter 14 ▪ Imaginative Fitness Games 170
Fast-Moving Action Games
    Tag
    Cops and Robbers
    Hide-and-Seek
    Follow the Leader
    Keep Away
    Tug-of-War
    Simon Says
    Rock and Roll
    Kangaroo Jumping
    Parachute Game
    Logrolling
    Relay Races
    Obstacle Course
    Fitness Circuit Training
    Dodgeball
    Aerobic Soccer
    Aerobic Volleyball
    Frisbee Football
    Home Run Aerobics
    Fast-break Basketball
    Aerobic Kite Flying
    Tom Sawyer Adventure Hikes
    Shuttle Run
    Body Slam
    Ocean Wave Running

Winter Games
Snowball Tag
Uphill Sledding
Sled Pulling Races
Making Tracks
Snow Baseball
Snow Shoveling

PART FIVE: LIFETIME AEROBIC FITNESS ACTIVITIES

Chapter 15 ▪ Aerobic Fitness Activities   183
Selecting Your Activities
Cross-Country Skiing
Roller-Skating and Ice-Skating
Tennis, Handball, Racquetball, and Squash
Canoeing and Rowing
Jumping Rope
Dancing
Aerobic Dance Exercise
Aerobics for Kids

Chapter 16 ▪ Biking   196
Safety Guidelines for Biking
Bikes for Kids
Safety for Children
Adult Bikes
Biking the Right Way
Getting Fit with Biking
Competing
Touring
Family Biking
Clothing and Accessories
Stationary Bikes

Chapter 17 ▪ Running   207
Running and Children
Starting the Kids Running
Pre-school Running Tips
Elementary School Age Tips
Tips for Teenage Runners
Training for Elementary Age and Teenagers
Where to Run

How Fast?
Parental Competition
Running the Right Way
Equipment
Injury Prevention
Getting Fit with Running
   Start with Walking
Beginner Runner
   Method 1: The 20-Minute Run-Easy Program
   Method 2: The One-and-a-Half–Mile Run-Easy Program
   Method 3: The New York Road Runners Club Run-Easy
     Program
Advanced Beginner
Intermediate Runner
Fun Racing and Competition
Competition for Kids
Running-based Fitness Programs for Kids

Chapter 18 ▪ Swimming   226
Swimming for Kids
Competitive Swimming
Water Exercise
Safety Guidelines
Getting Fit with Swimming
   Swim-for-Fitness Training Program for Beginners and
     Intermediates
The Warm-up and Cool-down
Swimming the Right Way
Equipment and Facilities

Chapter 19 ▪ Walking   236
Walking for Kids and Families
   Special Supplies
   Games Along the Way
   Exploring: Tom Sawyer Adventure Walks
Groups
Equipment
How to Walk
Getting Fit with Walking
When to Walk
Where to Walk
Increasing the Challenge

Racewalking
Marching
Hiking, Tours, and Vacations
Walking Events

PART SIX: FITNESS AND SPORTS

Chapter 20 ▪ **Pre-schoolers   253**
Birth to One Year: Age of Self-Discovery
  Birth to Three Months
  Three to Six Months
  Six to Nine Months
  Nine to Twelve Months
Ages One to Two: Walking and Running
The Terrible Twos
Ages Three to Five
Pre-school Exercise Programs
Exercise Equipment, Records, and Videos
Physical Education

Chapter 21 ▪ **Teenagers   263**
What Can We Do?
  Watch Our Kids
  Pay Attention to Them
  Eat with Them
  Exercise with Them

Chapter 22 ▪ **Girls and Women   269**
History
  Why Do Girls Quit Exercising?
  The Parents' Role
Should Physical Activity be Coed?
  Before Puberty
  After Puberty
  Adult Coed Sports
  The Results
Obstacles
Male vs. Female: The Differences
  Injuries
  Equipment
  Coaching

Chapter 23 ▪ The Health Impaired and Physically Disabled   281
Mainstreaming
The Achilles Track Club
The Achilles Track Club Youth Program
Fitness for the Handicapped
The Orthopedically Impaired
The Hearing Impaired
The Visually Impaired
Arthritis
Asthma
Cancer
Cardiac Rehabilitation
Diabetes
Epilepsy
Obesity
The Emotionally Disturbed and Mentally Handicapped

Chapter 24 ▪ Youth and Sports   294
Participation
When Should Kids Start Playing Team Sports?
Choosing a Sport
Dropouts from Sports
Getting Cut
Sports-related Stress
Winning and Losing
Sportsmanship
The Parents' Role in Youth Sports
Codes of Ethics for Athletes, Parents, and Coaches

Chapter 25 ▪ A Model Youth Sports Program   314
Starting a Sports Club
Success-oriented Philosophy
Sports Club Baseball
Sports Club Basketball
Family Sports Day

Chapter 26 ▪ Injury Prevention and Treatment   320
Sports and Youth Injuries
Youth Injury Causes
Preventing Injury
Pre-exercise Health Evaluation
Physical Conditioning

Nutrition, Drugs, and Sleep
Protective Equipment and Facilities
Supervision
The Overuse Syndrome
Caring for Your Own Body
Emergencies
Listen to the Warning Signals
Heat Injuries
Cold Injuries
Colds and Flu

PART SEVEN: WELLNESS

Chapter 27 • The Holistic Approach to Health and Fitness   335
Wellness Quiz
Smoking
    Kids and Smoking
Alcohol and Drug Abuse

Chapter 28 • Stress Management   349
What Causes Stress?
What's Stressful?
Stress and Adults
Stress and Children
Dealing with Stress

Chapter 29 • Nutrition   364
The Four Basic Food Groups
Nutrients
Junk Foods
Cholesterol and Triglycerides
Fiber
Good Eating Habits
Kids and Nutrition
Nutritional Tips for Children
Families and Meals
    Breakfast
    Lunch
    Dinner
The Family Meal

Chapter 30 • Weight Management   380
Calories

Weight
Body Composition
Losing Weight
Weight for Children
   A Formula for Children's Body Weight
Summary

Appendix ▪ Fitness, Health, and Sports Resources **391**

Index 409

Foreword

In the 1950s, public attention was first focused on the fact that the nation's children were deplorably unfit. It was discovered that they were watching TV instead of participating in active games, riding in buses and cars instead of walking—in other words, viewing instead of doing.

At first, good physical education seemed like the answer. However, P.E. became and remained mired in games. Games help those children who need help least and make viewers of the ones who are unfit to join the teams.

The Swiss program, if adopted, might provide a possible remedy: one hour of fitness work every day, with team sports optional. The program favors carryover sports like bicycling, tennis, and swimming.

Few schools have made the necessary change. But even if the Swiss program were to be adopted, this would be only part of the answer.

It is also necessary to encourage good exercise habits and to restrict TV time; this is the parents' domain. Physically active parents can set a good example for their children to follow.

In this respect Bob Glover's book fills a long-standing need. His past experience in physical education, his work as an instructor in the "Y's Way to a Healthy Back" program, his leadership in the New York Road Runners Club, and last, but not least, his success in raising an active youngster give him all the qualifications needed to write this book.

In following Bob Glover's career, I have seen him develop into an outstanding fitness expert. His balanced program begins with relaxation, limbering, warming, and stretching before proceeding to aerobic workouts; it then reverses to cool down his students.

The author describes in detail how to make such programs palatable and even attractive to youngsters. He also discusses ways of influencing schools, teachers, and other groups.

Bob Glover's book is must reading for parents interested in their child's well-being. Fitness in the young can help prevent sickness in the adult. It forms the basis for an emotionally and physically balanced person.

—Hans Kraus, M.D.
Medical Consultant to President's Council
on Physical Fitness and Sports
Youth Fitness Advisor to
President Eisenhower and President Kennedy

Introduction

This is a book about—and for—parents, teachers, and kids.

In the 1930s, my father walked more than two miles to school every day in rural Canaseraga, New York. At lunchtime, he walked home to eat and then walked back to school. After school, he hiked that two-mile road for the fourth time in the day. He didn't call it exercise, he called it transportation. That was the way most rural American kids in the 1930s got to and from home and school. My mother, growing up in South Dansville, New York, walked three miles to a one-room schoolhouse and then after school walked three miles home in time to help with farm chores. Asked what they did for family fitness in her youth, my mother laughed and said: "In our days, and for my parents and grandparents, farming was the family exercise."

I grew up after World War II, when technological improvements were rapidly changing the way we lived. Although I walked a mile to school as a six-year-old, many children in those days rode to school in a car or on a school bus. I remember riding my bike after school all over town and playing cops and robbers or hide-and-seek for hours at a time. My brother and I played sports all summer, almost from the time we woke up until it was too dark to see the ball anymore.

We were part of the postwar "baby boom" that lasted until 1960 or so. Millions of children were born during a time of major sociological changes, including the rapid mechanization and urbanization of America.

Little by little, my brother and I saw our playing fields bulldozed for housing, shopping malls, or highways. Junk food became widely available. Affordable cars, movies, television, and the start-up of big-time college and professional spectator sports all combined to make us more sedentary. Our parents and we ourselves began to fall victim to what my friend and mentor

Dr. Hans Kraus calls "hypokinetic disease"—caused by lack of exercise. We needed to put regular exercise back into our lives.

During the 1970s, increases in cardiovascular disease, stress, and a growing awareness of the health dangers of excess weight, smoking, and the sedentary life created an exercise revolution. Millions of American men and women started down the road to fitness. Dr. Ken Cooper led the way with his series of *Aerobics* books. In the late 1970s, three running books placed high on the *New York Times* best-seller list—including my first book, *The Runner's Handbook,* which became a classic in the field.*

One convert to fitness was my father. With increased mechanization in his life, he got less exercise than he had as a boy and had more time and money to eat and live "well." He gained weight and his blood pressure shot up beyond the safe range. I encouraged him to watch his diet and to start a walking program, and now he is almost as trim as he was when I, as his young son, looked up to him as a role model.

Although many adult Americans are still not physically fit, progress has been made since the early 1970s in decreasing incidents of heart disease and overcoming our sedentary lifestyle. The "wellness revolution" of the 1980s helped educate millions of adults about the need for exercise combined with eating wisely, managing stress, and eliminating tobacco, drugs, and alcohol.

But that's us—the current generation of adults. Between 1945 and 1960, more than four million of us were born on average each year. We, including myself, are now parents or are becoming parents at a rapid pace. Encouraged by a strong economy, just as our parents were hopeful following the war, many of us are now starting families. Our nations's pre-school and lower elementary school population is the largest in twenty years.

These children—our children—are being born into a society that is now firmly trapped by its own technological advancement. Most physical exertion has been taken out of our lives. We can travel great distances, communicate with people anywhere in the world, be entertained—all without walking very far, let alone breaking into sweat. Our children ride to and from school; when they get home, they are entertained by a variety of electronic gadgets.

With the arrival of Christopher Ross Glover in 1981, a second fitness revolution took place—in our family. No longer do I train ten to fifteen miles a day for competitive racing. I exercise for personal fitness and to create a model for Christopher, as does my wife and his mother, Virginia.

---

*Since then, my Runner's Handbook trilogy—*The Runner's Handbook, The Runner's Handbook Training Diary,* and *The New Competitive Runner's Handbook*—has sold more than 500,000 copies.

Several times a week Christopher and I exercise together. I even helped start some youth fitness/sports programs at Christopher's elementary school so that I could exercise with him and his friends.

Kids change us. They make us recall our own youth. We seek ways to help them get more from life than we did. When I think of Mike Wiley, to whom this book is dedicated, and my own family, I realize that I want to help create the second fitness revolution among the new generation of America's sons and daughters. As the opening chapter details, they have been left behind.

To do this, I've drawn on my own experiences—growing up and playing in the small town of Dansville, New York; coaching youth teams; and directing YMCA programs in Enterprise, Alabama, and in Rome, New York, for thousands of youngsters. I've also drawn on words from my mentors in physical fitness, particularly Dr. Kraus, who was promoting the need for youth fitness before I was born. He often told me when I worked with him in adult fitness that we were merely doing "reclamation" work—that to make a real impact on our nation's poor fitness levels we needed to start with our children. That is the hope of this book.

To develop a program for kids I needed to work with one. Therefore most of the research and concepts for this book were developed day-to-day as my son, Christopher, became more and more a part of my exercising life. My experiences working with him and with his school's physical education program confirmed my sense that this book is necessary and can make a difference.

Christopher has been a very enthusiastic co-author: he helped create many of the activities detailed here and served as an inspiration to me that children might indeed learn to enjoy exercise. The joy of sharing exercise with one's own child is something that should be cherished by everyone. Not only am I helping him develop a healthy body and mind for life, but he is also helping me feel young again in a special way. Together, we hope we have created something for other parents and their children to enjoy.

This book is primarily designed for children between five and twelve years old—kindergarten through about the sixth grade. This is where, as Dr. Kraus suggested, we should most seek to improve fitness and develop sound fitness habits. Guidelines for pre-schoolers and teenagers are also discussed. The book's objectives include:

- To create a parent's and teacher's guide for improving the fitness level of children using a variety of imaginative, practical, and success-oriented activities.
- To involve the parent as a role model by encouraging him or her to

participate in both an individual fitness program and in a family fitness program.

- To enhance the family unit—under siege now for almost twenty years—by helping families to enjoy physical activity and good health together. I hope you will discover that exercise with your kids is a lifelong gift of love.

Part 1

THE UNFITNESS REVOLUTION

The Epidemic
of Unfitness

Is fitness passing our children by?

If you are an American between the ages of thirty and seventy, and you read fitness books, chances are you are participating in one of the greatest health revolutions among adults in this country's history. During the 1970s and 1980s, men and women in the United States began exercising aerobically—running, biking, swimming, and walking—in unprecedented numbers. Researchers are now confirming a parallel reduction in the diseases of inactivity among active adult Americans.

But we have left our children at home. Oddly enough, they are not exercising as much as we. The fitness boom among adults is passing them by. According to two major fitness surveys in the 1980s,* at least half of all U.S. school-age children do not participate in enough vigorous exercise. That is, most of our kids don't work up an aerobic sweat for at least twenty minutes, three times a week—the minimum required to maintain an effectively functioning cardio-respiratory system.

"We are under the impression that youth are the most vigorous segment of the [U.S.] population," wrote Dr. Robert Gold, project director of the 1984 National Children and Youth Fitness Study (NCYFS). "However, young and middle-aged adults are probably as fit or more fit than what appears to be the case among [U.S.] school children."

* The 1984 "National Children and Youth Fitness Study" by the United States Department of Health in association with the American Alliance for Health, Physical Education, Recreation and Dance; the 1985 "School Population Fitness Survey" by the President's Council on Physical Fitness and Sports and the University of Michigan.

THE UNFITNESS REVOLUTION

The results of this inactivity are dismaying:

- Half of our girls between the ages of six and seventeen, and 30 percent of our boys ages six to twelve, cannot run a mile in less than ten minutes—a task that can be accomplished by most of their parents, average middle-aged joggers, and many senior citizens.
- Among two hundred California schoolchildren—indicative of nationwide unfitness—in 1988, more than half could not finish the thirty-meter swim test used in the Soviet Union's school system.
- Dr. Kenneth Cooper, whose book *Aerobics* started American adults down the road to fitness, directed a ten-year study of 167,000 U.S. kids ages five to seventeen through his Institute of Aerobic Research. The outcome: compared to kids in the same age bracket in 1975, the kids were in worse shape, and 40 percent of the children of the 1980s scored below the national fitness norms.

The Amateur Athletic Union (AAU) found similar results: 57 percent of four million U.S. children ages six to seventeen failed to meet AAU fitness standards for an "average healthy youngster" in 1979–80. A follow-up in 1984 showed that 64 percent couldn't meet the "average" standard. By 1987, the fitness failure rate among nine million U.S. youngsters had reached 71 percent. In brief, our kids today are in worse shape than those of a decade ago.

- Forty percent of boys ages six to fifteen cannot reach beyond their toes—a minimum standard for flexibility in the sit-and-reach test.
- Forty percent of our boys and 70 percent of our girls can do only one pushup. Forty-five percent of our boys ages six to fourteen and 55 percent of our girls cannot hold their chins over a raised bar for more than ten seconds.
- Twenty-five percent of all U.S. youngsters, according to Dr. Kraus, cannot do a single bent-knee sit-up because they lack sufficient abdominal strength.

What do these figures mean in terms of our children's health? A 1985 President's Council on Physical Fitness and Sports survey pointed out:

> The low levels of trunk flexibility revealed by boys indicates a good chance of developing back problems in later life. Low back problems are generally

caused by either weak abdominals, tight hamstrings, or both, and are one of this country's leading problems in the workplace.

Upper arm and shoulder muscle girdle strength and endurance for both boys and girls was poor. It remains a significant weakness in our youth. *Many have insufficient strength to handle their own body weight in case of emergency and were judged as being often unable to carry on daily work or physically demanding recreational activities successfully or safely.* [Emphasis added.]

Our kids are not only dangerously out of shape and unable to "carry on daily work or physically demanding recreational activities," but they are also fat: the two go together. According to the Center for Adolescent Obesity at the University of California, as many as twenty million American youngsters, including almost one-third of children ages six to eleven, may be overweight. Researchers Steven Gortmaker of the Harvard School of Public Health and Dr. William Dietz of the New England Medical Center in Boston found that by 1980 the number of obese kids in the United States had increased 54 percent since 1963; the number who fell into the "super obese" category had risen 98 percent. According to the National Center for Health Statistics, about 80 percent of overweight teenagers will remain overweight as adults.

These two characteristics—low fitness levels and obesity—are having a serious impact on our kids' health. The President's Council reported in 1985: "There was a low level of performance by large numbers of boys and girls on cardio-respiratory endurance tests. Low levels in this component are related to early fatigue in physical activities. High levels of cardio-respiratory endurance have been shown to be related to a reduction in heart disease and to a longer life span." The conclusion: Our kids are in worse shape than those ten years ago, and this is endangering their health.

- According to the Department of Health, more than 40 percent of U.S. children ages five to eight already show risk factors for heart disease.
- A University of Michigan study indicates that 50 percent of all children in kindergarten through grade twelve have at least one risk factor for heart disease. Risk factors include smoking, elevated blood cholesterol, high blood pressure, obesity, and inactivity.
- Additional data from the University of Michigan found that 25 percent of children in kindergarten through grade twelve have elevated cholesterol levels (above 180 milligrams per deciliter).
- A 1984 study of elementary school children in Jackson County, Michigan, by Charles Kuntzleman, creator of the "Feelin' Good" program for kids, reflected the nationwide effect of unfitness:

* Twenty-eight percent had above normal blood pressure;
* Forty-one percent had high levels of cholesterol;
* Thirteen percent had five or more risk factors for heart disease.

Dr. Gerald Berenson of Louisiana State University Medical Center is conducting a long-term study of more than five thousand children in the small town of Bogalusa, Louisiana. "We're finding that risk factors, which include high cholesterol as well as obesity and high blood pressure, track into adulthood. That is, what you see in children predicts what you'll see in them as adults. If we want to prevent heart disease we'll have the most success with the children."

"It's discouraging," said Dr. Kenneth Cooper. "I'm afraid that as these kids grow up, we will see all the gains made against heart disease in the last twenty years wiped out in the next twenty years."

FITNESS HISTORY

Is this new? Are today's kids any different from their parents when they were children in the 1950s and 1960s?

Concern over the fitness levels of U.S. children was evident at least half a century ago. In 1940, Dr. Hans Kraus, working with Dr. Sonja Weber at the Posture Clinic of Columbia-Presbyterian Hospital in New York City, became concerned about poor posture as "the result of a muscular inability to move properly." Their patients were increasingly complaining about back pain, and Drs. Kraus and Weber wondered "if many people had become weak and tense because now they were leading lives that were largely sedentary." To explore their theory, they devised a battery of six tests that became known as the Kraus-Weber tests.*

In 1952, they tested more than five thousand healthy U.S. urban and suburban children between ages six and sixteen. They found the youngsters "amazingly weak and tense." When they tested about three thousand children in the same age group in what were then less-mechanized European countries (Austria, Italy, Switzerland) "the difference was startling."

Here are the results of those *minimal* fitness tests:

* 57.9 percent of the U.S. children failed one or more of the six Kraus-Weber tests. Only 8.7 percent of the European children failed. (Follow-up research in 1962 revealed that the rate of failure in Austria almost doubled as that country became more mechanized and prosperous.)

* The six tests are detailed in Chapter 4.

- 44.3 percent of American children failed the flexibility test, while only 7.8 percent of the European children failed.
- 35.7 percent of the U.S. kids failed one or more of the strength tests, while only 1.1 percent of the European children failed.

Not surprisingly, Dr. Kraus's finding caused an uproar in the United States. The opening paragraph of the August 15, 1955, *Sports Illustrated* article "The Report that Shocked the President" sounds embarrassingly true now:

> There is a problem in the United States today, one which goes far deeper and has more serious implications for the future of the nation than many of those which haunt the headlines daily. It is the problem of the physical fitness . . . or rather unfitness, of U.S. youngsters.

In response to Dr. Kraus's findings and report, President Dwight D. Eisenhower issued an executive order establishing the President's Council on Physical Fitness and Sports. Vice President Richard Nixon headed the council, and all over America school kids started doing more push-ups and jumping jacks and working up a good sweat. But the fitness surge lasted less than three years. In 1958, Nixon turned over the chairmanship to Secretary of the Interior Fred Seaton and the program sagged into inactivity. In an interview, Seaton suggested bird-watching as a painless way to gain fitness and remarked that the ordinary American spectator got a lot of exercise at a football game by walking from his car to the stadium and then climbing the stairs to his seat.

The election of John F. Kennedy in 1960 created a brief resurgence in the fitness movement in the United States. In two major articles in *Sports Illustrated*, President Kennedy blamed "technology and automation" for making life easier and becoming "the instruments of the decline of our national vitality and health." In 1962, President Kennedy noted that a fitness survey he ordered showed that "more than ten million of our forty million school children are unable to pass a test which measures only the minimum level of fitness, while almost twenty million [are] unable to meet the standard set by more comprehensive tests of physical strength and skills. . . . These figures represent the vast dimensions of a national problem which should be of deep concern to us all." As a result of President Kennedy's interest, for a while in the early 1960s U.S. school kids got more physical education: more calisthenics, more running, more strength training. In 1965, President Lyndon B. Johnson spoke about the "wholesome and welcome" gains in youth fitness, but warned that "the job [is] far from finished." In fact, tests that year of U.S. schoolchildren showed significant improvement over previous tests—but for the *last* time. Soon lost in the distraction of the Vietnam War, the youth fitness crusade stumbled to a halt.

Dr. Kraus, whom President Kennedy consulted for his back problems, states that the youth fitness movement essentially collapsed after JFK was assassinated in 1963. Twelve years later, I met Dr. Kraus for the first time. I'll never forget the moment when he pointed up to an autographed picture of himself and Kennedy, and stated with deep frustration: "It all died with him. We had such hope."

TODAY'S PARENTS VS. THEIR KIDS

So the kids of the 1950s and 1960s were, for the most part, out of shape too. But what changed was the so-called fitness revolution of the 1970s and 1980s. These adults, largely the children of the 1950s and 1960s who probably learned some valuable lessons from government-inspired fitness programs, took to the roads with vigor. Those lessons are now seen every day as America's adults exercise. But, paralleling fitness gains among adults in the last decade, *youth fitness programs have decreased.*

This book is a step toward changing that pattern. It recognizes a paradox: that today's adults who are running down the road toward fitness were yesterday's out-of-shape American kids. They were probably like their children are now.

The concern about fitness among America's schoolchildren, so alive in the Eisenhower-Kennedy-Johnson era, has not revived. While America's adults began, in the late 1970s, to improve their health and conditioning, little effort was made during that or the next decade to improve the fitness of their children. Perhaps the adults were responding to the "Me Generation"—with its interest in self-improvement—or perhaps they were recalling the lessons of their youth, when they were children and their teachers and parents, urged by three presidents, increased physical education and fitness training in and outside their schools. Whatever the reasons, two facts exist side by side today: we adults—the children of the 1950s and 1960s—are exercising in large numbers (although still too many do not exercise adequately) and reaping the health benefits from doing so. Our children are not. As *Newsweek* headlined in 1985: "Failing in Fitness: The health and exercise boom eludes America's kids." The *Wall Street Journal* in 1988 proclaimed that "American children are getting fatter and more and more out of shape. . . . Surprisingly, the fitness craze that sent their parents into the streets in jogging shoes and into health clubs in leotards has passed them by."

CAUSES OF UNFITNESS

What is causing the unfitness epidemic?

The decline in youth fitness and the advance in hypokinetic diseases among American children today are directly related to the way we live. Technology and cultural changes have turned our children into watchers instead of doers, undermined their nutrition, and created a stressful, hectic lifestyle. We've even added a new term to the dictionary: couch potato. We are paying the price for the conveniences our ancestors didn't have—and the price is the health of our children.

Yet many adults and their children are healthy despite these changes. It is possible to enjoy the conveniences of modern life and also be fit. The blame, therefore, falls on us, the parents, and on the institutions that we select and allow to influence our lives and the lives of our children. Let's call those institutions Lifestyle, Parents, Schools, and Community.

Lifestyle

We sit almost all day. We ride everywhere. After school, too often children come home to a parentless house. They may be "latch-key" kids, who open the door to an empty home or are looked after by a baby-sitter. Exercise is not high on anyone's list at that time of day; quiet inactivity is. Fewer parents are home, and fewer kids are allowed or urged outside to play. The (in)activity of choice is watching television or the VCR, attending sporting events, or playing video and computer games. The loser is the child.

Passive forms of entertainment compete with vigorous activity for our children's time, and take the place of exercising. Television is the most serious culprit. When I was six years old, my parents purchased our first TV. The number of programs was limited (and they appeared in black-and-white on a small screen), but still my parents restricted the hours I could watch. Today, many kids have their own television set (and personal computer) in their room. Thanks to tape and software rentals, and to cable TV or satellite dishes, they may sit alone for hours playing with their computers or watching television programs selected from more than two hundred channels. "Children are living vicariously," says Dr. Joseph Zanga, chairman of the American Academy of Pediatrics' section on school health. "Instead of playing sports, they watch sports. Instead of dancing, they watch rock video."

What is this doing to them? According to a National Children and Youth Fitness Study made by the U.S. Department of Health in 1987: "Children who watch greater amounts of television tend to have lower activity levels and are less likely to participate in organized sports or to engage in physical activity through community organizations. Television watching takes away directly from time that could be spent in other, more constructive activities, including exercise."

How much television do our children watch? The National Children and Youth Fitness Study (NCYFS) surveyed 4,435 parents of children in grades one through four:

- On school days, 72.3 percent of those grade-school children watch up to two hours, 27 percent watch between three and five hours.
- On weekends, 28.3 percent watch up to two hours, 61 percent watch three to five hours, and more than 10 percent watch six or more hours a day.

The average TV time for American kids in grade school? Two hours and two minutes a day during the school week and three hours and twenty-six minutes a day on weekends. A far more pessimistic estimate of the number of hours U.S. schoolchildren spend watching television comes from the National Assessment of Education Progress. This organization, which tracks trends in young children's behavior, notes that 32 percent of America's fourth-grade children reported watching six or more hours of television every day.

"The amount of time a child spends in watching television seems to be related to how active the child is," says the NCYFS study. "The less television a child watches, the higher the parent's rating of the child's physical activity level. In addition, the less television a child watches, the more likely the child is to be involved in organized sports and a variety of other activities through community organizations. Thus, television watching is an important indicator of how physically active our children are."

It is my guess that as studies are made about the amount of time that a youngster spends playing with a computer or playing video games, the results will be similar. Apparently, when given the choice, America's youngsters prefer to spend large amounts of time in passive inactivity rather than taking a portion of that time for exercise. Certainly, much of that two to four hours of daily television-watching time could be spent in more productive and creative play, including exercise.

Television viewing and poor diet also tend to go together. The 1987 NCYFS study also showed that youngsters who watch large amounts of television tend to be fatter and to perform worse on distance run tests. This investigation is backed up by 1985 studies conducted by Steven Gortmaker of the Harvard School of Public Health and Dr. William Dietz of the New

England Medical Center, who found that kids who watch several hours of television a day are fatter than kids who watch fewer hours. Add to this the high-fat, high-calorie diets of most Americans and the emerging picture is of an overweight, inactive kid eating and watching his or her way to a health disaster.

Chapter 29 offers guidelines for family nutrition.

Our lives and those of our children are stressful; doctors are now seeing stress-related health problems among our kids. Exercise has been shown to often alleviate stress among adults. Chapter 28 details guidelines for managing stress in the family with exercise.

Parents

We, the parents, can change our children's habits of unfitness. We must first acknowledge the fact that our children are under-exercised and suffer from hypokinetic disease. We have to agree that there is a problem. Despite alarming evidence to the contrary, most parents think their children are active enough. A 1986 Harris Survey reported that nine out of ten U.S. parents thought their children were physically fit. A 1987 *USA Today* report stated that 71 percent of parents thought that the exercise their kids got was "about right." Only 21 percent thought it was "not enough" and 8 percent reported that it was "too much."

Students tend to reflect their parents' attitudes. When physical educators administering the Chrysler Fund-AAU fitness test were asked why students did so poorly, student apathy toward exercise was given as a primary reason. Some 35 percent of the instructors thought this reflected parental attitudes as well.

Despite the highly touted "fitness boom," few adults in the United States today get enough physical exercise to increase their cardio-respiratory fitness levels. The National Institutes of Health report that 25 percent of adult Americans are more than twenty pounds overweight; thirty-four million American adults need to lose thirty-five pounds or more. More than 25 percent of U.S. adults still smoke cigarettes; alcohol abuse affects one-third of all U.S. homes.

But parents are relatively young adults and should be quite active. Do they differ from the national average? The 1987 National Children and Youth Fitness Study found that fewer than 30 percent of parents take part in moderate to vigorous exercise three days a week (the minimum generally recommended by fitness experts). Even more alarming, approximately 50 percent of parents *never* engage in vigorous exrcise, and more than 58 percent of all U.S. mothers and 61 percent of all U.S. fathers say they *never* exercise with their children in a typical week.

Schools

During the 1950s and 1960s, our schools were packed with "baby boomers" and money was made available to improve the schools' physical education programs. But then the Vietnam War took funds away from education, the baby boomers grew up, and there were fewer kids in the public schools. In times of financial belt-tightening, physical education is one of the first school programs to be cut.

In 1987, the American Alliance for Health, Physical Education, Recreation and Dance (AAHPERD), a trade association of physical educators founded in 1885, conducted "The Shape of the Nation: A Survey of State Physical Education Requirements." After looking at school kids from kindergarten through the twelfth grade, the AAHPERD researchers concluded that the United States is experiencing "a youth fitness crisis" because of a lack of physical education programs in the schools. "There are simply not enough quality physical education programs across the country to enable our children to learn how to keep themselves healthy and maintain a basic level of fitness."

Here are some of their findings:

- Only four states—Illinois, New Jersey, New York, and Rhode Island—require all students to take a specific amount of physical education in all grades (kindergarten through twelfth grade). Only Illinois requires all students to take physical education every day, though other states are considering adoption of similar standards.
- Only five states require elementary school students to take physical education for 150 or more minutes per week—the equivalent of only thirty minutes per day.
- Only 12 percent of states require high-school students to take physical education for all four years of high school; almost half the states require their students to take physical education for only one year of high school.
- Eight states—Arizona, Colorado, Maine, Michigan, Mississippi, Oklahoma, South Dakota, and Wyoming—have no minimum requirements for physical education for children in kindergarten through twelfth grade.

The 1984 NCYFS study discovered that only 36 percent of students in grades five through twelve—the years when kids are growing most rapidly—take physical education daily. Many elementary students have only one or two P.E. classes per week. The NCYFS follow-up in 1987, with grades one through four elementary school children, found that barely one-third take physical education daily; 37 percent take P.E. only one or two days per week. This means that schools expect the majority of students, kindergarten through grade twelve, to sit passively through an eight-hour school day without any exercise other than the occasional walk to another classroom or to the bathroom.

Yet even those taking physical education classes may be getting short-changed. The 1987 report added:

> The study also revealed the conflict [between] the physical curriculum-competitive sports and motor performance vs. development of patterns for life-time (health-related) fitness. The results show that classes and testing programs are focusing on motor performance and not [on] lifetime fitness activities. In addition to not enough testing of the five fitness components [see Chapter 2], the emphasis, instead, is on sports skills in the curriculum, and this increases from grade to grade.

> Also, as many as one-third of physical education specialists do not hold current, valid certifications in physical education.

Clearly, parents need to lobby to improve physical education courses in their schools and to get the programs to stress more lifetime fitness classes (such as running, cross-country skiing, bicycling, and swimming) rather than primarily competitive sports. The emphasis on competitive sports, especially in high schools, means that the active few entertain the passive many.

"We have to conclude that not enough time is spent in school or outside school on activities that would maintain a high level of cardio-respiratory fitness, such as running, swimming, bicycling or walking," wrote Dr. Gold of the NCYFS study. "The majority of activities are team and competitive sports and informal games, which don't promote fitness and are not the kinds of activities that will be pursued throughout life."

Chapters 5–9 on Physical Education and Chapters 24–25 on Sports will offer guidelines on how we can give our children the best of both worlds— the fun and controlled competition of sports with the aerobic benefits of fitness activities.

Community

School physical education programs are only one small part of the fitness mosaic. Your community organizations can play a major role in your children's fitness programs. But you, as parents, are going to have to get after them and participate yourselves.

Children have plenty of time for exercise after school, weekends, and summers. For example, the 1984 NCYFS study found that the average student gets more than 80 percent of his or her physical activity outside of the school physical education programs. In the Rome, New York, Family YMCA, where I was physical education director during the early 1970s, we had thousands of kids, from toddlers to teens, working up a sweat all over the Y.

But too few community programs offer fitness programs other than competitive sports. Little League Baseball and Pop Warner Football get the kids involved, but neither offers much more than minimal fitness and no lifetime activity benefits. Other community programs simply keep the balls pumped up and the grass mowed. Without health-related fitness activities tied in with sports, community activities fall short of what is needed to help improve the fitness level of young Americans.

Some communities lack facilities. When my son Christopher was six years old, I took him back to my old hometown to show him the things I did when I was a kid. One of my favorite ballfields is now a parking lot for a shopping mall, another is a housing development, and a third is a fast-food restaurant. This is progress? My favorite biking route is now interrupted by a four-lane highway. In big cities and small towns across the country, the playing fields are disappearing.

The old ritual of playing outdoors after school has also almost disappeared. Children now rush home to watch television and play video games; in most cities, parents cannot allow their children to play in the parks unattended by an adult because of fear for their safety. Indeed, Christopher is robbed of the spontaneity of after-school exercise that I enjoyed as a kid. Instead, I have to rearrange my work schedule so we can get out to play after school a few days a week. Few parents, working or non-working, take the time or trouble. (Ironically, in many U.S. homes, the parents rush out for exercise after work while the children stay safely inside watching television.)

YMCAs and YWCAs, the Scouts, religious groups, town recreation programs, and other similar organizations should include fitness testing and fitness conditioning programs along with their usual sports offerings. Communities need to do more than erect playgrounds, baseball fields, and tennis courts to improve the overall fitness level of their members.

YMCA executive Lynne Vaughn summarized the challenge to the Ys: "YMCAs need to apply the same commitment they have for adult fitness to the area of youth fitness," she wrote in the organization's magazine, *Perspective*. "We need to pick up where the schools leave off and teach children about good health habits and positive health styles. We need to incorporate health and fitness concepts into our ongoing youth programs such as progressive swimming, gymnastics, youth sports and child care."

In addition to community programs, the medical profession should be encouraged to participate in youth fitness programs. Between 1973 and

1982, the tables of contents of the *American Journal of Diseases of Children*, the *Journal of Pediatrics*, and *Pediatrics* listed only two articles concerning America's youngsters and their physical fitness. An editorial in the March 1981 issue of *Preventive Medicine* criticized the medical profession for a "noteworthy failure to implement health promotion in clinical practice or to offer advice concerning exercise, nutrition, substance abuse, stress, and health habits." Dr. William Castelli, director of the Framingham Health Study, added: "Physicians aren't into preventive medicine and that's our problem. We teach preventive medicine in all the med schools, but they just give it lip service. It all becomes diagnostic treatment."

Concern for the physical (and mental) condition of our children should begin with the pediatrician. In recent years, the American Academy of Pediatrics (AAP) has become increasingly active in promoting physical fitness and sports safety for our youngsters. The AAP has published a parent's guide to sports for kids, cooperated with the AAHPERD in a nationwide survey of physical education programs in schools, and initiated a nationwide public relations campaign to promote youth fitness. An article in *The Physician and Sportsmedicine* suggested that physicians make fitness checks among their young patients, record body weight and body fat, and get families to hold each other accountable for their fitness activities. AAP physicians have suggested that "pediatricians should encourage parents to see that all family members are involved in fitness-enhancing physical activities, so that these activities become an integral part of the family's life-style."

"Poor fitness in childhood increases the likelihood of heart attacks and other ailments in adulthood," wrote Charles Kuntzleman, who conducted the Jackson County, Michigan, study. "Cardiovascular disease starts by the first grade. . . . It's clear that our patterns of activity, eating and outlook are established early in life. That's the time to help a child develop sound habits."

Parents, and particularly parents who are physicians, could play a special role in combining school, community, and family to work on improving levels of fitness among children and adults in their towns. Dr. William Strong and Jack Wilmore, Ph.D., wrote in *Contemporary Pediatrics*: "In addition to encouraging their patients to be physically fit, pediatricians should work with the school system and community programs to promote increased emphasis on physical fitness."

Parents can make a difference. Take the case of New York City's Asphalt Green, which developed out of one of the most seemingly hopeless situations parents face: no play space combined with astronomically high real estate values. Twenty years ago when an asphalt plant closed down, developers planned to use the block it had occupied for more high-rise luxury apartments. Just what the city needed! But then Dr. George Murphy and his Neighborhood Committee for the Asphalt Green sprang into action. "This really is an oasis, with all these high rises around," said Dr. Murphy, "and they wanted to take away our last open space. What a vulgarity."

The committee gained control of the land and raised the funds to develop a recreational center and a large, bright-green artificial field for sports and recreation. Now Christopher and his neighborhood friends can exercise and play on this green oasis in the middle of New York's asphalt jungle.

THE CHALLENGE

The President's Council on Youth Fitness and Sports, in its 1985 survey, concluded that "Every youth serving agency, institution and organization at all levels, federal, state and regional, in both the private and public sector, should look critically at their responsibilities to improve youth fitness. Families can also provide encouragement and motivation towards good fitness habits. Youth must be self-motivated to develop physically and learn how to maintain at least a minimum of fitness throughout life."

But fitness is a learned lifestyle. Parents cannot assume that children will exercise on their own. In a study of boys and girls ages seven to nine, Patty Freedson, Ph.D., an assistant professor of exercise science at the University of Massachusetts, found that despite apparent high levels of activity the children did not exercise enough to improve their cardio-respiratory fitness.

Nor can parents simply rely on the schools and community—on others—to teach their children the fitness habit. They must supplement this educational process with family fitness activities themselves. According to the 1987 NCYFS study: "The frequency with which mothers and fathers exercise with their children can be presumed to communicate to the child something about the parental value associated with exercise. As a result, it could contribute to the child's immediate physical activity level and long-term adherence to exercise programs."

Children have four potential sources for exercise: free play, school physical education classes, community after-school and summer programs, and family activity. To reverse the tide of the "unfitness revolution," we need to improve the opportunities for our children in each of these four exercise areas. You, as parents, can immediately make a difference in two areas—family exercise and free play—and your efforts, and those of other parents, can change the other two.

The results will surprise you. The Institute for Aerobics Research tested 16,449 U.S. schoolchildren in 1984–85 and again in 1985–86, and then compared the results. They found both boys and girls, motivated by the test, improved their performances in the mile run and in doing sit-ups. Kuntzleman's "Feelin' Good" program in Michigan compared students before and after fitness/wellness exercise classes at several elementary schools. The results were also encouraging: improvements in lowering sugar and calorie consumption, fats in the diet, blood pressure, and cholesterol levels. Physical activity among the schoolchildren increased by an average of 46 percent.

Nationwide, the President's Council report warns: "The United States has more physical educators, more health educators, more gymnasia, more swimming pools, and more recreational opportunities than any other country in the world. Buttress this with the best medical science system in the world, not only in quality of care, but [also] in medical research, equipment, facilities, and the like. Yet we lead the world in degenerative diseases." To reverse this equation will take serious, persistent, and long-term effort. But the result will be improvement in the health of all our children. Most important, the habit of exercise begun in childhood is the gift of a lifetime.

The Benefits of Fitness

The decline in physical fitness among our children is shocking and dangerous. Their unfitness now and what that may mean in terms of health problems later is reason enough for serious concern, but there are additional ramifications to consider.

As those of you who exercise know, fitness improves mental alertness and academic performance. For unfit children, the reverse may be true: unfitness may be causing poor academic performance. In 1985, Senator Richard Lugar (Republican–Indiana) spoke at the National Conference on Youth Fitness, and warned: "There is a strong connection between the decline in academic test scores and the sorry state of fitness and health among our young people. We have to indicate that physical education is one of the important studies. Not everyone has to become a great athlete. But mental alertness and feeling good about oneself are dependent to some degree on physical activity."

Let's turn the problem around 180 degrees: What might be the benefits to your children, and your family, of regular and sustained exercise?

WHAT IS PHYSICAL FITNESS?

If a child or adult is very active, well-coordinated, or performing well in sports, does this mean that he or she is physically fit? Most parents and teachers confuse being athletic with being physically fit.

At any age, a person may be very athletic but not be very fit. Just watch a big, overweight kid hit a long ball in baseball and huff and puff trying to run around the bases. Or, for that matter, watch many major leaguers try to run for an extended distance—like from first to home. This is one of the serious weaknesses of competitive team sports so revered in our schools: a few good athletes play; the fit and the unfit may watch. More-over, in many schools the same athletes play all the sports.

On the other hand, one can be very fit but not very athletic. A youngster who is not good enough to make the varsity team in a sport may be in better shape than his or her more athletically gifted friends.

I am surprised every time I return to my hometown to see the sedentary former baseball, basketball, and football stars of my high-school years. Many retired overweight and out-of-shape athletes can easily rekindle memories of the glory days, yet they cannot run comfortably for twenty minutes with their less athletic, former classmates. Sadly, the skills they acquired and the glory they received did not prepare them for a lifetime of fitness. Meanwhile, most of us distance runners who labored in ano-nymity on the high-school track team are still running and in good health.

I see a similar pattern among my son's friends. Many of Christopher's classmates may be able to throw a ball farther and outsprint him in a short race, but very few can run a mile non-stop, stretch their muscles easily, or perform a moderate number of sit-ups. Which skills define fitness? Although Christopher enjoys playing sports very much, he is also aware that fitness means much more than the ability to perform at sports. In his school and family exercise programs, Christopher enjoys the benefits of both athletics and fitness exercise. He was as proud of passing all the health-related fitness tests for this book as he was of hitting his first home run in our baseball league.

Popular team sports like baseball and football are generally not good fitness developers. Yet the National Children and Youth Fitness Study shows that motor skills and competitive sports are strongly emphasized in the typical school physical education and community programs, at the expense of lifetime or health-related fitness activities.

This is slowly changing. Before 1980, fitness testing offered in schools primarily measured athletic ability. Tests such as the softball throw, stand-ing long jump, shuttle run, and fifty-yard dash measured skills that are largely determined by genetic endowment and the child's level of physical development, but not fitness. In 1980, the American Alliance of Health, Physical Education, Recreation and Dance (AAHPERD) developed the "Health-Related Physical Fitness Test" and identified five basic fitness com-ponents later endorsed by the American Academy of Pediatrics. (Chapter 4 details youth fitness testing.)

The AAHPERD defined physical fitness as "a physical state of well-being that allows people to perform daily activities with vigor, reduce their risk of health problems related to lack of exercise, and establish a fitness base for participation [in] a variety of physical activities." In the mid-1980s, the

American Academy of Pediatrics, building on the AAHPERD, further defined physical fitness:

> During the last decade our concept of what "physical fitness" means has undergone a major change. Traditionally, the "physically fit" child was one who had obvious motor (or athletic) abilities, ordinarily defined by such parameters as muscle strength, agility, speed and power. But the high levels of power, speed and agility necessary for success in most competitive sports have little or no relevance in the daily lives of most adults. Today, the words "physical fitness" imply optimal functioning of all physiologic systems of the body, particularly the cardiovascular, pulmonary, and musculoskeletal systems. Physical fitness is now considered to include five components: muscle strength and endurance, flexibility, body composition (i.e. degree of fatness), and cardiorespiratory endurance.

The development of motor or athletic skills is still an important part of a balanced physical education program. So, too, as we shall see in a moment, are team sports, which can instill psychological as well as physical benefits. But parents, teachers, and school administrators should first emphasize lifestyle-fitness habits and encourage children to participate in frequent and vigorous aerobic exercises—walking, running, biking, swimming—both in and out of school. In addition to promoting health-related fitness, we as parents and adults should also integrate exercise into a comprehensive healthy lifestyle for our children. "The ultimate goal," says Dr. Russell R. Pate, Ph.D., director of the Human Performance Laboratory and professor of physical education at the University of South Carolina, "is to help kids become regular, lifetime exercisers." In addition to exercise, this includes "wellness" for the child and family, which in turn means proper nutrition and stress management (see Chapters 27–30). In sum, the primary emphasis should be on improving health-related fitness among our kids—the central theme of this book.

HEALTH-RELATED FITNESS

What are the components of physical fitness and what are their benefits to us? Let's look at the American Academy of Pediatrics list: cardio-respiratory endurance, body composition, flexibility, muscular strength and endurance.

Cardio-respiratory Endurance

Without the proper functioning of this important muscle—your heart—life wouldn't exist. Your heart pumps the equivalent of eight thousand gallons of blood through twelve thousand miles of tubing every day. To do this, it must beat about one hundred thousand beats every day. The efficiency of this process depends on this special pumping muscle; its efficiency in turn depends on regular conditioning. Yet, the heart is one of the most neglected muscles we have.

Cardio-respiratory fitness is measured in terms of aerobic capacity. The AAHPERD defines that as the ability to perform large-muscle, whole-body physical activity of moderate to high intensity over extended periods of time. Research shows that by engaging in regular vigorous exercise that improves aerobic capacity, you can reduce many risk factors of coronary heart disease. This kind of exercise—called aerobic exercise—helps the heart get bigger and stronger, which allows you to be more active, have more energy, and remove stress from your cardio-respiratory system and your life.

Simply put, aerobics means "promoting the supply and use of oxygen." Dr. Kenneth Cooper popularized aerobic exercise beginning in the late 1960s with a series of best-selling books. In one of them, *The Aerobics Program for Total Well-Being*, Dr. Cooper writes:

> Aerobic exercises refer to those activities that require oxygen for prolonged periods and place such demands on the body that it is required to improve its capacity to handle oxygen. As a result of aerobic exercise, there are beneficial changes that occur in the lungs, the heart, and the vascular system. More specifically, regular exercise of this type enhances the ability of the body to move air into and out of the lungs; the total blood volume increases; and the blood becomes better equipped to transport oxygen.

There are many kinds of aerobic exercises, including running, swimming, biking, walking, and cross-country skiing when done vigorously. The basic idea is to exercise your body steadily over at least a twenty-minute period, to make your heart work within your "aerobic zone." (Chapter 12 details this idea.) This is a goal, and you should build up to it gradually. Chapter 12 also details ways to improve your aerobic capacity, and Chapters 15–19 offer guidelines for using the "Big Four" aerobic activities—walking, swimming, running, and biking—to build endurance in your heart and lungs.

Body Composition

Your body can be divided into two basic parts: lean weight (muscle, bone, internal organs) and fat weight. For good health and fitness, you should maintain a proper ratio of one to the other. But what is that proper ratio?

By assessing body composition, it is possible to determine if a person is underweight, lean, overweight, or obese. Estimates of body composition are easily determined by measuring skinfold with calipers. This is reported as percentage of fat, which means that out of a total weight a certain percentage is estimated to be fatty tissue. Thus, if your percentage of fat is 20 percent, the remaining 80 percent is lean weight.

Controlling caloric intake—what you eat—is one way to control your weight and, combined with regular aerobic exercise (caloric expenditure), is also an ideal way to achieve a balance between lean weight and fat weight. Chapter 30 sets forth guidelines for weight management and weight goals for adults and children.

Flexibility

As defined by the AAHPERD, flexibility is the ability to move muscles and joints—hip, elbow, shoulder, knee, ankle, back—through their full range of motion. Flexibility is important for injury prevention. But this requires regular stretching to increase the range of motion. Children generally have good flexibility, but it can be quickly lost by physical inactivity. In Chapter 1, we discussed the lack of flexibility discovered among our children: few can touch their toes with their knees kept straight. Sitting for long periods of time—such as in an office or classroom—contributes to the loss of flexibility.

Jerry R. Thomas, Amelia M. Lee, and Katherine T. Thomas discuss the importance of flexibility, especially among those who are exercising regularly, in their book *Physical Education for Children: Concepts into Practice:*

> [Flexibility] is joint specific: a person can have a good range of motion at one joint, yet a very limited range at another. Girls usually have greater flexibility than boys at all ages.

> Exercise can influence flexibility either positively or negatively. Activities that build strength frequently limit the range of motion of the joint associated with the increased strength. But strength training that uses the total range of movement and emphasizes stretching will not reduce flexibility. Regular stretching to increase range of motion has a positive effect on flexibility. Increased range of motion in a joint allows it to give somewhat under stress, thereby reducing the chance of injuries in physical activity. Teaching children how to maintain flexibility and encouraging its development is an important part of elementary physical education.

Despite the obvious importance of flexibility, adults and children who regularly engage in vigorous exercise often neglect it. They do not stretch before and after exercise. Yet a supple, flexible body, while of no direct benefit to your cardio-respiratory function, does allow you to exercise aerobically with greater ease. It also reduces your chances of injury. And if you are injured, you cannot exercise.

Most American men and women, at one time or another, encounter back problems, according to Dr. Kraus. I had a chance to work with him on a nationwide exercise program for adults suffering from back pain. What I saw from Dr. Kraus's studies is that about 80 percent of lower back disorders are due to weak and/or tense muscles. These can be greatly minimized with a regular relaxation and stretching program.

Guidelines for safe stretching exercise are detailed in Chapter 11. The most important areas of flexibility in the body are the lower back and hamstring muscles. The flexibility of these muscles is easy for you to determine by the standing toe-touch test and the sit-and-reach test (Chapter 4).

Muscular Strength and Endurance

Strength is the ability of your muscles to produce force at high intensities for short periods of time. An example might be lifting heavy weights. Endurance is the ability to sustain repeated productions of force at low to moderate intensities over extended periods of time. Timed sit-ups and push-ups are examples. Most youth fitness tests of strength and endurance use chin-ups and timed sit-ups and push-ups to evaluate muscular strength and endurance simultaneously. (See Chapter 4 for guidelines in administering these tests.)

Muscular strength and endurance enhance athletic performance. Abdominal muscle strength and endurance, measured with sit-ups, helps you achieve good posture and decreases the incidence and severity of low-back pain. Upper-body strength and endurance help us perform daily tasks like taking out the trash, mowing the lawn, changing a tire, moving furniture, and lifting, pulling, or pushing objects. "In an emergency," says the AAH-PERD, "the ability to apply force with the upper body can mean the difference between a serious injury and escaping harm."

Chapter 11 details the role of muscular strength and endurance in physical fitness.

THE BENEFITS

There are three ways to exercise: in a group, by oneself, or on a sports team. The benefits of getting physically fit will come only with regular exercise and good nutrition. This book stresses the role that parents, teachers, and other adults should take in helping children achieve and stay in good physical health. This process includes parents and other adults working out *with* the kids. It certainly does not endorse parents and other adults standing around in designer gym suits blowing whistles while kids run windsprints.

It is unlikely that children up through high-school age will enjoy exercising by themselves, although my friend and co-author Jack Shepherd knows runners on the Hanover (New Hampshire) High School track team—perennial state and New England track champions—who enjoy solitary long-distance running through the hills of New Hampshire and Vermont. More often, however, the team runs with its gray-haired coach, and the pack chatters away in animated conversation as it rolls up and down the hills. For the most part, exercise for youngsters is going to be done in groups or on organized teams. This will, and should, include parents and adults.

The most logical group is the family. Parents (and other adults) who exercise with their youngsters serve as role models. Kids who see adults exercising accept the idea that exercise and its benefits should be a part of their lives too. This is your gift to these kids. Parents exercising with their children are achieving several things: the fun of doing something together, the benefits of exercise, and the lifetime gift of good health. The family that exercises together, moreover, creates a situation in which kids and parents talk with and enjoy one another outside the physical setting of their home. Conflicts, tensions, and the pressure of modern living are put aside for this period of doing something beneficial together. The benefits are mutual: "The family that exercises together," says Dr. Kenneth Cooper, "or at least shares and supports one another in individual exercise programs, frequently possesses a much greater level of well-being and unity."

The physical and mental benefits of exercise are already well known among adults who work out regularly. But what are the benefits to our children? For one thing, *any* exercise for the majority of our children will be revolutionary; it will halt, if not reverse, the unfitness process. For another, regular exercise, as I've mentioned, will create a lifelong pattern conducive to good health. But there are also immediate benefits—gifts, if you will—that you can give your children.

Physical Benefits

During childhood, growth is fairly continuous. Regular exercise can assist in that growth in terms of increasing muscle size and strength, muscle flexibility, leanness, and aerobic power. "This means," write Dr. Mike Samuels and Nancy Samuels in *The Well Child Book*, "that children who exercise regularly will be stronger, more flexible, thinner, have greater aerobic power, and have larger muscles and bones than similar children who do not exercise regularly."

There are well-documented, measurable benefits from this. Kids (and adults) who are physically fit are at lower risk for hypokinetic diseases such as hypertension, cardiovascular disease, tension syndromes, diabetes, gastrointestinal stress disease (ulcers—yes, our high-stress kids get ulcers), and emotional problems. These degenerative diseases all begin in childhood.

In the regularly exercised body of a child or adult the heart volume increases, heart capillaries proliferate, heart-rate decreases (your heart beats less often but more efficiently), efficiency at utilizing oxygen while at work increases, and strength of bones and ligaments increases. The capacity of your child's lungs improves; some studies now show this increase in "vital capacity" indicates greater longevity. High-density lipoproteins (HDL)—the good "Roto-Rooter" guys—increase, thus reducing the risk of hardening of the arteries or coronary heart disease.

The physiological results are wonderful. Medical research shows that the exercising child or adult has improved posture, sleeps better, and bounces back from illness more quickly than the unfit child. Aerobic exercise improves digestion and controls constipation. Exercise also helps diminish hyperactivity and control disruptive behavior. Perhaps best of all—given recent national testing results—your exercising child has more endurance when engaging in strenuous physical activities. He or she can carry on daily work and play safely and successfully; equally important, your child can handle physical emergencies more easily.

Exercise plays an important role in both physical and psychological development. Dr. Samuels suggests that exercise creates "learned pathways" in our children's neuromuscular system, which play an important role in developing agility, balance, coordination, and reaction time. "These skills can only be learned and perfected with practice," he says. Everyone is aware of the rapid neuromuscular learning that takes place in babies between birth and two or three years of age. But, says Dr. Samuels, that growth does not stop when the baby learns to walk. "It continues through the teenage years of rapid growth and body changes, and can even be continued into adulthood. Such neuromuscular circuits are thought to be important for intellectual and emotional development as well."

There is a connecting pattern here. First, children (and adults) who exercise regularly tend to keep their body weight in check. Exercise controls body composition (the percentage of body fat) by helping to maintain or increase muscle mass while reducing fat. The result is a slimmer, firmer body that can do more physically than a heavier, fatter body. The consequence of *that* is increased self-esteem. Studies show that we regard fat people as physically and mentally lazy. When a child (or adult) looks good to others, self-confidence improves.

Psychological Benefits

Children (and adults) who feel good about themselves are, consequently, happier. Studies indicate that happier people are also more productive in the classroom and on the job; they are also much less absent from school and work. The cyclical pattern emerges: the fit child sees himself or herself improving and gains in self-esteem; that translates into being happier; that, in turn, increases skills both inside and outside the classroom, which gives the child greater self-esteem.

As the booklet *Sporting Chance*, produced by the Girls Club of America, points out, exercise is also helpful to children and adolescents suffering from anxiety and depression. One reason—and there are several—is that regular aerobic exercise increases self-esteem and the management of stress. "Fitness," says Dr. Paul Dyment, chairman of the Department of Pediatric and Adolescent Medicine at Ohio's Cleveland Clinic and chairman of the American Academy of Pediatrics's Committee on Sports Medicine, "leads to a heightened self-concept due to factors like a favorable body image, a sense of personal accomplishment and the pride of self-discipline."

Intellectual Benefits

As mentioned, there is evidence that self-esteem translates into better intellectual performance. Yet classroom time is at a premium and demands for daily physical education classes are generally rejected on the grounds that they would detract from academic work. The two, however, go hand in hand. Physical education, according to the AAHPERD, improves a child's mental alertness, academic performance, readiness, and enthusiasm for learning.

A six-year Canadian study that ended in 1977 indicated that exercise enhances academic performance. More than five hundred students in two elementary schools were assigned to an experimental program in which they exercised supervised by a gym teacher for an hour every day. During the first two years, basic motor skills were emphasized. In the next three years, the schoolchildren developed cardio-respiratory fitness and muscle strength. In the final year, they played a variety of vigorous team sports.

After six years, the exercising schoolchildren were compared to a control group at the same two schools. These kids had the same classroom teachers, but took only forty minutes of physical activity twice a week. Moreover, that activity was not well designed nor was it taught by a qualified physical education instructor.

The results? The experimental group increased its cardio-respiratory fitness and strength. And, despite the fact that they logged fewer hours in the classroom—they exercised for one hour a day instead of spending that time in class—the experimental group earned higher grades in French, mathematics, natural sciences, and English. Dr. Roy Shephard, director of the School of Physical and Health Education at the University of Toronto, and scientific director of the Canadian study, reached the following conclusion: "Through its impact on psychomotor learning, physical activity enhances the total process of intellectual development. Greek philosophers were correct to insist on the importance of a healthy body to a healthy mind; body and mind are closely linked at all ages, and an individual's potential can be realized only through the development of both."

A study of French schoolchildren during the 1980s concurred. It also showed that children who had eight hours of physical education—that is, sustained exercise for eight hours a week—achieved better academic results than control groups who had only forty minutes of physical activity per week. They also matured more quickly and were more independent. In the United States, in 1986 the U.S. Department of Education issued "First Lessons: A Report on Elementary Education in America," which was, in part, a scathing indictment of the U.S. educational system. The report stated:

> Physical education programs belong in elementary schools not only because they promote health and well-being, but [also] because they contribute tangibly to academic achievement. Researchers in France, Australia, Israel and the United States have all found that youngsters who partake in structured programs of vigorous exercise possess greater mental acuity and stronger interest in learning than those who do not.

FITNESS ACTIVITIES AND COMPETITIVE SPORTS

If, somehow, schools across America suddenly wished to incorporate five hours of weekly physical education for their children, what would be best? Some parents feel that organized competitive sports are best for their children. Others prefer that their kids undertake only non-competitive fitness exercise. I suggest that competitive sports and fitness exercise are both worthwhile. I believe that exercise could, and probably should, combine both competitive and fitness goals. In fact, my philosophy is that human beings should seek to balance fitness, sports, and fun. Exercise should be all three.

The problem with organized sports for children today is that too often they have been taken over by adults whose overcompetitiveness steals a lot from the youngsters. Little League baseball, country club tennis, Pop Warner football, and elementary school basketball leagues often put competition ahead of fitness and fun. Most coaches in these sports think someone else is conditioning their players. The kids stand around shagging ground balls or learning set plays. In many cases, the players, under stress from coaches, parents, and even teachers to perform well, aren't having fun.

We—adults, parents, children—should balance sports, fitness, and fun in exercise programs. Team sports can indeed be fun and teach kids a lot. While youngsters are learning to play, says Fred C. Engh, president of the National Youth Sports Coaches Association, they should also be playing to learn. "Sports gives the opportunity at an early age to learn discipline, training, desire to succeed and the ability to work with others."

BENEFITS OF TEAM SPORTS

I believe that competitive sports and fitness together teach qualities and skills useful in other areas of life and work. Together, they teach youngsters about competition and success, striving for well-defined goals, deferring gratification, and being rewarded for hard work. Kids learn to attribute success to ability, persistent work, and team effort—not to luck or chance—and thereby increase their self-esteem and motivation. Playing team sports and participating in regular fitness exercise can improve goal-setting abilities and help develop perseverance, industriousness, and motivation—all of value in later life. There are important lifelong concepts that your children will learn from playing sports and from regular exercise that contain clear health goals:

- to accept criticism;
- to practice and repeat skills;
- to take risks;
- to think strategically and make plans;
- to treat opponents as opponents, not as enemies;
- to train their bodies (discipline);
- to recognize rules and regulations;
- to recognize a contest as a game and leave it on the field when it's over;
- to support teammates when mistakes are made;
- to be responsible for themselves and others;
- to learn to be humble in victory and gracious in defeat;
- to work cooperatively toward a common goal.

Among the most valuable skills team sports teach is how to work together as a group for a common goal. John Madden, a successful coach of a professional football team and now a knowledgeable and humorous television sports commentator, never took himself or his teams too seriously. That is, he maintained the perspective that even in professional sports, these are young men playing a boys' game—and it is *playing*. Madden did not make the macho, and erroneous, observation that winning is everything. Winning, in fact, is a small fragment of playing. But John Madden did make a profound observation about the experience of competition:

> Being part of a team, you're part of a group that's bigger than you, and you're in it with people who think it's as important as you do.
>
> You're seeking to achieve as a unit, and that's a very civilized thing to attempt, very human.

Achieving something together is indeed a very human endeavor. It involves identifying goals, planning ways to achieve those goals, encouraging and motivating others to strive toward those goals and defending against attempts by others to block goal achievement. Having goals and planning and striving for them make the team, in Madden's words, larger than any single individual. Within this unit, individuals may take on various roles in which they will learn things of value later in their lives. Not all those roles are as leader, but each role does teach each player much about himself or herself as a person. The substitute used in key situations understands the importance of training, being ready, following the flow of events, and doing a brief task well in a short period of time. All the players learn the value of preparation and the efforts and rewards of teamwork, cooperation, and sharing. The leader or captain learns the value of every player to the success of the team. All these skills and approaches have significant carryover values that will enable your child to be better prepared in any walk of life.

Many parents and educators believe that sports also teach children moral behavior. They learn our society's values for success, achievement, and conformity. These lessons also come from non-sport activities, but on sports teams kids should be taught to achieve something together, with clear rules and clear, fair authority figures guiding them.

Beyond all this, organized sports can inculcate not only leadership skills, physical well-being, and moral behavior, but also self-concepts—a strong identity—and independence. Rainer Martens, in *Joy and Sadness in Children's Sports*, says:

> Sports and games are thought to give children an opportunity to resolve the psychological conflicts they encounter as they are growing up by exposing them to the emotional and cognitive polarities of these conflicts.

For example, through sports children experience the emotional highs and lows associated with victory and defeat. Sports also confront children at times with the cognitive dilemma of having to choose between being honest or dishonest competitors.

At the heart of all this lies the essence of fitness: to learn and perform the process of improving your body and your self. As Dr. Mike Samuels and Nancy Samuels write in *The Well Child Book:*

> The connection between the central nervous system and the muscles of the body should not be neglected during childhood. Physical activity creates circuits that help us develop so we function as a whole. Scientists now know that the two lobes of the cerebrum serve different functions.
>
> In almost everyone, the left brain is involved with verbal, analytic-mathematical, and time-oriented thought; the right brain with images, orientation in space, body image, and grasping whole concepts from parts. The right brain is also crucially involved with dreaming and creative thought.
>
> . . . Optimum health surely involves training both sides of the brain. Since schools tend to concentrate so heavily on left-brain, academic skills, it is doubly important that parents see that their children pursue body learning, which stimulates the right brain.

That body learning can take any form of exercise: competitive sports or fitness. In our home, Christopher combines both team sports and fitness. He understands that to be physically fit, he will most likely have to train outside of team sports competition. For all of us, fitness benefits come to those who exercise aerobically for at least twenty minutes at a time, three times a week. For this lifetime habit to take root among our children, we need to combine fitness, sport, and fun. For me, the fun comes first.

Now, let's get started.

Part 2

CHILD/ PARENT/ FAMILY

The Role of the Parent and Family

There are many factors that influence the physical activity of our children. None is as powerful as the role of the parent and family. The 1987 National Children and Youth Fitness Study II examined the relationship between the exercise habits of parents and the fitness of their children. The study concluded that youngsters who have physically active parents, especially parents who spend time exercising with their children, are leaner and more physically active. Why? The "modeling effect"—your children copy your behavior.

The Melpomene Institute (an organization devoted to research involving women's and girls' sports and fitness) issued a preliminary research report in 1988 that showed that the most significant influence on a child's involvement in physical activities and sports is the "parents' physical activity patterns (role modeling), lessons and classes and community recreation programs (educational opportunity and peer role modeling), and the time mothers and fathers spend with their children doing physical activities (role modeling and behavior facilitation)."

These simple facts are important to you and your child—and central to this book. From my own experience I believe that the most critical factors influencing a child's participation in fitness activities are: (1) the parent's level of fitness activity and (2) the child's family involvement.

WHERE TO START

As parents, we focus intensely on almost every aspect of our children's early life. We do not forget to give them vitamins, proper food, books and bedtime stories, vaccinations, love, and hugs. But regular exercise is seldom placed in the same important category of parenting despite the fact that lack of sufficient exercise in childhood is the primary cause of tension and back pain, obesity, and heart disease in adult life. As Dr. Hans Kraus has warned: "Geriatrics starts in the cradle"; adult fitness programs are "reclamation projects."

We, as parents, turn over to others—or to chance—one of the most important aspects of our children's upbringing. What happens is inevitable. Pre-school children seem to be born to move and they continuously clamber around their little worlds. They climb, jump, sprint, roll, and fall in bursts of energy that go on all day long—unless they are restricted by adults who want them quiet, "out of trouble," in the "play" pen, or in front of the television set. We parents, the baby-sitters we select for our kids, and later, their schools, play a powerful role in our children's fitness development. Along the way, as Mary Howell, M.D., wrote in *Working Mother*, something happens:

> For most children, there comes a time when that exuberant, unplanned and wholehearted physical activity is curtailed. Different children "get the message" at different ages, depending on the example of adult models, the personality and interests of the child and his or her experiences at school. Some children become physically quiet at four or five, when they are first engaged in formal schooling. Others quiet down in the elementary years, or in early adolescence. By the time of high school, most children have curbed the spontaneous expression of physical activity.

We can do something about how "damped down," in Dr. Howell's phrase, our children's activity level gets. But this commitment is going to cost us. The first step is for us as parents to encourage, by our own example, physical activity in our children. We should teach ourselves—and, therefore, our children—to value both the effects of physical exercise and the exercise itself. We should honor, as Dr. Howell writes, "our child's physical being and to teach the child to honor herself. . . . This means respecting the child's need to be physically active and encouraging her to keep listening to inner signals that say, 'Time to get up and move around a little'— or 'a lot.' "

As our children grow, we should not sit back and relegate their physical fitness to the schools. For example, we as parents do not simply turn over to our schools our child's education or diet. We should be as vigilant about our children's physical well-being. School, by definition, requires that our children sit and concentrate on academic work. Ideally, this should be balanced with daily physical activity. Moreover, as the studies detailed in Chapter 2 show, physical activity has educational benefits. Dr. Kraus urges us toward a simple truth: "If you are a parent, you must see to it that your children engage in vigorous physical activity not only at home, but also at school, whether it be kindergarten or college."

As I said in Chapter 1, your child has four potential sources for exercise: family activity, free play, school physical education classes, and community after-school and summer programs. You control them all. You should be familiar with and monitor school and community recreation programs taken by your child, whose fitness you entrust to these programs. If these programs fall short of the recommended standards in Part III of this book, you and other parents should lobby for improvement. We can never assume that someone else is doing the fitness job. Too often they are not, and the result is that your child's health may suffer.

Also, you should evaluate and monitor your child's present physical activity and health habits. Look for signs of trouble:

- *Poor stamina*. Your child is out of breath walking up a few flights of stairs or continually tires playing organized games. (Warning: If your child shows signs of persistent fatigue, have him or her examined by your family doctor.)
- *Lethargy*. Your child seems to get bored easily and lacks enthusiasm in general. He or she may spend more time watching television or in subdued play. School grades may slip.
- *Poor posture*. Your child's poor muscle tone results in slouching when standing or sitting.
- *Excess weight*. Your child is well above the normal weight compared to height and has excess "baby fat." (Warning: Sudden weight *loss* is also cause for your concern.)
- *Poor coordination*. Your child does not try to run, jump, throw, or catch and shows little skill at these basic activities. This is probably due to poor fitness and a lack of practice at motor skills.
- *Irregular sleeping patterns and lack of appetite*. These, too, may be due to inadequate exercise.
- *Complaints*. Your child complains about school or community physical education classes or sports being too hard or boring. He or she wants to drop out of activities that require any exercise. This may be caused by embarrassment at being overweight or not fit or skilled enough. Or it may be caused by poor physical education instructors. In either case, you should monitor the activities to observe for yourself.

Next, evaluate three things: your child's play environment and physical activity, your physical activity, and your parent-child activity. Then using the fitness tests in the following chapter, evaluate your and your child's present fitness levels. Work with your child so he or she will understand the reasons for taking these tests, and then over a period of several months work with him or her to improve the test scores. Help your child set and move toward a fitness goal—while setting a good example yourself—in measureable and clear ways. Reset these goals for the next step.

All of this must be done in a positive, supportive way, with understanding, love, and praise for your child's attempts to accomplish an agreed-upon task. There are some very valuable lifelong lessons here, in goal setting, and in striving to achieve and accomplish goals. Use the testing and fitness conditioning not only for teaching physical fitness lessons and benefits, but also for these other lessons of life.

THE PARENTAL ROLE MODEL

You as a parent must show the way. The National Children and Youth Fitness Study II concluded that few parents set good examples for their children: nearly half of all parents of young children *never* participate in vigorous exercise; less than 30 percent exercise vigorously three times a week—the recommended minimum level of physical activity.

"The best and easiest way to motivate your child to stay fit is to stay fit yourself," wrote Paul H. Gabriel, M.D., a child and adolescent psychiatrist. "The main reason children are out of shape is that they have poor role models. By making fitness a part of your life, you teach your child to value it."

Your children don't always do what you tell them, but they will be quick to do what you do. You should be aware, therefore, of the model that you present to your child. You should be an honest example of the type of person you would like your child to become. We all know that as parents even our best efforts are often not good enough. But there, too, there are good lessons for your child. When she or he sees you trying your best—win or lose—you demonstrate goal-setting, effort, and perhaps even coping with failure or frustration. Your child sees that the lack of immediate success does not mean quitting, but re-directing goals and learning to handle challenges better in the future.

Setting a good example for your child is not a casual thing. If you are overweight, eat too much junk food, watch too much TV, smoke, or shun exercise, you're sending very clear messages to your child. Virginia and I exercise regularly, watch our weight, don't smoke or allow smoking in our home, and practice reasonably good nutrition. We do watch too much TV and have a weakness for chocolate-chip cookies. Christopher says that smoking is "yuckie," and he knows that exercise is good for him and that certain foods are better than others. He also understands—as we do—that

TV can be habit-forming (and needs to be controlled) and that chocolate-chip cookies are delicious!

The Exerciser's Triangle

It is important to balance the three sides of what I call the "Exerciser's Triangle": career (or school), family, and exercise. When you spend too much time in one of the three areas, the triangle gets out of balance. Too much time working, and your exercise and family suffer. Too much time exercising, and your family and work suffer. What you do in this triangle also shapes your child's life: you can (and should) include her or him in this triangle. For example, if you are training for a marathon—deliberately creating an imbalance in favor of exercise to attain some goal—include your whole family. Let the kids do part of your training routine with you: the stretching and warm-ups, or a mile or so of the running. Share your training and race strategy with them. Bring them along to watch you in training races and certainly bring them along and involve them as your support crew during the event. I've heard a lot of runners tell the same story about the New York City Marathon: "My family wouldn't have put up with my training program if they didn't get an exciting trip to the city out of it."

One other thing. Sometimes each member of the family has to let his or her triangle get out of balance for a while. Your youngster might need to study a lot during exams and temporarily interrupt or neglect his or her regular exercise pattern. Your spouse may need to train for a race, leaving you to run the family for a while. Temporary imbalance is all right as long as each family member understands the reason and is willing to adjust for it.

Don't set a negative image. If you complain too much about the fatigue, injuries, and other obstacles you face in your exercise, you risk painting the wrong picture: you will turn off rather than turn on your children to exercise. Missing too many family meals or activities because it conflicts with your exercise routine may result in your children feeling deprived of your time and love and hating exercise as a result. Keep your triangle in balance.

FAMILY INVOLVEMENT

What do I mean by *family?* We all know that the American family has changed dramatically since the 1960s. It continues to change. High divorce rates and the trend toward having fewer or no children are making the old-fashioned, intact nuclear family—Mom, Dad, kids—increasingly rare.

If you are a parent today, you might very well be a single adult raising a child or children largely on your own. According to the Bureau of Census, the divorce ratio (the number of people who are divorced at any given time compared to the number who are married) more than doubled between 1960 and 1980. That resulted in more than six million children living in one-parent homes. In addition, more than 40 percent of all mothers with children under age six are working—including Christopher's. A 1976 Roper Organization poll of families with young children showed that 72 percent ate dinner together frequently. Ten years later a similar poll showed that the figure had dropped to 63 percent. We have become a society on the go. Even the extended family—parents, children, grandparents—is getting smaller. Grandparents typically live at some distance from their children and grandchildren.

What does all this have to do with a book about parents, kids, and exercise? For one thing, there's yet another trend: the aging "baby boomers" are settling down. We are creating a "baby boomlet" ourselves. For the first time since the 1970s, the number of married couples with children under the age of eighteen has increased. More babies were born in 1988 than in any year since 1965. I have run in New York's Central Park almost every day for fifteen years. Maybe it's because I have a young child now, but for the first time I am noticing parents and kids together. In 1988, while running a six-mile loop of the park, I counted twelve parents running while pushing baby carriages, twenty-five parents biking with their children, hundreds of parents skating at the park rink with kids, and countless more strolling through the park or playing ball with their families.

An unlikely example of this change comes from Club Med, the international resort that for decades was synonymous with swinging singles. Now it's into the family market. As Andrea Brox wrote in *Club Industry* magazine: "It is a little bit like *Playboy* merging with *Parents Magazine*. . . . But times have changed, even for Club Med: its swinging singles have met, mated, and are now bringing the kids along on vacations."

So we seem to be re-forming the old family. We may be marrying later and having fewer kids, but we are making more of a commitment to our families than parents did during the 1960s and 1970s. And we are playing with our kids more: a 1987 *Parents Magazine* poll showed that 67 percent of us play with our children more than our parents played with us. That's a good sign, both for this book—which seeks to create a lifetime pattern of fitness among parents and their children—and for our kids. Mom, Dad, and kids together create the best support for maintaining a healthy diet and regular aerobic exercise. That, in turn, creates a closeness and harmony that strengthens the family.

The Aerobic Family

What can we create for parents—with or without strong nuclear or extended families—so that we can put the programs and goals of this book into action? I think Dr. Kenneth Cooper has the right idea. He advocates "aerobic families." These aerobic families are linked "by a concern for their mutual health and well-being." They "exercise together, share their daily progress in moving toward individual health goals, and feel free to share their problems and release their tensions and stresses in a constructive, healing way in one another's presence."

The aerobic family can be put together through your local runner's club, YMCA, YMHA, church or synagogue group, or even informal fitness clan. It should have both parents and children of roughly the same ages; teenagers exercising with toddlers probably won't work well. It could consist of just your nuclear or extended family, a single parent and children, or it could mix nuclear families and single parents. Both adults and children should share a single goal: fitness and health with fun. These family members should act as cheerleaders, monitors, reminders, sympathizers, and partners to help each member reach his or her goals. Achieving those goals will be sweeter because it will mark a family victory. "Family members who exercise individually or together," writes Dr. Cooper, "have much more to share, and better communication and relationships are the inevitable result."

Aerobic families come together for exercise. They exchange information about fitness programs for their adults and children. They teach each other the basics of fitness, nutrition, and health. They listen to each other and encourage each other. In brief, the aerobic family can substitute for or strengthen the nuclear family. It seeks to create the same support system and encouragement that a nuclear family would give to its members. It benefits, as does the nuclear family, from this bonding and the close contact with its parents and children in a mutually beneficial goal: lifetime fitness and health.

When I use the term *family*, therefore, think of it as either your nuclear family or your aerobic family. In terms of physical fitness and its rewards, they are the same.

"The family makes a lot of sense as a vehicle for bringing about changes in diet and exercise," says Karen L. Senn, MPH, Ed.D., chair of the Department of Health Science at San Diego State University. "We know that children's early habits translate into risk factors for cardiovascular disease. We know that support—family support—is probably the key factor in promoting changes in habits. Unless the people trying to change have that support, there's little hope they will succeed." Family members seeking to improve their fitness, trying to stop drinking or smoking, or getting treatment for obesity, high blood pressure, or other medical problems do better with support from other family members. Additionally, one family member may be exhibiting symptoms, but the whole family might be next. Thus the entire family needs to be involved in behavior modification.

FAMILY EXERCISE

It's encouraging that today's parents play with their kids more. But do we exercise with them? The National Children and Youth Fitness Study II found that among children ages six to nine, 58 percent of their mothers and 62 percent of their fathers never exercised with them. On the average, parents exercise with their children less than one day a week.

It's one thing to play with your pre-school or grade-school children. But what about teenagers? Parents tend to lose contact with their teenage children because both adults and children are changing rapidly, have different interests and stresses, and often find it difficult to communicate. Dr. Cooper, who struggled through his kids' teenage years, advises: "Family members who exercise individually or together have much more to share, and better communication and relationships are the inevitable result. In many cases, I've seen parents maintain good, close relationships with their kids even during the difficult teenage years—simply because both parent and child have a deep interest in good health and physical conditioning."

A good way to keep lines of communication between parent and child open is by scheduling regular fitness and sports activities together. Along with getting you both in shape, the exercise eases the tension and gives you a common ground for discussion. From the mutual effort of exercise and its common theme, you and your child may build a fragile but working sense of trust and a tentative dialogue. Listen more than talk. Ask questions. Don't try to make the experience too profound or important—just a time for both of you to share some exercise and talk. Let the closeness grow slowly from the encounter.

Family fitness can mean exercising together as a unit or as parts of a unit, exercising at the same time—such as at a family fitness center—or exercising separately but sharing the experience with each other.

The Three F's: Fun, Fellowship, and Fitness

I'm often asked, "How can I get my kids to exercise?" My answer is always the same: If you emphasize fun and fellowship, fitness will follow. By using your imagination and being very enthusiastic about your child's exercise play, you will demonstrate that not only do you approve of physical activity, but that you think it is fun. Forcing children to exercise in order to improve their health will never work. Fake 'em out, I say, get them exercising by making the experience enjoyable. Few kids think exercising alone is fun. The fellowship of their friends or family members can turn a boring activity into a fun-filled adventure. Christopher won't ride his bike alone, but if his dad or a buddy—or preferably both—come along, then he'll ride for hours. In this respect kids are all alike, whether a pre-schooler or a teenager: they do not possess the adult motivation to exercise "because it is good for you." If you want children to exercise in order to promote physical fitness, they must first be motivated by fun and fellowship.

Learn to Play Like a Child

You can best involve your children in exercise by lowering yourself to their level of play rather than trying to force them to exercise by adult rules and behavior. If you have a two-year-old, play like a two-year-old, not a forty-year-old. Be silly, have fun, let yourself go! Encourage them to be uninhibited by your behavior. If you act uptight and seem not to really be enjoying yourself, your child will pick this feeling up and it will affect his or her attitude about exercise. Play shouldn't be the property of just young children. Frolic with your older children too, including the teenagers.

Parents are always amazed at how well I relate to their kids. My secret is that I can immediately focus on their interests, lower myself (or perhaps I should say raise myself) to their fun level behavior pattern, and enter their world. I don't invite them into my adult world of exercise, but rather tune in to their child's world of fun and then I can shift the activity toward fun and fitness.

Play like a child: roll in the grass with them, wrestle on the bed, laugh, hug, be silly, have fun. Once you have learned to act like a child, a fun attitude about fitness and sports will naturally evolve from the parent-child relationship.

Tips for Family Exercise

- First, make a commitment to get in shape with your kids. Put aside time to exercise with them. You may not believe it, but you do have the time. The investment is worth any sacrifice of time you may make.
- Schedule weekly family activities. In Sweden, it is a tradition on Sundays for the entire family to go off to the lakes or mountains for the day to enjoy exercise together. We should emulate this model by planning an active family day once a week—or at least once or twice a month. Pick activities that will allow all your family members to get

into the action: bike rides, walking, hiking, cross-country skiing, skating, tennis.

- Set aside vacation time for family fitness trips. The best way to sightsee is not out the window of a bus or car, but on foot or bike. My family likes to hike together, and we climb everything in sight during our vacation trips: I love to climb to the highest spot in town and look around. Some choices: a hike up a mountain or backwoods trail (plan this carefully and include a map, water, and food); a canoe trip; bike or cross-country ski tours. Some states—Vermont, for example—have tours that let you canoe (in summer) and cross-country ski (in winter) from country inn to country inn; your gear is taken to your next destination by van. Use your imagination. Explore, hike, climb. In Arizona, we hiked and rode horses and even trail bikes through the desert. When families visit us in New York City, Christopher likes to take them for a climb up the steps of the Statue of Liberty.

- A good recommendation is to start a family tradition of annual active vacations. Let the whole family plan the trip, making sure to allow each person space for individual interests. For example, a vacation at a family resort will allow for plenty of group activity but also provide for individual activities such as tennis or scuba diving. The annual active family vacation allows parents and children to spend valuable time together away from the hassles of home and work, and develops a common pool of memories to reflect on over the years. Some families bring along the children's grandparents, making it a three-generation vacation.

- Join a family-oriented fitness club or the YMCA or YMHA. People join for two reasons: (1) to do things as a family, such as swimming, volleyball, aerobic exercise classes, paddleball, or squash; (2) to have a place to leave the children—in a nursery or youth program—while they work out themselves.

- Schedule some activities for the entire family—but save others for just you and one child. This will give you both the chance to share an exercise experience together. I do most of the exercising with Christopher, but Virginia enjoys ice-skating and I leave that activity for the two of them. My brother Don has four sons, including twins, and he does his best to exercise with Mark, Matthew, Michael, and Danny. But what they really like is to have their turn alone with Dad for ball playing or one-on-one exercise.

- Support each other. When someone in the family is trying to lose weight, stop smoking, or get in shape, everyone should help. If family members exercise at widely different fitness levels, which makes it difficult to work out together, use the aerobic family. If you exercise together, but at different levels, always exercise at the level most comfortable for the slowest, least-fit member of your family. This may mean sacrificing your aerobic workout sometimes in exchange for family companionship.

One trick I use is to run or bike with Christopher and Virginia at their pace. Then when we finish I continue the workout at my own pace. Zooming up ahead and coming back, or always running a step or two ahead, gives the others the feeling that they are being dragged along. Think of your family first, your ego last.

- Control the competition. Teach each individual to compete only against himself or herself—to improve only against his or her own fitness level.

Perhaps the best method of all is to eliminate any adult-child competition. Then, as your kids get older, you can turn competitive instincts into such neutral fitness events as seeing how long the two of you can keep a volley going in tennis or volleyball. Such "fitness team" concepts involve you and your family without emphasizing competition between family members, which too often leads to disharmony and a child's quitting exercise workouts. Save competition for school and league activities and save family fitness time for fun and fellowship.

- Even if you can't exercise with your children for medical reasons, or are so far out of shape that you can't keep up with them, think of ways to go along and provide support. You could ride a bike while your child runs (if you're in a wheelchair, you can ride when they run) or provide them with water along a running path, or sit at poolside or trackside and cheer them on.

- Look for ways to involve your children in your own exercise routine, and for ways to join in their games. Christopher often stretches with me before I go out for my runs. I often come home from work and watch him play tag with his friends; sometimes I join 'em! Let your children see that you enjoy playing with them. Let the kids make up the rules.

- Use your imagination. Participate as a family in charity fun runs, bike- or walk-a-thons for exercise, and fund-raising. (Others pledge the money, you get the exercise.) See Chapters 15–19 for more ideas on using these and other aerobic activities for family workouts.

Here are three examples of how you can be physically active with your children:

- You run or walk; your young child pushes along on a scooter or play motorcycle. When Christopher was two years old he pushed his vehicle half a mile to school as I ran along every morning. Then I carried it home. Sure, some parents thought I was loony—and I am!—but we enjoyed it and he was a lot more fit than his classmates we passed as they rode to school in strollers or a taxi. Later, this exercise evolves to include a tricycle or a bike.

- Wrestling or "toughing" on a bed or other padded surface. The Freudians will debate this until they collapse from cardio-respiratory failure: What does it mean when daddies or mommies wrestle with their boys and girls? As long as it's gentle and fun, to hell with them. Christopher and I love it. I pick him up and toss him into the air, let him bounce, and he comes back for more. We go at it for up to fifteen minutes—an aerobic workout. He also gets strength training as I apply resistance to his holds. He is usually "Hulk Hogan" and I am the bad guy (Freudians, please note). The exercise is not suggested to let a parent demonstrate his strength over a child: Christopher *always* wins.
- Rock-and-roll aerobics. Turn on a record, radio, or rock show on TV and dance away with your child. Involve the whole aerobic family. Christopher likes to do this on the bed so he can jump around like rock star Michael Jackson.

Chapter 14 details several imaginative fitness games you can play with your children.

PARENTAL RESPONSIBILITIES

There are other things you can do as a parent who takes responsibility for the health and well-being of your child.

Education

- Help your child evaluate her or his own abilities. This means measuring only against past levels of fitness or performance.
- Help your child face failure in a positive way and reset his or her goals in a realistic manner. Everyone has setbacks. As Dame Agatha Christie said: "We cannot enjoy the sunshine without experiencing the shadows." Failure is part of life and part of life's lessons. We should allow our children to deal with both success and failure and teach them how to move on.
- Help children understand the purpose of play and games. Your child should learn why exercise is important and how fitness—along with good nutrition and stress management—can be incorporated into daily life. As your child grows, he or she should get a balance of free play,

then family activity, and school and community programs that promote motor skills important to developing coordination, balance, and agility. You and your child should learn lifetime sports that will promote fitness: swimming, brisk walking, skating, running, cross-country skiing, and so forth. These should be mixed with activities that involve success-oriented, controlled-competition team sports.

This is tricky. You want your child to become aware that exercise is good for him, but you don't want to harp on it. I can only suggest a personal example. It is difficult for me to get Christopher to brush his teeth regularly although he understands that it is good for him. But he doesn't particularly care at his young age about tooth decay that may not occur for years. Toothbrushing isn't a very exciting event in his life. If I made him do push-ups and sit-ups every morning along with brushing his teeth, he wouldn't want to do them either. Instead, we do sit-ups and push-ups together a few times a week and he enjoys the fun of it. He also likes adventure walks and other imaginative ways I try to sneak fitness into his days. Most of all, he enjoys physical activity because I believe it is fun and not something he has to do because it is good for him.

The surest way to avoid the "good for you" blues is to participate and bring your kids along for the fun of it. This is not an easy task. Swimming, running, or cross-country skiing with your child all take time. But they also return benefits to you, both as individuals and in your parent/child relationship.

Nutrition

Watch your child's weight and food consumption. Nutrition is an easy place to teach and learn about fitness—and an equally easy battleground between parent and child.

Good eating is mostly a matter of acquired tastes. Apples, oranges, or raisins, for example, are far better snack foods than potato chips, Fruit Loops, or candy, and are just as easily purchased. The same is true of fruit juices and milk, as opposed to colas or other canned beverages with high levels of caffeine and sugar.

Here, too, your example as a parent matters most. Children like to imitate adults. Give them something worthwhile and healthy to model. You won't have any success restricting your children from munching on unhealthy food if you do it yourself. Set a good example. At meals, forget the idea that leaving food is a waste; food from one meal can be saved to be eaten either as a snack or at another meal. Eating more than you need or want does more harm than good. Even a trip to the grocery store can be educational for your child: Why purchase certain foods but not others? What cereals, for example, are high in cholesterol or salt, and what are the long-term effects of these ingredients?

You can grant some leeway for bad habits—such as our chocolate chip cookies—if you are fair and honest with your children. But you also control what you and your kids eat, and you can (and should) eat healthy foods. Munching, by the way, isn't always bad. Friends of mine with teenage and adolescent children find that some of them need to eat constantly; they are "grazers." So the parents put out lots of snack foods like raisins and other dried fruits, apples, oranges, low-salt popcorn (made at home), yogurts, seeds, and nuts around the house. The kids suck 'em down.

The point here is simple: Don't become exercise/nutrition *fanatics*. Teach but don't lecture. Practice good health with your family, but make it fun.

Start Early

"You can start with the baby," says Dr. Kraus. "Instead of imprisoning him in a confining playpen, stick him out on the lawn and let him move around. Let him try out his muscles; let him develop them at a natural pace. If your baby does not walk as soon as others in a neighborhood, don't worry. The crawling about does him a great deal of good; it gives him the opportunity to develop strong trunk muscles." See Chapter 20 for guidelines on physical activity for pre-schoolers.

When your child outgrows the playpen and lawn/park scramble, start rolling a ball toward him or her. Move gradually into gentle games of rolling-ball catch and then catch itself to develop hand-eye and eye-foot coordination. Some kids who don't learn these simple skills—catching, throwing, and kicking a ball—later avoid sports and, thereby, fitness. You can encourage them to improve these skills by playing with them. This gives them fun time with you and, as they develop, confidence in their own physical skills. I believe that skills in both team and individual sports give a child and especially a teenager both exercise and self-esteem.

Eliminate Shortcuts

Encourage your children—and set an example—to minimize the use of labor-saving devices. Avoid making life too easy for them. Let them earn extra money by shoveling snow, raking leaves, or mowing the lawn—and turn these chores into fitness workouts.

I always walk with Christopher to his doctor's office a mile away. He is used to it and thinks nothing of the excursion. Meanwhile, his friends take taxicabs or the bus to go two or three city blocks because that is what their parents do. Set an example yourself. Walk anywhere you need to go if it is within a mile. (Time plays a role here. You might use the walk as your fitness exercise, thus saving time later in the day.) Send the kids out on errands or to activities on bikes or on foot rather than driving them everywhere. (Safety, of course, is a serious factor in deciding when and where to send your children.) The point is, leave the fitness-stealing devices at home. Exercise any way you and your kids can.

I remember Christopher coming home from school in shock one day because his class had walked across Central Park to visit a museum. He said the other boys were all complaining about the walk; they wanted to take the bus although the museum was less than a mile away and the path went through a lovely section of park. He couldn't believe it. "Dad," he said, "what's the big deal? We walk across the park together all the time."

I even refuse to use the elevators in our building. We live on the fifth floor and Christopher and I are the only people in the building—including those who live on floors below us—who walk up rather than ride. Again, Christopher gets the message that walking stairs is good for you and that mechanical contraptions aren't needed when you are fit.

Control TV Watching

Let's admit it and agree: Television is a lot of fun to watch, but it steals fitness from us. It robs both kids and adults of time that could be spent exercising. Action for Children's Television (ACT) suggests that kids watch no more than ten hours of television a week. Most kids in the United States now watch at least twice that. ACT also suggests that we parents teach our youngsters to watch specific quality shows, not just turn on the TV and sit.

This is easier said than done. Christopher, like all his friends, loves to watch cartoons and adventure movies. He would watch TV for ten hours straight if Virginia and I allowed it. We noticed something else. When he does watch it at great length, he turns into a short-tempered, irritable little boy.

"Television programs build up tension in a child," says Dr. Kraus, "at the same time that they keep him from having a physical outlet. You should no more let your child saturate himself with television or similar sedentary distractions than you should expose him to a contagious disease without inoculation. This may sound harsh, but it is the truth."

The American Academy of Pediatrics developed a thirty-second public service announcement that warns children against watching too much TV. It was made available in 1988 to the three major television networks and over 400 local stations. The cartoon depicts a boy and girl turning into "couch potatoes" while they watch television, with the message: "Avoid this dread disease; be choosy in what you watch."

The habit of watching TV too much, if started young, can be a lifelong habit. You need to set the example: Limit your own TV watching. Never use the TV as a baby-sitter. Seventy per cent of 1,800 women readers surveyed in 1988 by *Working Mother* magazine admitted to using TV as a baby-sitter so they could do chores or sleep later on weekends. Set firm limits on TV watching for your kids and hold to them. I attempt to get Christopher to turn off the set after a maximum of an hour. (I'd prefer it to be half an hour.) My rule is that he is allowed to watch a reasonable amount of TV as long as he gets a reasonable amount of exercise, and does his homework and chores. As the homework load increases, I'm counting on the TV watching to decrease. Stay tuned.

Often the only way I can get Christopher away from the TV on weekends is to take him out and play with him myself. As an only child in a city, he gets lonely easily and seeks companionship in television. After his Saturday morning cartoon marathon (which I do concede to him grudgingly), I drag him outside to play ball or go for a walk. At first he is irritable and claims to be tired. By the time we return, however, he is full of energy and in a great mood. Just as adults need to drag themselves out to exercise after a long and perhaps stressful day at work—or in front of the television set on weekends!—so too do our children need to be dragged away from TV for play and fun. But when you drag them away, be prepared to offer them not isolated free time with their toys but physical activity with you.

Jack Shepherd tried a different method with his children while his family lived in New York City. You might want to try this too.

When he realized that his kids were watching television every night and all weekend he gathered the family together. He talked with them about how too much TV made them irritable and stole valuable time from them. He explained that, if they agreed, the whole family would do the following:

- Have only one TV set in the house.
- Watch only three hours of television a week. Special programs the whole family watched together would be extra and not count as part of the three hours. Hours watched at friends' houses counted against the three-hour maximum.
- All programs to be watched would be marked by each family member in the TV listings during the weekend before viewing. His children were just learning to read, so he thought he would get a "two-fer": increased reading and a cutback in TV watching.

The family agreed, and they drew up a contract, dated it, and each of them signed it. There was no argument and no turning back.

The transformation was immediate and remarkable! The kids had to read the TV listings to find their programs, evaluate how they wanted to "spend" their three hours, and make plans. They learned how to budget and use their time. They scurried upstairs to do their homework—all homework spaces were TV free and isolated—and took breaks by watching their pre-selected TV programs. Three hours meant as many as six half-hour shows spread over the course of the week. Moreover, they became more selective and evaluative about television programs.

The control mechanism here is the contract, coupled with a calm and detailed discussion about television watching and what it does to us. There were some slips—at first, the kids tried to sneak in a few extra half-hours at friends' houses. When the first slips occurred, the kids were asked to help determine what "punishment" would be fair. They agreed that if someone went over the three-hour limit, the overtime would be deducted from the coming week's hours. Each person monitored himself or herself. An unforeseen benefit occurred: the kids started making plans over several weeks' time so they could watch shows that were special to them. (One other rule emerged: They could not accumulate hours for a TV binge later. Spend it or lose it was the rule.) As things turned out, they watched less and less TV as they grew up. As high-school students active in college-prep academics and varsity sports, they watched no TV at all. They had kicked the habit.

Cheryl and Jerry Ralya of New York City tried a more drastic measure in their family: They never owned a television set. Both parents think TV is a waste of time. Their son, Martin, claims he doesn't miss it. Other parents ask Cheryl and Jerry: "How will he ever learn to read without watching 'Sesame Street'?" Their answer: He has plenty of time to read because he isn't sitting in front of a TV set.

Here's a typical day without TV in the Ralya home: Martin walks one mile to school every morning with his father, then walks one mile home. Playmates who come home with him are shocked; some cannot walk the mile. Usually, Martin relaxes for half an hour when he gets home and then does his homework until dinner. After dinner he plays board games with one of his parents or goes out to exercise. Cheryl, a top runner with my elite Atalanta women's team, and Jerry run a six-mile loop of Central Park. Martin rides along on his bike. Once a week, Martin takes gymnastics classes. He also gets plenty of exercise at his school. Once or twice a year he will train for a two- to four-mile race and run it with his parents.

What is the Ralya Rule for creating a happy and fit child? Throw out TV and replace it with plenty of family intellectual and physical activities. You can start now: turn off the TV set; turn on exercise.

Think Long Term

Your primary responsibility as a parent who cares about your child's physical health is not to create a jock in your family. You simply want to teach your child the benefits of exercise and good nutrition. Christopher, a seven-year-old as I write this book, wants to be a baseball player for the New York Mets when he grows up. I go along with his dream as we play together. But in the meantime I make sure he enjoys all kinds of physical activity. Whether or not he grows up to be a major leaguer—and the odds are slim—he will enter adulthood physically fit and able to select various ways of keeping himself fit. That is the bottom line for me—and for you and your children.

ENCOURAGE YOUR CHILD

Parents should create an atmosphere at home that encourages children to want to participate in physical activity. They should not try to impose a specific program—including the exercise routines in this book. Let children be children. That is, let the kids play, explore, and seek activities on their own. The goal for parents of pre-schoolers and young grade-school kids is to plant a good attitude about fitness rather than whip the kids into shape. You can do this by providing an environment for exploration, including a variety of types of play. Older grade-school youngsters and teenagers will need more structure, more of a push, and will thrive only in an encouraging atmosphere.

It would be ideal if your children got into good enough shape to pass all of the fitness tests detailed in the next chapter, and if they exercised aerobically at least three times a week. But we don't live in an ideal world. If we simply help our children to enjoy exercise and make some progress toward improved fitness, we can establish a foundation for a lifetime of good health. As adults, our children will be more inclined to exercise for fun and fitness, rather than recall exercise as something they learned to hate when they were young because it was forced on them. Make a firm commitment to helping your children get in shape, but be flexible and loving, keep it fun, and most of all participate with them.

Don't stress the negative: heart attacks, obesity, permanent status as a "couch potato." Stress fun. Kids are smart—smarter than us. They know that running, jumping, chasing, rolling, and tumbling are fun. Later, they can become aware of and understand the reasons why exercise and good nutrition are important for them.

Christopher responds quickly to the technique of equal participation. I announce: "Dad wants to go out and have some fun exercising. Anyone around here want to come?" Or, "Dad has a bunch of boxes that have to be carried. Is there anyone around here strong enough to help?" Just carrying a big box upstairs with his dad makes Christopher feel good about his strength and fitness, and he enjoys sharing a physical activity with me.

He also gets a sense of his importance in the family by helping out with its work, as well as participating in its fun.

It's better to avoid making exercise a "have to do" assignment. Force never graduates to fun; it becomes hatred and rejection. Never bribe a kid to exercise by promising a reward such as more television, a new toy, or an ice-cream cone. That gives him or her the wrong message: that exercise is in itself not a worthwhile task unless there is a tangible reward attached to it.

Give Your Kids a Place to Play

Don't give them too many restrictions. It is far more important to have happy, active kids than a house in which everything is neatly in its place— at least that's what I tell Virginia after Christopher messes up our bedroom while "toughing" with his dad. Kids need a place to run wild. That doesn't mean turning the living-room sofa into a trampoline. But why not their bed—or even yours—if the beds are sturdy. Christopher enjoys wrestling and doing "rock and roll" on our bed. He is also allowed to dive from the dresser onto our bed in a "flying somersault." His bunk bed doesn't allow this exercise. If possible, erect a basket in your child's room and let him or her shoot away. I shoot baskets with Christopher in the bedroom with a six-foot-high basket and a mini-basketball. I put away all breakable things and guard the windows.

Ideally, one room in your apartment or house can be set aside as a real "romper room." Let the children play as rough as they want (within safe bounds). They can wrestle, bounce on one of those round padded trampolines (or a bed), play football or basketball, and so forth, during impromptu bursts of energy. Kids need to release energy in an unrestricted but controlled way. That is not contradictory: fighting or breaking beds or hurting someone else is not the same as bouncing around a room in controlled exercise.

That goes for the backyard or park where your kids play. Don't place a lot of rules on what can or cannot be done because you don't want the flowers stepped on or the grass worn out. In many city neighborhoods, kids can even play safely on the street; stickball, ring-a-lario, stoopball, and other city sports are good exercise and fun.

Don't Hold Them Back Too Much

Too many parents hold back their children for fear the kids will get hurt. As I tell Virginia: Little boys are made for getting dirty and roughed up. So are little girls. Boys and girls should be allowed to zoom full blast through rough physical activities. A New Hampshire family Jack Shepherd knows loved ice hockey. Long before such things were even dreamed of, they outfitted everyone—Mom and Dad, sisters, and brothers—with sticks, pads, helmets, and mouthguards. They hit the ponds near their home during the heart of winter and later rented ice time on the Dartmouth College hockey rink—even when the only time available was from one to two in the morning! Everybody played. Friends and dates filled out the sides and the girls checked the boys into the boards with equally resounding thunks! One daughter became an outstanding ice-hockey player at Middlebury College in Vermont.

Let 'em play, I say! I admit that I get nervous when Christopher crawls full speed across a playground obstacle high above the ground or climbs a tree. But I hold it in and remember how reckless I was at his age and how that benefitted me. Even when he was accidentally pushed off a playground structure and seemed badly injured, I struggled to stay calm. Once I knew that he wasn't seriously hurt, just scared, I held him close and waited it out. Soon, he zoomed back into action with his friends. We both learned a valuable lesson: Freedom and caution are two sides of the same coin, and both should be used.

Most young children can and should play all day. Dr. Ernst van Aaken, the late German fitness enthusiast, once measured the total distance covered by a seven-year-old boy at play. The lad covered five miles in ninety minutes with four hundred breaks—no surprise to his exhausted mother! That's why we should stand back and let kids be kids, within set limits. When our own anxieties discourage our children from playing, we send the message that physical activity is dangerous or harmful.

Encourage, Don't Compare

It is important to praise your child honestly. False praise gives the child a false image, but honest praise helps the child progress toward a goal by competing only with himself. Encourage your child by expressing your interest in his or her attempts, no matter how small they are.

Christopher could hit a baseball very well at a young age, but he was slow in developing his ability to catch a ball compared to the other boys he played with. I devised games where he could set a "world record" for catching throws and compared him only to his own progress. This took the pressure off him, made him feel more confident, and resulted in improvement in his catching.

Let your child grow at his or her own speed. Allow your child to have the opportunity to improve. Avoid any comparisons with other children. Instead, make sure your child increases his or her activity level. Encourage participation, not competition. Like adult runners, bikers, swimmers, and walkers, a child should compete only against his or her own past self, not others. Improvement becomes a reward in itself.

Establish Incentive Goals and Rewards

You will want to establish some fitness goals, such as running non-stop for a mile, biking around the park, or accumulating a certain number of minutes of aerobic activity in a month. You may want to reward your child with fitness-related prizes.

Any fitness goals should be reasonable and mutually set. Do not set goals *for* your child, but *with* your child.

A friend of mine helps his children set two goals: one likely to be obtained with good effort; the other a "reach goal" to be attained with extra effort. When his kids reach the first, they celebrate and then set off to reach the second. Even if they fail, they win: they will have attained the first goal, and they will have learned how to set a goal, achieve it, set another goal, and deal with failure and frustration.

Rewards are somewhat more tricky. Sometimes the goal attained is itself a reward. That same friend taught his kids the two-goal attainment pattern when they tried out for teams. Their first goal was to try to make the lowest level team—for example, to make the freshman team if they were freshmen, or the B team. Their second goal was to work hard enough to not only make the freshman or B team, but also to make the next team up, perhaps even the varsity or A team. The same two-level attainment can be used for any goal objectives. These are usually incentive enough.

But if you want to reward your child, be certain that the reward is fitness related and that both you and the child define the reward specifically and clearly beforehand. For example, if your child sets a goal to run so many minutes at an aerobic level per month, the reward might be a new pair of running shoes. (Name the shoes and the price before your child starts.) Do not reward your child with non-fitness-related prizes like candy bars, ice cream, soda, and so forth. The message is contradictory. If food is a reward—and I don't think it should be (reward implies its counterpart, punishment, and I do not advocate withholding food from a child)—you might agree on a fun, carbohydrate-loaded dinner at a good spaghetti restaurant. Other than that, stick to fitness-related rewards. And when the kid wins, reward quickly. Never be slow or go back on your word.

ENCOURAGE A VARIETY OF ACTIVITIES

Children need variety, and you can make sure that through family activity, free play, community programs, and school physical education classes your child's fitness program is properly balanced. "Under age twenty, all we're trying to do is get youngsters interested in a life that includes physical activity," says Paul Dyment, M.D., chairman of the Sports Medicine Committee for the American Academy of Pediatrics. "Any activity that is enjoyable and that the family does together is of value."

Those activities should, as your child grows to school age, gradually provide:

- Motor skills (coordination, balance, agility, speed, power);
- Cardio-respiratory endurance, muscular strength and endurance, flexibility, body composition;
- Skills in lifetime sports such as swimming, tennis, running, and biking;
- Experience in success and failure, teamwork, and goal-setting through controlled team competition.

Kids love unstructured play in natural surroundings. They turn a pile of dirt into a mountain climbing expedition or a wooded lot into active hide-and-seek. Let your kids use their imagination and the environment to exercise freely. Later, children can also use structured time to learn those motor skills, fair play, sharing, flexibility exercises, new games, and so forth. As they grow you will want to encourage your children to use after-school gymnastics programs, sports teams, and the like, combined with school physical education classes. These should continue to add skill development, but they must be fun for the kids.

Young children like a variety of activities. Be prepared to switch gears and move them from one activity to another to hold their interest. This is also true over the course of a week. Christopher may play baseball on Monday, but on Tuesday prefer to go on an adventure walk with me. Then on Wednesday we might play baseball again or take a run in Central Park. Wherever you live, the lesson is simple: Mix up your family's fitness activities both within the individual session and over the course of the week. Allow your children to select activities they enjoy. This will keep their interest high.

Playgrounds and Parks

Children need unsupervised play time along with structured activities. Just turn children loose at a playground and watch them run, climb, chase each other, and have fun. Christopher makes up all kinds of tag games with the kids at the playground, and those become informal fitness exercises.

An ideal playground includes plenty of places to climb, run, and jump safely. Christopher prefers—and so should we as parents—"active" playgrounds that include all kinds of imaginative fitness lures, such as ropes and chain-link fences to climb, wiggly bridges to run across, obstacles to be scrambled over to reach the top of a slide, rubber tires to jump and swing on, poles to shimmy up and slide down, and so forth.

Give Your Kids Active Toys

Blocks, balls, non-motorized scooters, bikes, jump ropes, and other such equipment encourage fitness activities. Let the kids push their toys and use their imagination. One day Christopher and I were out walking in New York City's Central Park when we were passed by the ultimate lazy child: a four-year-old gliding along effortlessly in a motorized play car! That kid's parents were robbing him of exercise!

When Christopher was only a few months old, Virginia and I bought a Jolly Jumper and rigged it up in a doorway of our city apartment. The contraption hangs in any doorway and straps around a small child, who then can jump up and down as though on a spring. Christopher loved it and we believe that the exercise strengthened his legs and was a significant reason why he took off running before he was ten months old.

You don't need expensive equipment. In fact, we drain our kids' imagination by showering them with toys that do all the thinking and work for them. Kids often like best everyday things they convert to toys; even parts of toys, like bicycle wheels, are fun. When one couple I know tried to toss out their old broken double bed with its "deep valley" mattress, the kids cried for Daddy to retrieve it from the dump. He did, and they used it for the next ten years as a huge, wonderful trampoline. A broken baseball bat topped by an old sheet tucked tightly into the mattress created a mysterious tent on long summer days.

Encourage After-School Activities

As your children grow and enter school, begin to look around for good after-school activities for them. These are especially important if your child is getting less than thirty minutes a day of physical exercise during the school week. Consider the alternative: your kid sits in front of the television set, monitored by a baby-sitter who usually has no interest in physical activity, until you come home from work. There is no gain here; and there is, as we discussed above, considerable loss.

If possible, start with unstructured physical activity after school. This means you, a fitness-conscious baby-sitter, or a play group. When I grew up, I rushed home and hit the streets to bike, run, and play sports with my neighborhood friends until my parents made me come inside for dinner. If you live in the suburbs or a city, lack of space to play safely—and the lure of video games and TV—may put you and your child at a disadvantage. Here's an early parental battleground. You should work with other parents—perhaps your aerobic family—and the schools or community organizations to create after-school programs and play space. You might "pool" your kids with other parents a few times a week and let them get together and play and exercise. Rotate the parent supervisor and you've got several afternoons off while your kid is getting his or her workout and fun. Homework comes after dinner. Pawn the TV set.

Balance Lifetime Sports with Competitive Sports

Team sports, when they are fun, can contribute to your child's education and fitness. Not all children like them, however. No child should be forced to play a team sport. In fact, the so-called lifetime fitness sports are of far more value. Not many forty-year-olds get together for a football or basketball game, but they certainly go out running, swimming, biking, rowing, mountain climbing, ice or roller skating, and so on. All of these are fun for kids, too. Lifetime sports are building blocks and long-term investments that your child can use as he or she grows into adulthood.

Unfortunately, we as adults tend to stress only competitive team sports for our children. If a child is not very good at sports, he or she is often ignored by those who enjoy sports. If you want to test this, the next time you attend a gathering of adults and kids see which kid gets the most adult attention. It will most likely be the high-school football player or his equivalent.

Jack Shepherd in Vermont raised a son, Caleb, who was captain of his high-school lacrosse team in both his junior and senior years. He was also a solid student at an outstanding high school, and when he applied to college the adults began acting very foolish over him. After one college interview, for example, the dean of admissions told him in a loud voice that could be heard by every other parent and child anxiously waiting for an interview: "We are really looking forward to your application. You're going to be an outstanding player here at ol' Slipshod U." Luckily, the boy was also bright and interested in going to a college where academics had more value than athletics.

For your own child, search out a team sports program that rewards all participants equally and where everyone gets to play a lot. In addition, teach your child lifetime sports and let him or her try as many as possible.

The primary goal is not to have an athlete in the family. That's okay as long as the athlete enjoys the team sport and doesn't get a distorted image of himself or herself from playing in front of adoring adults. But the goal here is a lifelong interest in good health and fitness. This lasts a much longer time than the cheers.

4

Family Fitness
Evaluation Tests

There's an old saying that a journey of one thousand miles begins with a single step. The first step you and your children take on the road to fitness is—like all the other steps I suggest here—small, easy, progressive, and important. You need to answer this question: How fit are my children and I? To do this, you need to establish a baseline of fitness for each member of your family.

The tests in this chapter will help you evaluate your family's fitness level. The tests may be given at home or in your child's school. (See the Appendix for details about various school fitness testing programs.) Then, after a period of fitness training—at least eight weeks—you may re-test yourself and your family to measure your progress. (In a school physical education program, testing is usually done in the fall for a baseline and repeated at the end of the school year.)

These tests are designed to enable you to measure the basic fitness components—flexibility, muscular strength and endurance, and cardio-respiratory endurance—defined and discussed in the previous chapter. Additional fitness testing and goal setting should be established for body composition. Chapter 30 establishes guidelines for body fat percentages, weight goals, and so forth.

Two cautions:

- Adults over the age of thirty-five who have been inactive should have a thorough medical examination prior to taking these vigorous tests and before starting a fitness program. Even children who are inactive, especially if they are overweight, should be checked out by the family physician or pediatrician before taking these tests or starting a fitness program.

- Practice the tests before taking them. Practice, for example, doing sit-ups at a relaxed pace a few times a week prior to taking the timed one-minute test. After getting your doctor's approval, jog slowly a few times a week for a few weeks prior to taking the running test. Before taking the tests, warm up; cool down afterwards. Be conservative in your first fitness test. Don't go all out. (After all, you want to leave some room for improvement!) View the tests as an opportunity to know more about yourself and set a baseline from which to start your journey.

Use the tests in this chapter as motivating tools. Although I have detailed in the previous chapters the level of unfitness in the United States, do not feel as though you are competing against that mark. *Do not compete against other family members or peers.* Instead, focus on competing against yourself. Every step you make toward fitness is made along a path only you follow: you compete only against the "old" you. The same is true of your children. Don't let them get into competition with one another. This is fitness, not sports competition; they compete only against their "old" selves along their own, individual paths.

Don't be discouraged if you score poorly on all or some of the tests. In our unfit society, most children and adults fail these tests. Don't think the tests are too hard; they measure where we should be. They are goals. Use your test returns to improve the level of fitness in your entire family. You may score "excellent" in one category but "poor" in another. To be physically fit, you should score at the average-good level of fitness in all fitness components. I tested Christopher at age six on all the test items as I started this book, and then again just as he turned seven, as I finished the book. He improved from "average" to "excellent" in all categories. It was a toss-up over who was more proud, the excited boy or his dad.

After testing, follow the training guidelines in the following chapters to improve fitness levels in each of the key components. If you (or your child) score poorly, set a goal to reach average levels. If you score "average," aim to meet "good" standards, or perhaps health-fitness standards established by the AAHPERD. Once you (or your child) reach these standards you may want to see if you can score in the "excellent range" and perhaps qualify for the President's Challenge Award by reaching the eighty-fifth percentile. This was a goal Christopher set, and met, for all categories. Unfortunately, only 2 percent of youngsters in the U.S. can qualify for this award. These levels, however, are beyond fitness requirements for good health, and are performance goals rather than fitness goals.

The following family fitness evaluation program includes information from a variety of testing programs. I have selected and pieced together (thus there is some overlap of standards) highlights from many programs to provide your family with a comprehensive, simplified evaluation requiring a minimum of equipment. More detailed information on the individual testing programs is available from the indicated sources.

So, let's get started! How do you and your family score in flexibility, muscular strength and endurance, and cardio-respiratory endurance? You can take these tests alone or together as a family event. Here's what you should do:

1. After getting your doctor's go-ahead, find a good place to do the tests. Then, after properly warming up, *take the tests one at a time*. You should take breaks between the tests.
2. Establish fitness *baseline scores* for each family member and record them.
3. Determine individualized *fitness goals* for each family member in each test.
4. Follow the *fitness training programs*, as detailed in the following chapters, to achieve your individual goals.
5. After eight or more weeks, *re-test* on all items to monitor progress and record your scores. *Continue* with your fitness program.

You may want to establish rewards for each family member who achieves his or her goals and who continues. Christopher's award for running his first non-stop mile was one of his dad's old running trophies. He cherishes it more than anything I could have bought him.

TEST #1: KRAUS-WEBER

Kraus-Weber Tests, introduced in Chapter 1, were first administered to U.S. schoolchildren in 1952. The awful results were given to President Eisenhower and then to President Kennedy, which led to a vigorous—but short-lived—national youth fitness crusade. These tests determine whether your muscles have the strength and flexibility to handle your weight and height. The same basic fitness tests apply to both sexes, and to all age, weight, and height groups because they are self-correlating: they test your strength against your own body weight and size.

I was trained by Dr. Kraus and Alexander Melleby, author of *The Y's Way to a Healthy Back*, to administer the Kraus-Weber Tests to all students entering our beginning fitness and back-exercise classes. I was shocked at how many adults couldn't pass these seemingly simple tests. Indeed, Melleby reports that 61 percent of back-pain sufferers entering his national "Y's Way to a Healthy Back" program fail the toe-touch test for flexibility and 48 percent can't perform a single bent-knee sit-up for abdominal strength.

The K-W Tests are *minimum* tests of fitness. If you can't pass them, you may still begin an easy comprehensive fitness program to get you started toward fitness. Passing all of these tests doesn't mean that you are physically fit. Continue with more advanced tests to better measure your fitness level.

Do the following Kraus-Weber Tests in order. Do not warm up beforehand. They should be completed as slowly and smoothly as possible. Avoid jerky movements. Don't strain. Stop and rest briefly after each test. When you take the tests, make sure that you are comfortable. Take off your shoes and socks, and wear loose-fitting clothing that allows you to move freely and easily.

Here are the six Kraus-Weber Tests:

Kraus-Weber Test No. 1: Hip Flexor Minimum Strength
Lie on the floor on your back with your legs out straight. Put your hands behind your neck. Raise both feet (knees straight and feet together) until your heels are about ten inches off the floor. To pass this test, hold your legs in this position for ten seconds. (The test measures minimum strength in your hip flexor muscles.)

Kraus-Weber Test No. 2: Abdominal and Hip Flexor Minimum Strength
Lie on the floor on your back with your hands at the side of your head, feet out straight. Have your partner hold your legs at the ankles. To pass the test, roll into a sit-up position. (The test measures the combined strength of your hip flexors and abdominal muscles.)

Kraus-Weber Test No. 3: Abdominal Muscle Minimum Strength
Lie on the floor on your back with your hands at the side of your head. Bend your knees, feet flat on the floor, with your ankles close to your buttocks. Have someone hold your ankles. To pass the test, roll up into a sit-up position. (The test measures the strength of your abdominal muscles.)

Kraus-Weber Test No. 4: Upper Back Minimum Strength
Lie on the floor on your stomach. Place a thick pillow under your hips. Put your hands behind your neck. Your partner should put one hand on the small of your back and another on your ankles. To pass this test, lift your upper body just enough to clear the floor and hold that position for ten seconds. (This test measures the strength of your upper back muscles.)

Kraus-Weber Test No. 5: Lower Back Minimum Strength

Lie on the floor on your stomach with your forehead resting on your hands. Keep the pillow under your hips. Your partner should place one hand on your shoulders and the other on the small of your back. To pass this test, raise both legs from the hips, keeping your knees straight, just enough to clear the floor and hold for ten seconds. (This test measures the strength of your lower back muscles.)

Kraus-Weber Test No. 6: Minimum Flexibility of Back and Hamstring Muscles

Stand erect, legs together, ankles touching, arms at your side. Put your chin on your chest, bend over, slowly reach toward the floor with your hands without bending. Don't force the stretch or bounce. To pass this test, touch the floor with your middle finger. (This test measures the flexibility of your back and the muscles in the backs of your legs.)

TEST #2: FLEXIBILITY

Carefully warm up for all flexibility tests. To improve your flexibility for these tests, use the stretching exercises in Chapter 11, particularly exercises #1 and #9. Two simple tests for flexibility of the low back and hamstring muscles—which relate to back pain—are described here. Choose one test. It should be noted that females are naturally more flexible than males.

Test: Modified Sit-and-Reach

Take your shoes and socks off and sit on the floor with your legs extended. Put the bottoms of your feet against a wall with your heels about six inches apart. Keeping your legs straight, slowly extend your arms forward, hands together, and try to touch the wall and bring your forehead as close to your knees as possible. Stop and relax when you feel a mild pulling sensation, then try to stretch a bit farther until you feel another pull. Hold for three seconds. Scores:

Poor: Fingertips four or more inches from wall.

Fair: Fingertips one to three inches from wall.

Passing Score: Can hold fingertips touching toes or wall for three seconds.

Excellent: Can touch fists or palms to wall.

Test: Trunk Flexion

Place a yardstick or measuring tape on the floor. Take off your shoes and socks and sit near the zero end of the tape, legs straight and flat on the floor. Your heels should be twelve inches apart and even with the fifteen-inch mark of the yardstick. (A strip of tape at the fifteen-inch mark will make it easier to line up your heels.) A partner should hold your knees down by gently pushing on your thighs.

Slowly reach forward with both hands overlapped with palms facing the floor. Do not jerk or bounce—that's cheating and you might injure yourself. Exhale slowly and drop your head as you reach forward. Reach out with your fingers and touch as far up the yardstick as possible without lifting your knees. Record, to the nearest inch, your best score in the three trials.

Charts A and B list standards for boys and girls ages six to seventeen. These standards were developed for the Chrysler Fund–AAU Physical Fitness Program. Your goal should be to reach at least the "national average" figure. Christopher at age seven scored eighteen—much better than average.

Chart C lists general standards for adults. Your goal should be to reach at least the "average" figure.

TEST #3: MUSCULAR STRENGTH AND ENDURANCE

Muscular strength and endurance are generally tested simultaneously. The two most important areas of strength in terms of fitness are the abdominal muscles and the upper body. Your abdominal muscles relate to

CHART A

Boys' Youth Flexibility Test: Trunk Flexion

AGE	6	7	8	9	10	11	12
STANDARD							
National Average	15	16	15	16	15	16	16
Outstanding	17	18	18	18	18	18	18

AGE	13	14	15	16	17
STANDARD					
National Average	16	16	17	18	17
Outstanding	18	19	20	20	20

CHART B

Girls' Youth Flexibility Test: Trunk Flexion

AGE	6	7	8	9	10	11	12
STANDARD							
National Average	17	17	17	17	17	18	19
Outstanding	19	20	20	21	21	21	21

AGE	13	14	15	16	17
STANDARD					
National Average	20	20	21	21	21
Outstanding	23	23	23	23	24

All measurements are in inches.
Fifteen inches is the baseline at the heels.
National average is the average score for the 1986–1987 Chrysler Fund–AAU Physical Fitness Program.
Outstanding standard is the eightieth percentile for the Chrysler Fund–AAU Test.
Data compiled for the Chrysler Fund—AAU Physical Fitness Program. Reprinted by permission of the Amateur Athletic Union.

CHART C

Adult Flexibility Test: Trunk Flexion

	Men	Women
Excellent	21–23	23–25
Good	16–20	20–22
Average	15	17–19
Fair	12–14	13–16
Poor	5–11	9–12

lower back strength (and pain) and your upper body concerns good posture and your ability to lift, carry, and push objects.

The following tests are divided into scores for boys and girls ages five to eighteen, and for adults. Abdominal strength and endurance are measured by sit-ups. Upper body strength is measured by push-ups and pull-ups. (See Chapter 11 for guidelines for sit-ups, push-ups, and pull-ups.)

Test: Boys' and Girls' Modified Sit-ups

Lie on your back on the floor with your knees flexed at about ninety degrees, feet, buttocks, and back flat on the floor, heels about twelve inches from your buttocks. Fold your arms across your chest with your hands on the opposite shoulders, arms close to the chest. Hold your arms in contact with your chest throughout the test. Have a partner hold your feet or anchor them under a solid object, such as a couch.

Curl to a sitting position, breathing out as you come up, until you touch your elbows to your thighs (keeping your arms tight to your chest). Then lower your body until your midback makes contact with the floor. Do not bounce off the floor or arch your back in an attempt to do more sit-ups. This might cause injury.

Goal: See how many sit-ups you can do within a timed minute. You may rest at any time and start again within the one-minute timed period. Count and record only those sit-ups completed correctly within the one-minute period.

Charts D and E list standards for children and youths ages five to eighteen. Your goal is to reach the "health fitness" standard (established by the AAHPERD). The President's Challenge level (eighty-fifth percentile) is included if you wish to aim toward that higher performance goal. Christopher reached that goal with fifty sit-ups (despite stopping twice to scratch a mosquito bite), surprising and pleasing me.

CHART D
Boys' Muscular Strength and Endurance Test: Modified Sit-ups

AGE	5	6	7	8	9	10	11
STANDARD							
Health Fitness	20	20	24	26	30	34	36
President's Challenge		33	36	40	41	45	47

AGE	12	13	14	15	16	17	18
STANDARD							
Health Fitness	38	40	40	42	44	44	44
President's Challenge	50	53	56	57	56	55	55

CHART E

Girls' Muscular Strength and Endurance Test: Modified Sit-ups*

AGE	5	6	7	8	9	10	11
STANDARD							
Health Fitness	20	20	24	26	28	30	33
President's Challenge		32	34	38	39	40	42

AGE	12	13	14	15	16	17	18
STANDARD							
Health Fitness	33	33	35	35	35	35	35
President's Challenge	45	46	47	48	45	44	44

*Modified sit-ups in one minute.

Health Fitness standard established by AAHPERD's 1988 Physical Best program and refers to the fitness level needed to be healthy.

President's Challenge is the eighty-fifth percentile score for the 1985 President's Council Survey and represents the high level of fitness required to qualify for the Presidential Physical Fitness Award.

Adult Test: Sit-ups

Lie on the floor flat on your back, knees bent, feet about eighteen inches from your buttocks. Clasp your hands behind your head.

Exhaling, curl up to a sitting position. Alternately touch the inside of one knee with the opposite elbow—left elbow to right knee, right elbow to left knee. Inhaling, slowly recline to your starting position flat on the floor. Each curl-up is one adult unmodified sit-up. Using a timer, score the number of sit-ups you can complete correctly within one minute.

Caution: Do not attempt to grind out more sit-ups than you can do with reasonable comfort, especially if you haven't been exercising with sit-ups frequently. If you cannot do the minimum (ten for men, two for women), start instead with the modified sit-up described in the boys' and girls' section above. As your stomach (abdominal) muscles become stronger, shift to this adult sit-up form.

Chart F lists standards for adult unmodified sit-ups as developed by the YMCA.

CHART F

Adult Muscular Strength and Endurance Test: Sit-ups*

	Men	Women
Excellent	40–45	35–39
Good	31–39	26–34
Average	25–30	20–25
Fair	18–24	11–19
Poor	10–17	4–10

*Sit-ups in one minute.
Source: Clayton Myers, *The Official YMCA Physical Fitness Handbook*, 1975.

CHART G

Muscular Strength and Endurance Test: Modified Push-ups

	Average	Outstanding
Boys and girls ages 6–9	10–15	20–30
Girls ages 10–13	20–30	30–40
Girls ages 14–19	20–30	30–40
Women ages 20–29	20–30	30–40
Women ages 30–39	15–25	25–40
Women ages 40–49	10–20	20–30
Women ages 50–59	5–10	10–20

Test: Push-ups for Upper Body Muscular Strength and Endurance

This is a simple test of strength and endurance in your arms, shoulders and chest for both children/youths and adults. The idea is to see how many push-ups you can do within a minute.

Modified Push-ups: The modified push-up is recommended for all women and girls, and for boys under age ten. Lie face down on the floor with your hands palms down under your shoulders, fingers pointing straight ahead, elbows bent, legs together. Keeping your knees in contact with the floor, but lifting your feet off the ground, push your upper body off the floor until your arms are straight. Keep your back straight at all times. Lower yourself to the floor until your chest lightly touches it. Breathe out as you push up. No rest periods are allowed. Do as many push-ups as you can until you can no longer do them with proper form, or until a minute elapses.

The following are general standards for modified push-ups. Christopher was able to improve from five to thirty between ages six and seven.

Regular Push-ups: All males above the age of about ten should do the regular push-up. Boys around ten may want to try modified push-ups until they can do the regular push-up with good form.

Start in the same position as for the modified push-up. Instead of pushing off from your hands and knees as in the modified push-up, you push off from your hands and toes. Lift your knees off the floor and keep your back and legs straight throughout the push-up. Arching of the back is not allowed. You should not touch your knees or stomach, only your chest, to the floor.

The following are general standards for regular push-ups.

Test: Pull-ups for Upper Body Strength and Endurance

This is one of the most controversial tests among physical educators. Many educators feel the pull-up is not a good indicator of upper body strength. Also, because the individual must pull his or her body weight upward, heavier children are penalized.

Many children and adults do not possess adequate strength to pass this fitness test. Instead of being graded "zero" for not completing one pull-up, their progress can be noted as scoring one-half or three-quarters of a pull-up—how much the person can pull himself up toward the bar. Use this to motivate you or your children, if you or they cannot do a pull-up.

Modified Pull-ups: You and your child might try the modified pull-up. This was developed by the AAHPERD with standards established for boys and girls ages six to nine as part of the 1987 National Children and Youth Fitness Study II. In the modified pull-up test, the youngster lies on his or her back on the floor. A bar is positioned—between two chairs, for example—at a height one or two inches above the child's shoulders but beyond the child's reach when his or her arms are fully extended. An

CHART H

Muscular Strength and Endurance Test: Push-ups

	Average	Outstanding
Boys ages 10–13	20–30	30–40
Boys ages 14–19	30–40	40–50
Men ages 20–29	30–40	40–50
Men ages 30–39	25–35	35–45
Men ages 40–49	20–30	30–40
Men ages 50–59	15–25	25–35

elastic band is placed parallel to the bar and seven to eight inches under it.

Grasp the bar, buttocks off the floor, arms and legs straight. Only your heels touch the floor. Use the overhand grip, palms facing away from your body. Now, using your arms, pull your body up until your chin is hooked over the elastic band. Then return to your starting position, still holding the bar, arms extended and only your heels touching the floor. Your hips and knees must remain extended throughout the test.

There is no time limit. Do as many modified pull-ups as you can do properly. Charts I and J list the suggested number of modified pull-ups for boys and girls six to nine.

Test: The Pull-up

You need to erect a horizontal bar in a doorway or at a playground, or even find a sturdy tree limb of the proper thickness. A secure horizontal bar is best. You should be able to hang with your arms fully extended without your feet touching the ground.

CHART I

Boys' Muscular Strength and Endurance Test: Modified Pull-ups

AGE	6	7	8	9
STANDARD				
National Average	6	8	10	10
Outstanding	12	15	17	20

CHART J

Girls' Muscular Strength and Endurance Test: Modified Pull-ups

AGE	6	7	8	9
STANDARD				
National Average	6	7	8	9
Outstanding	11	14	14	15

Standards represent the fiftieth percentile and eighty-fifth percentile from AAHPERD's 1987 National Children and Youth Fitness Study II.

Hang from the bar with an overhand (palms outward) grip and your legs and arms fully extended. Pull your body with your arms until your chin is over the bar without touching it. Then lower yourself completely back to the full-hang starting position.

Do as many as you can. There is no time limit. Do not swing your body, bend your knees, or kick your legs.

Standards for pull-ups for adults are unclear. The levels for teenagers are as good a goal as any: three to five pull-ups for men; one for women. Charts K and L list the standards for boys and girls ages five to eighteen. The goal is to reach the "health fitness" level established by the AAHPERD.

A more challenging goal: the President's Challenge standard at the eighty-fifth percentile. For seven-year-old Christopher this high standard is four pull-ups, which I considered impossible, since as a six-year-old he couldn't even move from the starting position. After meeting the President's Challenge with four full pull-ups, he informed me that he and his buddy Liam Millhiser do pull-ups at camp on a tree limb "all the time for fun."

TEST #4: AEROBIC TESTS

Next comes a series of three simple cardio-respiratory endurance tests. Choose one. These will help determine your aerobic fitness. *Warning:* If

CHART K
Boys' Muscular Strength and Endurance Test: Pull-ups

AGE	5	6	7	8	9	10	11
STANDARD							
Health Fitness	1	1	1	1	1	1	2
President's Challenge		2	4	5	5	6	6

AGE	12	13	14	15	16	17	18
STANDARD							
Health Fitness	2	3	4	5	5	5	5
President's Challenge	7	7	10	11	11	13	13

CHART L

Girls' Muscular Strength and Endurance Test: Pull-ups

AGE	5	6	7	8	9	10	11
STANDARD							
Health Fitness	1	1	1	1	1	1	1
President's Challenge		2	2	2	2	3	3

AGE	12	13	14	15	16	17	18
STANDARD							
Health Fitness	1	1	1	1	1	1	1
President's Challenge	2	2	2	2	1	1	1

Health Fitness standard established by AAHPERD's 1988 Physical Best program refers to fitness level needed to be healthy.

President's Challenge is the eighty-fifth percentile score for the Council's 1985 Survey. It represents the high level of fitness required to qualify for the Presidential Physical Fitness Award.

you are an adult and have not been exercising vigorously on a regular basis, check with your doctor before attempting these tests. Next, I suggest that you also prepare yourself for these tests with six to eight weeks of aerobic conditioning, following guidelines in Chapter 12.

Before doing these tests, you must warm up properly with stretching exercises and a brisk five- to ten-minute walk prior to starting the test. The ideal place to test yourself is your local high-school track, which is probably a quarter-mile in length (or four hundred meters, about three yards short of a quarter-mile). You can design a course anywhere, but try to keep it level. After finishing each test, be certain to cool down with a five- to ten-minute walk and a series of stretching exercises.

Aerobic Test #1: Continuous Vigorous Activity

You don't need precise measurements to get a good idea of how physically fit you are. If you can exercise vigorously—fast walking, easy jogging, lap swimming—for an extended period of time, you are at least minimally fit in terms of your cardio-respiratory endurance.

Using any of the aerobic exercises mentioned in Chapters 15–19, you

CHART M

Aerobic Fitness Test: Continuous Vigorous Activity

Ages 5–6	10–12 minutes
Ages 7–9	15–20 minutes
Ages 10–18	20–30 minutes
Adults	20–30 minutes

CHART N

Aerobic Fitness Test: One-Mile Walk

Ages 5–6	20 minutes
Ages 7–9	15–20 minutes
Ages 10–18	12–15 minutes
Adults	10–15 minutes
Ages 50 +	15–17 minutes

should be able to exercise continuously at a rigorous pace in reasonable comfort. Here are my guidelines:

To maintain aerobic fitness, you should exercise aerobically at least three times per week for at least the period indicated above.

Aerobic Test #2: Walking

Walking provides a safe, easy way to measure aerobic fitness. You should be able to walk fast enough to pass the following tests. *Note:* Start with this walking test if you have not trained enough to perform the other aerobic tests like running.

The following are approximate fitness goals for walking a brisk mile:

Youth Walking Test

To use this test, measure two miles on a relatively level surface (an oval outdoor track is best). Have your child walk the distance and record the time. Compare it to the times on Charts O and P.

These charts give minimal standards developed by the President's Council on Physical Fitness and Sports for the two-mile walk for children and young people ages six to seventeen. Minimally, your child should reach the national average score. This is not, however, the final fitness goal. The ideal would be to reach the President's Challenge level and maintain it. A good level of fitness would be to score somewhere between the two figures. Christopher, at age seven, walked seven miles at a fourteen-minute mile pace—easily bettering the President's Challenge Standard of fourteen-minute mile pace for two miles.

CHART O

Boys' Youth Aerobic Fitness Test: Two-Mile Walk

AGE	6	7	8	9	10	11
STANDARD						
National Average	34:07	32:40	32:10	31:14	29:56	28:52
President's Challenge	28:05	28:18	27:20	26:44	25:42	25:25

AGE	12	13	14	15	16	17+
STANDARD						
National Average	28:03	28:14	28:02	27:57	27:55	28:06
President's Challenge	25:07	25:01	24:50	25:08	25:16	25:20

CHART P

Girls' Youth Aerobic Fitness Test: Two-Mile Walk

AGE	6	7	8	9	10	11
STANDARD						
National Average	35:16	35:10	33:51	32:45	30:28	31:15
President's Challenge	28:09	29:57	29:19	28:04	26:46	27:11

AGE	12	13	14	15	16	17+
STANDARD						
National Average	29:15	29:01	29:34	30:06	30:30	30:10
President's Challenge	26:20	26:24	26:32	27:09	27:20	26:59

Times are in minutes:seconds.

National average is the fiftieth percentile score for the President's Council 1985 School Population Fitness Survey.

President's Challenge is the eighty-fifth percentile score for the Council's 1985 Survey.

Adult Walking Test

Chart Q lists adult fitness standards developed by the exercise physiology laboratory at the University of Massachusetts Medical School for the one-mile walk.

Aerobic Test #3: Running

Youth Running Tests

There are two charts here, and they overlap in terms of age. But both measure fitness standards for children and young people between the ages of five and eighteen based on running. Here, as in the previous section, you should find a safe and level measured mile to use for these tests.

Charts R and S list fitness standards for the one-mile run for children ages five to eighteen. The goal is to reach the "health fitness" standard established by the AAHPERD. If your child enjoys running, he or she might want to try for the President's Challenge, a high level of fitness. Christopher reached this level at age seven by running and talking a nonstop mile in eight minutes and twenty seconds.

Note: Walking breaks are permitted during both these tests. No child should be forced to tough these runs out. The idea is to be able to run a mile nonstop and with an even pace.

Chart T lists fitness standards for boys and girls between the ages of six and nine for the half-mile run. This distance was chosen because kids this age sometimes lack the attention span or motivation to complete a one-mile test. The half-mile offers an alternative to the one-mile test and will

CHART Q

Adult Aerobic Fitness Test: One-Mile Walk

	MALES	FEMALES
Excellent	10:12 or faster	11:40 or faster
Good	10:13–11:42	11:41–13:08
High Average	11:43–13:13	13:09–14:36
Low Average	13:14–14:14	14:37–16:04
Fair	14:15–16:23	16:05–17:31
Poor	16:24 and up	17:32 and up

Times are in minutes:seconds.
Developed by the University of Massachusetts Medical School.

CHART R

Boys' Youth Aerobic Fitness Test: One-Mile Run/Walk

AGE	5	6	7	8	9	10
STANDARD						
Health Fitness	13:00	12:00	11:00	10:00	10:00	9:30
President's Challenge		10:15	9:22	8:48	8:31	7:57

AGE	11	12	13	14	15	16
STANDARD						
Health Fitness	9:00	9:00	8:00	7:45	7:30	7:30
President's Challenge	7:32	7:11	6:50	6:26	6:20	6:08

AGE	17	18
STANDARD		
Health Fitness	7:30	7:30
President's Challenge	6:06	6:06

accurately measure fitness in children of this age. A good score will fall somewhere between "average" and "outstanding."

Adult Running Test

Chart U gives approximate fitness goals for men and women for the one-mile run/walk.

Note: If you have not been running regularly you should put in at least six to eight weeks of aerobic training before attempting this vigorous test. Use caution during the test and take walking breaks if you wish. Later, after proper aerobic training, you can push yourself more.

CHART S

Girls' Youth Aerobic Fitness Test: One-Mile Run/Walk

AGE	5	6	7	8	9	10
STANDARD						
Health Fitness	14:00	13:00	12:00	11:30	11:00	11:00
President's Challenge		11:20	10:36	10:02	9:30	9:19

AGE	11	12	13	14	15	16
STANDARD						
Health Fitness	11:00	11:00	10:30	10:30	10:30	10:30
President's Challenge	9:02	8:23	8:13	7:59	8:08	8:23

AGE	17	18
STANDARD		
Health Fitness	10:30	10:30
President's Challenge	8:15	8:15

Health Fitness standard established by AAHPERD's 1988 Physical Best program. Refers to the fitness level needed to be healthy.

President's Challenge is the eighty-fifth percentile score for the President's Council 1985 Survey. It represents a high level of fitness required for the Presidential Physical Fitness Award.

Times are in minutes:seconds.

CHART T

Youth Aerobic Fitness Test: Half-mile Run/Walk for Ages 6–9

	BOYS			
AGE	6	7	8	9
STANDARD				
National Average	5:23	5:00	4:22	4:14
Outstanding	4:35	4:22	3:41	3:42

	GIRLS			
AGE	6	7	8	9
STANDARD				
National Average	5:44	5:25	4:56	4:50
Outstanding	4:57	4:38	4:06	4:04

National Average for ages six and seven is the fiftieth percentile score for the AAHPERD's 1987 National Children and Youth Fitness Study II. National Average for ages eight and nine is the average score from the 1986–1987 Chrysler Fund-AAU Physical Fitness Program.

Outstanding standard for ages six and seven is the eighty-fifth percentile from the AAHPERD's 1987 NCYFS II. Ouststanding standard for ages eight and nine is the eightieth percentile score from the 1986–1987 Chrysler–AAU program.

Time is in minutes:seconds.

CHART U

Adult Aerobic Fitness Test: One-mile Run/walk

AGE	MEN	WOMEN
19–29	8:00	10:30
30–39	8:30	11:00
40–49	9:00	11:30
50–59	9:30	12:00
60 and over	10:30	13:00

Times are in minutes:seconds.

Here is a sample Family Fitness Evaluation form. Use this or copy it and make one for each member of your family or school fitness group.

Family Fitness Evaluation

Name:

Age:

	Test Date	Score	Fitness Level	Comments
Flexibility				
Test #1				
Test #2				
Test #3				
Abdominal Strength and Endurance				
Test #1				
Test #2				
Test #3				
Upper Body Strength and Endurance				
Test #1				
Test #2				
Test #3				
Cardio-respiratory Endurance				
Test #1				
Test #2				
Test #3				

Body Weight: Goal:

Write in weekly body weight.

Part 3

CHILD/
TEACHER/
SCHOOL

5

Physical Education in the School

Too many of us, as adults, remember gym as that part of the school day we hated most. Why? Because we were humiliated by being picked last for a team, chewed out by macho coaches, pushed through calisthenics by drill-sergeant–type instructors. We did push-ups or ran laps as punishment for such major infractions of gym life as not washing our white gym shorts every week, or wearing colored rather than white socks.

Today, we call gym *physical education*. But it hasn't changed much. Our children—who love to play, as we did—often hate physical education. In too many schools, P.E. remains a time of embarrassment, harassment, failure, and boredom. Nearly twenty million of our children participate in school physical education programs every year. About four million boys and two million girls also play interscholastic sports. Too few of our kids get enough quality exercise in these programs to meet fitness standards or receive an adequate education in fitness and wellness to prepare them for a healthy life. Not all of the blame rests with our schools.

Dr. George Sheehan, the running cardiologist, told a group of physical educators, "Today the training of the body has assumed its proper respect. That's the good news. The bad news: You teachers are not making the most of this opportunity. The subject of physical education is play. The process of physical education is learning to play better." The object, as Dr. Sheehan points out, is to learn what gets kids moving and keeps them moving. What is fun and how can fitness be fun? Too often, kids don't care about fitness after they leave school. Later, as adults, the motivation is fear: doctors warn of silent killers, shortened lives.

Why is physical education important? The AAHPERD says: "Physical education helps children develop fitness, become independent learners and develop social skills by interacting with other students. When children participate in a structured physical education program which provides opportunities for skill development and physical fitness, they use these skills in their spare time and integrate them into their lives."

Schools, says Dr. Sheehan, do not recognize physical education as equal to other subjects in the curriculum. "Yet," he says, "there are few things more valuable in life than learning how to play well. We should be first and always, man the player. The educator who helps us accomplish that can stand as tall as any other."

Most school districts and educators, however, face several handicaps:

- Budget cuts. Many schools don't have a full-time physical education staff, or if they do the director often isn't properly trained or certified. Even the most qualified P.E. directors are limited by low pay, lack of funds to hire good staff, inadequate facilities, bare-bones programming, and over-crowded P.E. classes.
- Low priority. Few school administrators, P.T.A.s, or school boards rank physical education alongside the three Rs of reading, 'riting, and 'rithmetic. When cutbacks in school budgets must be made, "frills" like P.E. feel the knife first.
- Lack of time to cover all that must be taught in the curriculum. Few teachers have the luxury of daily physical education classes. Most often, they have to attempt to cram in motor-skill development, sports, and other curriculum requirements in twice-weekly thirty-minute sessions. Then, in addition, they are asked to fit in all the components of physical fitness.
- Overemphasis on sports instead of fitness. Adult educators too often see fitness as sports, but the aim of sports is often winning, not fitness and fun. A sports-oriented physical education program turns out talented athletes and turns off the majority of less physically gifted students. A balance is needed to serve both the athlete and the student who needs fitness training.
- Lack of proper training and direction. Physical education teachers frequently emphasize sports and winning instead of lifetime fitness for all students. They may have no training at all in this field, other than their own experiences as athletes and as participants in sports-oriented P.E. classes.
- Lack of parental support. We parents too often send our children off to school and turn our backs on their physical education. At home, we don't think we have the time or the skills to guide our kids in exercise. The result is that, right or wrong, we leave fitness to the schools and we think our kids are being cared for properly. In fact,

fitness and wellness concepts taught in the schools need to be reinforced at home. We, as parents, need to be fully active in the fitness care of our children, much as we are in other aspects of their education and health.

TOOLS FOR PARENTS

Clearly, as parents, the problem and the solution are in our hands. We need to evaluate and lobby in this field. Take, for example, the role of the U.S. government in fitness education. In a 1980 report, "Promoting Health/ Preventing Disease: Objectives for the Nation," the U.S. Department of Health and Human Services called for improvements in the physical fitness of our nation. This included sound, health-related physical fitness programs in the public schools. The report identified three specific goals in the area of youth fitness:

1. That by 1990, 60 percent of America's students would take daily physical education classes. By 1989, however, no more than 30 percent of our children take physical education daily; more than 30 percent of our high-school students get no P.E. at all. Only one state— Illinois—requires that all its children, in kindergarten through grade twelve, take physical education every day.
2. That by 1990, 70 percent of our children would periodically have their fitness levels tested. By 1989, however, only half of our elementary students are regularly tested—and many of them are tested only for motor performance or athletic ability rather than health-related fitness.
3. That by 1990, school programs will expand beyond competitive sports and 90 percent of America's kids will participate in physical activities that contribute to their cardio-respiratory fitness. By 1989, however, our schools still emphasize sports, the P.E. curriculum honors the athletically gifted, and our less sports-motivated or less athletically gifted youngsters are getting bypassed. Very few students take fitness P.E. classes offering the minimum aerobic fitness levels three days a week for twenty to thirty minutes of continuous vigorous exercise each time.

To be sure, there have been serious, well-intentioned government studies and proposals to reach fitness goals for our children. These, like private studies mentioned in this book, provide good ammunition for parents to use when they are facing reluctant school boards and budget hearings. For example, in December 1987, the U.S. Senate passed House Concurrent

Resolution 97, which called for "high quality daily physical education programs for all children in kindergarten through grade twelve." Although the resolution, approved by both houses of Congress (and sponsored by Senator Ted Stevens of Alaska and Representative Beverly Byron of Maryland), does not have the force of law, it can be used to lobby state and local education agencies to mandate quality physical education in our schools. As Senator Stevens said: "This Resolution will be used by parents, educators and administrators alike to ensure that the physical education of our children is not seen as a frill to be cut from school budgets. It will work to reverse the erosion of health and physical education programs. . . . We must give our children's health and fitness an equal place in the classroom." Representative James Jeffords of Vermont added: "As we demand greater time to be given in our schools to the 'basics'—mathematics, English, science, reading—we should give consideration to encouraging schools to get back to the fitness basics as well. . . . We need to look at the whole child in our education process."

100TH CONGRESS
1st SESSION   **H. CON. RES. 97**

To encourage State and local governments and local educational agencies to provide high qualitydaily physical education programs for all children in kindergarten through grade 12.

IN THE HOUSE OF REPRESENTATIVES

CONCURRENT RESOLUTION

To encourage State and local governments and local educational agencies to provide high quality daily physical education programs for all children in kindergarten through grade twelve.

Whereas physical education is essential to the development of growing children;

Whereas physical education helps improve the overall health of children by improving their cardiovascular endurance, muscular strength and power, and flexibility, and by enhancing weight regulation, bone development, posture, skillful moving, active lifestyle habits, and constructive use of leisure time;

Whereas physical education increases children's mental alertness, academic performance, readiness to learn, and enthusiasm for learning;

Whereas physical education helps improve the self-esteem, interpersonal relationships, responsible behavior, and independence of children;

Whereas children who participate in high quality daily physical education programs tend to be more healthy and physically fit;

Whereas physically fit adults have significantly reduced risk factor for heart attacks and strokes;

Whereas the Surgeon General, in Objectives for the Nation, recommends increasing the number of school mandated physical education programs that focus on health-related physical fitness;

Whereas the Secretary of Education in First Lessons—A Report on Elementary Education in America, recognized that elementary schools have a special mandate to provide elementary school children with the knowledge, habits, and attitudes that will equip the children for a fit and healthy life; and

Whereas a high quality daily physical education program for all children in kindergarten through grade twelve is an essential part of a comprehensive education: Now, therefore, be it

Resolved by the House of Representatives (the Senate concurring), That the Congress encourages State and local governments and local educational agencies to provide high quality daily physical education programs for all children in kindergarten through grade twelve.

There are other useful tools for parents. One comes from AAHPERD. As a result of the alarming results of its study, "The Shape of the Nation: A Survey of State Physical Education Requirements," AAHPERD's members concluded that the schools could help overcome the youth fitness crisis. "There are simply not enough quality daily physical education programs across the country," said its follow-up report, "to enable our children to learn how to keep themselves healthy and maintain a basic level of physical fitness."

AAHPERD established the following *minimum* goals in 1988 for U.S. school kids:

- Elementary school children should receive thirty minutes of quality physical education every day.
- Secondary school students should get forty-five to fifty-five minutes of quality physical education every day.

By quality physical education, AAHPERD meant vigorous activity directed by a qualified instructor.

Members of the 1987 World Conference of the International Council for Health, Physical Education and Recreation also recommended daily physical education programs, not just in U.S. schools but worldwide. They recommended programs that would benefit cardio-respiratory health, muscle strength, and flexibility, and that students spend 150 to 300 minutes (two and a half to five hours) a week in physical education activities.

Using these studies and the Congressional resolution, we as parents can—and should—lobby for improved physical education classes in our children's schools. Individual states, not the federal government, set the laws that mandate physical education requirements. The following chart compares P.E. requirements (as of 1988) by state. Note that, as mentioned, only Illinois meets the AAHPERD's minimum goal and eight states have *no* physical education requirements for kindergarten through grade twelve. Parents in Arizona, Colorado, Maine, Missouri, Mississippi, Oklahoma, South Dakota, and Wyoming might want to get started lobbying today!

SHAPE OF THE NATION SURVEY: STATE RANKINGS

TOTAL NUMBER of minutes of physical education required per student career (K-12)

RANK	STATE	#Min/K-12	RANK	STATE	#Min/K-12
1	IL	96,300	26	HI	18,000
2	LA	71,136		MT	18,000
3	CA	64,800	28	NH	16,200
4	NY	57,240	29	NV	14,400
5	AL	55,800	30	IN	11,500
6	TN	54,180	31	VA	10,800
7	NJ	54,144		PA	10,800
8	MN	51,516	33	ND	9,468
9	TX	50,346		OR	9,468
10	RI	46,800	35	NC	9,000
	WA	46,800		KS	9,000
12	MA	37,800		MD	9,000
	WI	37,800	38	AK	8,1000
14	AR	37,467	39	CT	7,200
15	KY	35,550		IA	7,200
16	GA	32,400	41	NE	5,400
	SC	32,400	42	FL	4,500
18	MO	30,600	43	AZ	-0-
19	VT	30,240		CO	-0-
20	WV	27,945		ME	-0-
21	OH	27,432		MI	-0-
22	UT	23,202		MS	-0-
23	DE	20,376		OK	-0-
24	NM	18,468		SD	-0-
25	ID	18,360		WY	-0-

Source: AAHPERD's "Shape of the Nation Survey," 1988.

Typically, an elementary school child in the United States will have one or two twenty-minute physical education classes a week. A U.S. high-school boy or girl will get less: physical education is often an elective course in U.S. high schools. Even where the physical education curriculum mandates enough time, space, and equipment, there is often an inadequate amount of quality daily instruction.

What should our goals be for quality physical education of our children?

Again, I turn to AAHPERD, which suggests: "A good physical education program is sequential, and allows for the developmental needs of each child. The program should have planned objectives in a variety of activities, which allow for growth in motor skills (psychomotor), knowledge and understanding (cognitive), and attitude and appreciation (affective)." AAHPERD's members also suggest the following guidelines.

A good elementary physical education program:

- helps each child develop effective and expressive movement patterns and motor skills, and an understanding and appreciation of movement;
- encourages vigorous activity;
- emphasizes safety practices;
- fosters creativity;
- promotes self-understanding, acceptance, and social interaction;
- helps each child learn to deal with risk-taking, winning, and losing.

A good secondary school physical education program:

- offers a balance of fitness activities that are enjoyable;
- develops and refines a youngster's physical activities;
- offers a good aerobic workout;
- improves muscle fitness;
- explains and clarifies the meaning of physical health, the mechanics of movement, and the effects of exercise on the human body;
- develops personalized programs for fitness and health for life;
- explains the role of sports in society (to develop personal health and recreational skills);
- demonstrates appropriate and positive competitive behavior.

Along with the guidelines, we as parents should see that our children's schools offer physical education by qualified and trained teachers. These teachers should be regarded on the same level as the rest of the school's faculty, and be encouraged (and allowed) to improve themselves by taking additional seminars and training workshops, reading books and professional journals, and upgrading their own levels of education. Physical education instructors and sports coaches should also be trained and certified by organizations like the American Coaching Effectiveness Program (see Appendix) or AAHPERD. If the instructors do not have a degree in a related P.E. field, they at least should become certified and take college-level courses to improve their skills as coaches and teachers.

In elementary schools, classroom teachers are often called on to teach physical education classes—usually to supplement one or two P.E. classes a week, often because a school budget has been cut and the regular physical education staff let go. These classroom teachers need our support and guidance. They should be encouraged to read and study about fitness and they should be under the supervision of a qualified physical education specialist.

The physical education teacher needs to be more than a coach with a whistle. He or she must be innovative, motivated, and able to challenge and excite youngsters while balancing discipline with caring and sensitivity. Tough-guy coaches don't get kids interested in a lifetime of fitness and enjoyable recreational sports. The right person can inspire a P.E. class, and give your children the gift of a lifetime.

6

The Square Deal:
The Four Critical Cornerstones
of a Quality Physical Education
Program

You are lucky if your school offers your child a sufficient number of physical education instructors, good facilities, and equipment. But that is still not enough. Good instructors and equipment are of no value if the program stinks.

How can you tell? I believe there are four critical ingredients to a quality physical education program. They make up the four cornerstones of what I call the "Square Deal." If any one of these four ingredients is missing, or is inadequate, then the total value of your child's school physical education program suffers.

The four cornerstones of my Square Deal are:

1. Appropriate, year-round, quality physical education.
2. Fitness testing and reporting.
3. Wellness education in the classroom/lunchroom.
4. Parental involvement.

APPROPRIATE, YEAR-ROUND, QUALITY PHYSICAL ACTIVITY

In the typical school gym class, an overweight ex-jock throws out a bag of balls and sits back to watch the kids "exercise." Many of our nation's gym teachers are athletic coaches first, teachers second. These "ball rollers" know little about physiology, health, lifetime sports, wellness, and, least of all, child psychology. When they do teach, they spend their time coaching kids about sports skills. This doesn't do much for fitness. Charles Kuntzleman, director of the Michigan study mentioned earlier, has been tough in his criticism of the teachers running sports-oriented school P.E. programs: "They're more concerned with clean gym clothes than clean arteries. They develop volleyball techniques, but not heart-health techniques."

The first step in developing a quality physical education program then is to have quality instructors. Ideally these instructors should have a degree in physical education or a related discipline, be certified by programs such as the American Coaching Effectiveness Program (see Appendix), and keep current with developments in the field by reading the various publications of the trade organization, the American Alliance for Health, Physical Education, Recreation, and Dance (AAHPERD). Additionally, they should be good examples of personal physical fitness.

As children begin school, physical education instructors contribute significantly as role models to health behavior development. Yet, according to the September 1988 issue of the *Journal of Physical Education, Recreation and Dance* (JOPERD), studies indicate that physical educators score poorly in terms of body weight and cardio-respiratory fitness. According to a survey by L. Jerome Brandon and Raynette Evans, 57 percent of physical educators responding consider themselves to be overweight. The authors concluded that "to improve the poor physical fitness report that American youth continue to receive, elementary and secondary physical educators must become better role models by improving their own fitness levels."

In another report in the JOPERD, Jim Whitley, John Sage, and Mike Butcher summarized: "Ideally, every physical education teacher should maintain a high level of cardio-respiratory fitness and model it for his or her students. When compared to this desired professional standard, the major finding of this study is very discouraging: almost half (47 percent) of the instructors who responded to this survey reported that at the time of the survey they were not engaged in a personal cardio-respiratory fitness program. Since positive role modeling is generally accepted to be an effective means of creating desired behavior, the ability of these individuals to personally model and successfully promote fitness for their students can be seriously questioned."

As our children move from kindergarten to grade school to high school, the amount of time spent playing sports greatly increases until it dominates most P.E. programs. This weeds out kids who are not good athletes and favors those who are. A 1983 *Sports Illustrated* exposé on the failure of school physical education programs stated: "A strong school athletic program can develop sports skills, showcase excellence and generate student and community spirit, but it also has a way of gobbling up physical education. The problem is that administrators, parents and the local press are often more interested in what happens in the gym on Friday nights than during school hours. . . . In such programs, the talented few flourish while the many often grow discouraged and get turned off to all physical activity by age thirteen or fourteen." Jack Berryman, associate professor of kinesiology at the University of Washington, adds: "When you adopt sports as the curriculum for physical education, you're adopting things that go with it, such as the will to win. Then the cream rises to the top. But we must deal with all the students. What if we taught our math and English classes this way?"

My own school physical education focused entirely on sports, and I thrived on it. My high school won the county championships my senior year in *every* sport. Everyone, including me, assumed that we had a great P.E. program. But twenty-five years after graduation, an analysis of the fitness levels of my classmates proves that our program was a huge failure. Two classmates died of heart attacks before they reached forty. The stars of our sports teams are almost all fat and sedentary. Worse, they are setting a terrible example for their own children.

During the last few years, there has been a shift in the philosophy of physical education. It is slowly moving from emphasis on sports and athletic prowess—which has little value to the majority in the short term and no value to anyone in the long term—toward a health-fitness orientation. The new goal is to improve the physical fitness of everyone. This model, best exemplified by AAHPERD's Physical Best program (see Appendix), offers individualized fitness goals for all students and awards for improvement available to everyone.

Still, physical instruction educators cannot agree on what constitutes a good P.E. curriculum. Should teachers emphasize skills that may later pay off in interscholastic, intercollegiate, or professional sports? Should they emphasize competition with its valuable lessons about stress, working together for a common goal, preparation, trying hard, and learning to win and lose? Should lifetime sports, such as tennis, replace team sports, such as football, which is dropped after graduation? Should the major P.E. goal be to simply improve the fitness of each student?

In my opinion, a combination of fitness, team sports, and lifetime recreational sports—properly balanced—is the ideal physical education program. Chapter 8 details how a model school—my son Christopher's school—strives to maintain a delicate balance in physical activity between fitness, sports, and fun. Christopher is learning how and why to be physically fit. His school P.E. program is preparing him for a lifetime of health fitness. He gets aerobic exercise at least three times a week and his P.E. classes develop flexibility, muscular strength, and endurance. His school's P.E. classes are also teaching him to handle the stress of controlled competition, which may make it easier for him to handle other stresses in his life. In team sports, he is learning that cooperation is essential to achieve goals and that team players succeed—another lesson that will serve him well in school and later in life.

Christopher's school is also teaching him to ice-skate and swim, to play tennis and squash, and to enjoy walking and running for fitness and fun— all activities that will be of value to him later. Most of all, the fitness, team sports, and recreational activities are taught in a way that emphasizes the success of each individual, not just the gifted athletes. Woven into the school's curriculum are innovative fitness activities that are fun—such as "adventure walks" in the park, balloon relays, or games using a parachute.

According to *Physical Education for Children: Concepts into Practice*, there are two basic recommended goals of any school physical fitness program: fitness for *health* and fitness to *develop motor skills*. A good program "develops and maintains appropriate levels of physical fitness for health and teaches why fitness is important and how it is influenced by exercise." It also helps develop fundamental motor skills, "which lead to specific sport skills, and finally [emphasizes] lifetime sports."

Charles Corbin, a professor at Arizona State University, emphasizes that just getting our kids in shape is not enough. In the *Journal of Physical Education, Recreation and Dance*, he recommends a larger goal for physical educators and parents:

> Often overlooked is the fact that physical fitness, especially those components of fitness which have a strong relationship to good health, is temporary. To put it another way, just because elementary or secondary school youth achieve a desirable level of fitness does not mean that they will maintain fitness for a lifetime. . . . Higher order physical fitness objectives may be more important than temporary attainment of physical fitness. . . . Our job is not complete when children and youth are stimulated to be physically active in a physical education class, nor is it finished when we have helped students achieve good levels of fitness. Exercising and achieving fitness are lower level fitness objectives. If people are to be fit for a lifetime they must move to higher order objectives such as establishing personal exercise programs, learning to test their own fitness, interpreting their own test results, and learning to solve their own fitness problems. In this way they can become independent consumers of fitness and health rather than people who are dependent on others to get them fit.

The appropriate, year-round, quality physical education program includes daily classes of thirty minutes or more with professional, certified, physically fit teachers. It balances fun, fitness, and sports. It stresses the basic aerobic fitness of three vigorous workouts a week for at least twenty consecutive minutes. A quality program offers innovative indoor aerobic exercise routines (aerobic dance or the fitness routine detailed in Chapter 13), for wintry or rainy days, along with bundling the kids up for adventure walks. (Studies show that children lose fitness during the winter due to decreased physical activity.) It must include individualized, challenging goals that children feel they can attain, and offer activities that allow each child to demonstrate competence.

At its heart, the program must be fair and equal to all students whatever their athletic abilities. It should make sure they take with them from school not only the three Rs, but also a fourth: lifetime 'robics.

FITNESS TESTING AND REPORTING

Fitness testing is a key ingredient in a quality physical education program. A good and fair fitness test is a good tool to make our children aware that fitness is important and to involve us, as parents, in our children's fitness programs and goals. Also, a good fitness test sets a baseline for each child against which that child then competes. Third, the test helps us monitor our children's progress and, thereby, the effectiveness of each child's physical education program. Poor results generally mean that improvements are needed in the quality and quantity of fitness activities.

But what is a good and fair fitness test? The first U.S. national youth fitness test took place in 1958. It was conducted by the American Alliance for Health, Physical Education and Recreation (which later added the word *Dance*, making the acronym AAHPERD). Between 1958 and 1980, AAHPERD's Youth Fitness Test was the dominant fitness test in U.S schools. The test included some health fitness components, but was largely motor (athletic) skills: sit-ups, pull-ups, shuttle run, fifty-yard dash, six-hundred-yard walk/run, and standing broad jump.

In 1980, AAHPERD's members changed the test. They thought the 1958–1980 fitness test emphasized mostly innate athletic ability, which could not be improved significantly with training. It offered no incentive for kids to improve their levels of fitness. Instead, AAHPERD devised a fitness test for U.S. kids—revised and expanded in 1988—that was more health-related and added an "exercise prescription" that explains specific activities that each participant can do to improve weak areas. "The goal," says an AAHPERD article, "is to achieve personal goals that have been realistically set." A feedback sheet for each child allows him or her to share progress with the participant's family. The new test is the centerpiece of the Physical Best educational program and measures the key health-related fitness components described in Chapter 2:

- Aerobic endurance with a one-mile walk/run.
- Body composition with skinfold measurements.
- Flexibility with the sit-and-reach test.
- Muscular stength and endurance with modified sit-ups (for the abdominals) and pull-ups (for the upper body).

Other fitness-testing programs available to parents and schools are described in the Appendix. Unfortunately, the many groups providing services for youth testing cannot agree on a single coordinated assessment program. Most of the disagreement focuses on the conflict between health-related fitness testing and the inclusion of testing for motor (athletic) skills. I recommend the AAHPERD's health-related fitness test, Physical Best, for the following reasons:

- It measures all of the important health-related fitness components.
- It includes an educational program to help students establish and achieve individual goals. Fitness testing by itself is worthless if it doesn't motivate students to continue their conditioning and improve their fitness level.
- It does not encourage students to score high goals, but rather attain a standard of health fitness. That standard, in turn, helps the student to reach a level of fitness so that he or she will enter adulthood at low risk for degenerative and cardiovascular diseases.
- Its award system is designed to motivate all students. Its Fitness Activity Award is given for setting and achieving the goal of regular physical activity, both in and out of school. Its Fitness Goals Award is given for the student's setting and attaining goals; a student can be successful at this even if he or she cannot pass any of the tests. If children's fitness is measured according to standards which children have no chance of meeting, they will quit trying to achieve impossible goals. Its Health Fitness Award is given when the student attains a predefined health fitness standard goal in all five fitness components.
- Its report card allows the student to share his or her progress. It also increases the parents' awareness of their child's fitness level and seeks to motivate them to become involved in continuing fitness activity at home.

The ideal fitness program tests students in the autumn to establish a baseline, follows up with fitness training programs (designed to help each student meet individual goals) in the P.E. classes combined with fitness and health education in the classroom during the school year, and re-tests at the end of the year. The awards mentioned above and the final report card are then given to every participant.

The results of the fitness tests should be kept confidential. If other children find out how your child scored—and if he or she did poorly—he or she may be ridiculed by peers. Properly handled, fitness testing should enhance self-esteem rather than lower it.

WELLNESS EDUCATION IN THE CLASSROOM AND LUNCHROOM

It is important to teach our kids not only fitness activities, but also how to cope with life outside of school. In physical education courses, students must be taught about stress management (particularly the pressures of academics and sports), drug abuse, good nutrition and healthy diet, and the connection between caloric intake and burning calories with exercise as a key to managing weight. And they should learn how to balance all of this—exercise, diet, stress, and work—in their lives.

Health and nutrition ("wellness") education goes beyond fitness and should be part of our elementary and secondary school curriculum. School health and physical education programs should encompass such principles. Our kids need to learn how their bodies function, what foods are good for them, how to avoid illness, and what the disastrous effects of drug, tobacco, and alcohol abuse will be. They should also provide them with a nutritious school-lunch program. Our schools can provide our kids with fitness exercise programs, and beyond that, with the knowledge, habits, and attitudes that will sustain them through a fit and healthy life. A 1980 U.S. Department of Health goal was to establish nutrition education as a requirement in all states. By 1985, however, only twelve states had such a requirement.

The School Health Curriculum Project (SHCP), a cooperative venture of five federal agencies, surveyed more than eleven hundred fourth- to seventh-grade classrooms using four popular health programs. SHCP reported that "schools have much to contribute to the classic ideal of a sound mind in a sound body. Well-designed programs can affect subsequent student knowledge, attitudes, and—most important—behavior."

SHCP's survey also reached a logical conclusion: gains are greatest where schools devote more time to health and fitness education. Reaching this level of education, however, is a large task. A qualified health educator is almost essential to teaching and achieving this balance in our school programs. Unfortunately, few exist. There are, however, excellent programs, such as Fit Youth Today, Know Your Body, and Feelin' Good, that schools and parents can use. See the Appendix for information on these and other programs.

PARENTAL INVOLVEMENT

We parents cannot simply put the burden of getting our kids in shape on the schools and then walk away. It's not that easy. Getting in shape and staying in shape means commitments of time and energy for ourselves and the same commitment for our children. If the schools do a good job, you still need to reinforce that at home, just as you do with homework. If the schools are failing in fitness education, we parents must pitch in and exercise with our kids, involve them in community programs, and wrestle with the school boards and administrations to improve their programs.

Many schools, such as Christopher's, involve parents by encouraging them to join in adventure walks, fun runs, field days, parent-child sports contests, parent-child trips to sporting events, and so forth. There are also team events and recognition dinners.

You may ask, "Why bother?" Look at it this way: If someone said your child was getting a lousy education, you'd do something about it, and fast. And you'd stay with it until your child's education improved. Why do less for your child's lifelong physical well-being? Why shortchange this person, to whom you have given life itself?

Okay, now that I have made you feel guilty and committed, let's move ahead. The next chapter offers guidelines for parents on how to evaluate your school's physical education program and how to lobby for improvements.

A Parent's Guide to Evaluating Your Child's School Physical Education Program

How good is the physical education program in your child's school? Most parents don't know; many also don't care. They take it for granted that the physical activity needs of their children are being met at school.

You can (and should) learn the details of your school's physical education program simply by visiting the school and asking your child's P.E. specialist about the program, your child's fitness level, and how you can help at home. Just as the school should assess the fitness level of your child, you should assess the physical education program at your child's school. But how? The following questions will help you evaluate the school's P.E. programs. You should answer them yes or no.

ADMINISTRATION

In your child's school, is physical fitness considered a priority by both the administration and the physical education staff?

PHYSICAL ACTIVITY

- Does your child participate in daily physical education classes of appropriate length (a minimum of thirty minutes for elementary school kids; forty-five to fifty-five minutes for secondary school youngsters)?
- Are P.E. classes comparable in size to other classes, with no more than fifteen to twenty students per qualified instructor?

- Do qualified, certified P.E. instructors teach the classes?
- Are the P.E. specialists physically fit themselves in order to serve as good role models for the children they teach?
- Does the P.E. curriculum balance fitness, fun, and sports?
- Does your child enjoy the P.E. classes?
- Have your school's P.E. instructors abandoned the old-fashioned and destructive method of punishing behavior problems with running or calisthenics, and of humiliating students in front of their peers?
- Does your child's school provide for those students who need special consideration: the physically disabled, the obese, the unfit, and the unskilled?
- Does your child's school provide equal fitness and sports opportunities for both girls and boys?
- Is there sufficient equipment and facilities for every student?
- Does your child receive the minimum amount of weekly aerobic exercise: three days a week of twenty minutes' duration?
- Does your school adjust its P.E. program during the winter or inclement weather to continue its fitness levels and programs?
- Do the P.E. classes include relaxation, stretching, and strengthening exercises at least twice a week to teach flexibility and muscular strength and endurance?
- Are motor skills developed at an early age?
- Does your child receive instruction in lifelong fitness activities that he or she can use as an adult, such as swimming, tennis, walking, biking, skating, or running?
- Are team sports at your school introduced in the elementary schools in a relaxed environment with a success-oriented attitude?
- Can students who are less gifted athletically still play team sports? Is participation as important as competition? Also, do the school's teams have a no-cut policy so that those who want to play may do so?
- Does your child enjoy participation on school sports teams?
- Are the team coaches trained in the "athletes first, winning second" philosophy?
- Is the school properly equipped and the staff trained to handle injuries and medical problems?

FITNESS TESTING AND REPORTING

- Are all students tested for the key fitness components at least twice a year?

- Do parents receive a report of those tests with guidance about how to improve areas that may be deficient?
- Does the school provide an award-incentive program based on achieving reasonable health-related fitness goals?
- Does the school conduct annual medical screenings?

WELLNESS EDUCATION IN THE CLASSROOM AND LUNCHROOM

- Does the school provide a nutritious lunch program?
- Does your child receive classroom instructions in the reason for physical fitness to complement participation in P.E. classes?
- Does your child receive classroom health education in important life-long wellness topics as nutrition, substance abuse, and weight and stress management?

PARENTAL INVOLVEMENT

- Are the physical education specialists at your child's school willing and available to discuss the fitness status of your child and other individual students?
- Does the school's P.E. staff willingly give parents guidelines on appropriate physical activities outside of school, such as after-school programs and summer programs?
- Are school officials receptive to suggestions from parents about improving the P.E. program? Do they follow up on these suggestions?
- Does the school provide time during the year for the P.E. program director to meet with parents, explain the school's P.E. program to them, and answer questions?
- Do the school sports teams hold parent-orientation meetings?
- Are parents encouraged to attend school sports events, field days, adventure walks, and the like?
- Can parents become involved by attending parent-child events, dinners, and so forth?

Now, what can you do if the answer to the key questions above are "No"?

First you must decide whether or not your child's physical fitness and health are important to him or her and to you. How important? Do you want to work to reform the P.E. program at the school, change schools, or work on your child's physical fitness after school or through community programs? One way or another, you are going to commit a chunk of your time to this project.

If you decide to take on the school, here are some tips.

First, ask the school's P.E. director to review with you, in person, the questions above and your answers. Do not be confrontational, but directive. "Here are some issues that I see," you might say, "and I'd like to know how you see them."

Show the P.E. director this book—and highlight the areas you feel might apply to your child's school and that could be improved or incorporated into the school's P.E. program. Remember, at this stage you are merely seeking answers and encouraging the school to re-examine its program and perhaps start to make some changes.

The school's P.E. staff should support your reasonable efforts and concerns if they are interested in the fitness and health of the school's children. You may need to "educate" some of the staff on the values of health-related fitness programs versus the dominance of athletic and team sports programs.

Perhaps the physical education teachers will want to lobby for improvements within the system. Make them aware of the campaign directed by their trade organization, the AAHPERD, entitled "Fit to Achieve." The program includes a grass-roots action kit to be used by physical educators to get the message about the need for quality daily physical education to the public, school administrators, and school board members.

You should have a clear and simple agenda. What specifically do you want? If you want no-cut teams in the school so that all kids can play, you will have to take on a certain group of P.E. instructors and parents. (If this is a high school, you may even have to take on the principal, superintendent, and alumni—all of whom value and gain from the "winning is everything" attitude in high-school sports.)

If your objective is to re-focus the school's P.E. program toward more health-fitness-nutrition, then you may be asked to come up with specific references, books, and experts. This book will help you in all three areas. Also, research good programs in area schools and use them as a model.

If the P.E. director and his or her staff put you off, or seem uncooperative, repeat the above suggestions with the school administration. Go to the principal and then the superintendent.

At the same time, contact P.T.A. officers and school board members. Ask them to help you review the school's P.E. program and go over the checklist questions above with them. Remember, if you are committed to this, you must be prepared to spend time to get results. Fortunately, most school officials will be willing to make changes—particularly if they don't cost anything—to improve the education of the school's children.

At this point, it might help to enlist other parents. Let them answer the questions above, compare answers, fill them in on who you have contacted. You may have to start lobbying your school-board members to get changes made. You may have to take on the budget process, if your child attends a public school. Or, you may be faced with the ultimatum of take-it-or-leave-it if your child attends a private school.

Jack Shepherd, now living in an outstanding school district in Vermont–New Hampshire (the first bi-state district in the United States), lived in New York City for sixteen years. His kids went to private schools where the most aerobic physical exercise they got was scrambling for the cross-town bus. When he tried to get the school to start a P.E. program (the building came with a great gym, which was used for art classes and P.T.A. meetings), he was guffawed all the way out the door. If the school started a P.E. program, he was told, it would have to raise tuition. End of discussion.

The ultimate weapon in public and private schools is money. Be prepared. Shepherd, in Vermont, got lacrosse elevated from a community recreation sport to a high-school varsity sport by applying some very basic lessons.

First, have a specific and clearly stated agenda. What do you want? Make your answer precise. Example: I want every child to be able to play on a school team if she or he wants to.

Second, start with the coaches and P.E. instructors, and act dumb. Example:

YOU: Is it possible now for a child to play on a school team if he or she wants to?

COACH: No.

YOU: Well, why not?

COACH: We wouldn't win.

YOU: Is winning more important in the school's P.E. program than participating?

And so forth.

Third, after you give the P.E. people their chance, go to the top. See the school superintendent. He or she will tell you to see the school principal. When you see the school principal you can tell him or her that you have already seen the superintendent and were referred by the superintendent to see the principal. Watch the principal's eyes expand and attention level increase 100 percent.

Fourth, engage as many parents and their children as possible. Do not do this alone. You will be seen as a troublemaker and your child will get labeled by the school administration, teachers, and coaches as the son or daughter of a troublemaker. Make the idea appear to be grass roots, broad-based, and highly volatile. When you go to see anyone at the school after your first round, go with other parents and their children. Put together a little mass march.

Five, understand your school's finances, who pays for what, and how money is raised and allocated. This may be easier in a public than a private school. Do what you can. Then, fit your idea into a budget proposal. Example: You want no-cut teams? The school will tell you that larger teams mean more kids on the buses for away games, and therefore greater costs. You do the math ahead of time. You tell them that the buses hold forty-four kids, two fat coaches, and a very alert bus driver. But now the teams have only twenty-two kids, two fat coaches, etc. They can have this great idea—no-cut teams and every kid playing—with no additional cost. Free!

Six, when you get your money and facts ready, try them out on your strongest opponents, probably the P.E. instructors. Listen to their arguments, nod, go home, and re-work your ideas. Then go back to the superintendent, tell him or her whom you've seen, and get his or her support. Remember that superintendents love ideas that make the school look good and don't cost anything.

The keys here are clear focus on your idea, parent and child involvement, and beating the budget reply. Go for it!

Another path is to shop around for good school programs. You can do this easier in a city than in the suburbs or rural areas. For example, I switched Christopher from his first school because its physical education program didn't emphasize physical fitness. He is enjoying a sound sports and fitness program at his present school (which I detail in the next chapter).

One other thing: If your school is doing all it can now and the program is pretty good, praise it. See if they could use some parent volunteers to make the program even better. Supplement the program with community fitness activities and with your own family workouts. It's fine to demand that the school take on its share of the responsibility. But don't pass the buck.

A Model School Physical Education Program

What is the model physical education program for a school? There probably isn't one perfect program at one perfect school. But Virginia and I are happy with the one at the Allen-Stevenson School, a private boys school that Christopher attends only two blocks from our apartment in New York City. I'll detail the Allen-Stevenson program here, and you might want to adapt part or all of it to your own child's school P.E. program. Because Allen-Stevenson is an all-boys school, you may think that its activities are not suited for girls. Don't let the girls hear you say that! All of these activities should be equally good for girls and boys.

Let me emphasize two things. I will talk here about Allen-Stevenson's excellent physical education program. But make no mistake: Any good P.E. program is always found at a school where academics is stressed and comes first. Allen-Stevenson is, first of all, an excellent academic school. In addition to that, Allen-Stevenson has created and maintains a quality physical education program despite two obstacles. First, it is located in the middle of Manhattan, surrounded not by a suburban-type campus but by concrete sidewalks, busy streets, and high-rise buildings. Second, it has no playing fields, swimming pool, tennis or squash courts, ice hockey rink, or baseball diamonds of its own. The boys must walk to and from Central Park, a half-mile away, and make do with fields that are more dirt and stone than grass. Despite these obstacles, the program is a success.

Christopher, at this writing, is a spirited seven-year-old boy whose extracurricular enthusiasms include both sports and music. Virginia and I wanted a school with a strong academic curriculum taught by sensitive teachers, a physical education program that emphasized both fitness and competitive sports, and a quality music program. We also wanted a small school with lots of spirit and a sense of community—greatly lacking in a large city—similar to my hometown when I was growing up.

In New York City, parents have two choices: public schools or private schools. Some of the public schools are superb, but for your child to attend those, you must live in that school's district. The schools covering the district we live in have several obvious weaknesses, including awful physical education programs. Therefore, we opted for a private school. We selected from schools all over the city, and chose Allen-Stevenson, which happens to be close to our apartment. The school has a long history of blending a sound physical education program into its curriculum. Headmaster Desmond Cole and deputy head Jessie-Lea Hayes have themselves run and completed several marathons. "Physical fitness promotes mental fitness," says Cole. "We have no doubt that physically fit children are better students in the classroom."

Christopher adjusted quickly and loved the sports and music programs; he even sang a solo in the Christmas show. Success in these areas carried over into the classroom, where he has become a good student. Other parents we talked with had a similar experience: the sports and physical activity helped their children concentrate on their schoolwork and succeed in the classroom. They found that when kids have a lot to do, they tend to do it better.

As Christopher started first grade at Allen-Stevenson, I started to write this book. I reviewed the school's already excellent physical education program and offered suggestions that would make it an even better model for this book. Pat Lappin, director of physical education, added several suggestions to help us in this unusual project of writing a detailed model physical education program that schools across the United States could emulate. We thought that even though the program was already in good shape after decades of development, it could still be improved. We concluded that, although your child's school might not be able to provide everything included here, it should follow a philosophy similar to that of the Allen-Stevenson model.

THE ALLEN-STEVENSON MODEL

School Philosophy

In an ideal P.E. program, says Lappin, "fitness and enjoyment must come first, and the desire to do well in competition—a necessity in life—will evolve in a healthy and natural manner from this solid base." Lappin is a trained instructor for the American Coaching Effectiveness Program (see Appendix). He teaches and certifies all of his coaches and instructors. The ACEP philosophy of "athletes first, winning second" advocates that coaches and instructors focus on the best interests of their athletes. Lappin hires coaches and instructors who share that philosophy. They are enthusiastic about fitness and sports. Winning will come, but it is second.

Years ago, the Allen-Stevenson coaches stressed winning—to the detriment of the school's image and the boys' welfare. Winning was replaced by participation and fitness as the primary goal. That didn't mean that the school's teams went belly-up; in fact, they still win interscholastic games. But the teams play in a less pressured environment. They win because the boys have an excellent fitness base and are enthusiastic about their sports. "I grew up on competitive sports," says Lappin,

> and I appreciate that experience as I am now faced with working in a competitive society, and working with parents who work in very competitive jobs. I wouldn't ever want to compromise the desire to excel as an individual or as a team member. Getting beaten badly game after game isn't a necessary lesson in life. On the other hand, we have a responsibility to train our youth in fitness activities which will also help them cope with the stresses of a competitive society throughout their lifetimes. We try to achieve a delicate balance at Allen-Stevenson between fitness, fun, and competition.

The Four Cornerstones of Physical Education

As I detailed in Chapter 6, the four cornerstones of an effective school physical education program are: (1) fitness and sports activity, (2) fitness testing, (3) wellness education in the classroom and lunchroom, and (4) parental involvement.

The faculty at Allen-Stevenson work to interrelate all four cornerstones into the curriculum and school day. The Allen-Stevenson faculty know that not only do their students need to practice sports skills, but also they need a solid fitness base for whatever sport the student plays—and for adult life. Those skills and that fitness base are molded by nutrition—the student's daily school lunch, for example—and other wellness topics, including stress management, weight control, and avoidance of tobacco, alcohol, and drugs.

FITNESS AND SPORTS ACTIVITIES

The P.E. curriculum at Allen-Stevenson includes daily physical activity for all of the students from first grade through the school's top grade, the ninth. The elementary school students get 360 minutes a week of physical activity, more than double the AAHPERD's recommended weekly minimum of 150 minutes for this age child. The secondary school students have 450 minutes of physical exercise a week, twice the recommended minimum of 225 minutes.

The lower-school boys (first through third grades) have two to three 40-minute gym classes a week. They also enjoy three 80-minute field sports sessions a week. Many of them also register—on an optional basis—for a once-a-week 90-minute after-school sports program. Not counting the optional program, the boys average more than 60 minutes a day of physical activity, twice AAHPERD's recommended minimum.

The middle-school boys (fourth through sixth grades) have one 60-minute gym class per week, and three field sports days of 80 to 100 minutes each. This totals 360 minutes a week, or more than 60 minutes per school day.

The upper-school boys (seventh through ninth grades) take no gym classes. But they are required to select a team sport from a choice of three offered in each of three semesters. Their school day is extended to half past five to allow these boys time for fitness activity and athletic practice. This is highly unusual: every boy in grades seven through nine participates on an Allen-Stevenson athletic team each semester. Every boy exercises for 100 minutes three times a week and for 150 minutes on game day. (There are no workouts on Fridays.) This totals 450 minutes of athletic activity each week—an average of 90 minutes every school day.

Better yet, music, drama, and art programs are coordinated with the sports workouts so that the students can enjoy those activities without being forced to select one over the other.

Quality of Activity

Each gym class, field sport session, or team sport practice includes four types of fitness exercises: relaxation, stretching, strengthening, and aerobics. Even the baseball players—traditionally the least-fit school team—keep in shape by running one and a half miles before the balls and bats are unpacked. The theme of fitness first, sports second, is consistent throughout the P.E. program.

Relaxation exercises help the boys make the transition from classroom to playtime; this, in turn, teaches them that they can handle stress with regular exercise. Stretching exercises help flexibility and prepare the boys for physical activity. Specific stretches are done for specific sports. Push-ups, sit-ups, and other exercises are used in gym classes and sports-conditioning sessions to improve both muscular strength and muscular endurance.

Aerobic Activity

Except for a few gym classes, where emphasis is placed on strengthening and motor skill development, each P.E. session seeks to include cardio-respiratory endurance training—that is, twenty minutes of continuous aerobic activity at least three times a week (the AAHPERD minimum). This is done at Allen-Stevenson with a variety of activities, including walking, running, swimming, skating, racquet sports, aerobic dance, and aerobic sports such as soccer, cross-country running, hockey, and lacrosse, as well as aerobic imaginative games.

The Fitness Class

About once a week, the lower-school boys have a total fitness gym class. This includes warming up, twenty minutes of aerobics, and cooling down. A variety of fitness games, including aerobic dancing, are used to keep the boys interested and moving. The middle-school boys sometimes do this routine to supplement their field sport activities. Chapter 13 includes a sample youth fitness class developed with the cooperation of Christopher and his first-grade classmates.

Walking

A walking program was added to the school P.E. curriculum as a test project for this book. It was offered as an option to field sports and proved to be an outstanding success and great change of pace.

The lower-school boys went for adventure walks in Central Park each week throughout the entire school year. The middle-school boys also took walks. In the fall and spring, the lower-school boys watched the seasons change and explored the terrain of Central Park—climbing "mountains," rolling like barrels down hills, zooming through playground mazes, and chasing squirrels. As special treats, they visited the Central Park Zoo and then "walked like animals," or hiked to the carousel for a musical ride, or walked to the lake and paddled away in rowboats. In the winter, they escaped from the confinements of indoors to explore New York's winter wonderland by making tracks through fresh snow. Even in the coldest weather, they bundled up and walked briskly, returning full of energy to the warmth of the classroom.

For each walking session, the boys broke up into two or three groups of ten to twelve boys (according to fitness levels) led by an imaginative instructor. This way, the boys who walked fast or liked to take running bursts of joy were not held back by the less fit or less enthusiastic. And the slower boys did not feel dragged along and thus lose interest in the walk.

Chapter 19 details how walking can be used as an educational tool and provides examples of unusual walks that can be enjoyed by school groups.

Running

Can kids be conditioned and taught to enjoy aerobic running? Can they look upon it with fondness, even nostalgia? Let me tell you a story.

There is a great tradition of running at Allen-Stevenson, extended because Pat Lappin, the P.E. director, is a former national-class runner. For the last several years each autumn and spring the boys have taken up the challenge of running the one-and-a-half–mile loop around the Central Park Reservoir. The runs are festive occasions, with teachers and parents joining in or waiting to cheer for the boys when they finish. The event gives the boys a reason to get into shape and focuses their running exercise. It also motivates teachers and parents to take up a fitness program or activity.

When he entered Allen-Stevenson, Christopher's longest run had been three hundred yards in the New York Road Runners Club's peewee races. He enjoyed running fast, but not far. One day after school, he told me how he was training each week for the reservoir run, but he refused to run with me to demonstrate his new endurance. "I only want to run with my school friends," he said.

In the autumn and spring, the lower school boys run two or three times a week before their field sports activities. The goal is to finish the one-and-a-half–mile loop of the Central Park Reservoir. They start out running a quarter-mile and gradually build up to a full mile—saving the extra half-mile challenge for the event itself. The coaches pick a leader in practice runs and the boys must stay behind him at an even, slow pace until the last fifty to one hundred yards, when they are allowed to run as fast as they wish. The boys are encouraged to run nonstop, but if they get out of breath they may also walk briskly until they can run again—a run-walk pattern used by most adults to complete their own first races. Since they train at a conversational pace, they are also encouraged to talk with each other as they run along, which proves to be both a distraction from the ordeal of training and a special source of fellowship. (I emphasize to my adult runners that they should run and talk; it's fun and you meet all kinds of wonderful people.) Each lower-school boy participates in the reservoir run twice a year and receives a medal or other souvenir for finishing.

On the day of Christopher's first autumn reservoir run, I was as nervous as any parent on hand. Few of us believed that our sons could actually make it that far. They were, after all, only little first-graders! The boys, however, were full of excitement and confidence. There they were, thirty-six kids raring to go. They couldn't wait to run a distance that most of their parents wouldn't even consider walking.

Off they went. Coaches and teachers led the group for the first half-mile to keep the boys from starting too fast. Then they moved from boy to boy, encouraging each one. Some of the boys ran fast, some took their time, and most took walk breaks on occasion. But every boy met the challenge and crossed the finish line with a smile to the sound of spirited applause from parents, teachers, and classmates. When Christopher crossed the finish line, I had tears in my eyes. "He did it!" I exclaimed.

The boys had trained for the reservoir run in a non-competitive atmosphere of fitness and fun, and the event was held in that spirit. No times or places were recorded. Each boy was a winner by finishing and each boy got his finisher's medal at the post-run picnic as a souvenir of his accomplishment. The boys were proud of themselves and of each other; it was, after all, a team effort met by completing many team runs together in practice. The next day, most of the boys proudly wore their medals to school and showed them off to their friends. "Dad," said Christopher, "my medal is so precious." The next day he asked me if I would run the reservoir with him.

Christopher learned more than the sweet taste of getting in shape. He also learned to set a goal and achieve it. For the spring run, he decided that his goal would be to run the reservoir nonstop. He spent the winter and early spring training with his classmates and once in a while with me. On the day of the run, he let me join his classmates and some of their fit parents, and together we slowly took on the one-and-a-half-mile run. Christopher glided along this time, talking all the way, and finished without stopping. His pace was better than ten minutes per mile—well under the AAHPERD standard of twelve minutes per mile for six-year-olds. But beyond this, he had again set a goal, trained for it, and accomplished it.

Not to be outdone, in the autumn and spring the middle-school boys also run twice a week before field sports activities in preparation to run the reservoir loop. Once a week they also do a relaxed group fitness run. But the level of competition is heightened. For motivation, once a week the coaches record the top ten finishers over a mile, assigning a point value of ten for first down to one for tenth. The points are added up for both the autumn and spring running periods and the top ten scorers receive a special Allen-Stevenson running singlet. For each reservoir run, the top twenty finishers in each grade get a medal and all finishers get a ribbon.

The upper-school boys also run the reservoir twice a year, but with less competitiveness. They have enough competition and aerobic fitness training in their own sports-team programs. Instead, the reservoir run, which many of them have done together since the first grade, is now a social fitness run. They do it for fun and companionship and as a way of marking the years since that first scary run-walk over a distance that felt endless, in an autumn that seems long, long ago.

Activity Sessions

At Allen-Stevenson, the boys' physical activity is divided into three basic types of sessions: gym classes, field sports, and team sports. Additional activities include after-school sports (intramurals) and the annual Field Day.

Gym Class. The forty-minute gym class is directed by a professional physical educator. Each class contains between fifteen and twenty boys. The P.E. director personally teaches many of these classes in order to monitor closely the physical development of each boy.

Lower-school boys have two to three gym classes a week and the middle-school boys, who have team sports, have only one. The curriculum is designed to improve specific areas of physical development not covered by sports play or aerobic workouts. Specific attention is paid to improving muscular strength and endurance, and flexibility, as well as motor skills.

A typical lower-school gym class includes fifteen to twenty minutes of relaxation, stretching, and strengthening exercises, followed by games and drills that improve agility (such as shuttle runs) and coordination (such as kickball). Once a week, the lower-school gym class becomes a fitness class with aerobic creative movement such as "fitness freeze," "safari aerobics," or "Simon says fitness." These are explained in Chapters 13 and 14.

Field Sports. The goal of the field sports program is to introduce the boys to a variety of sports experiences. The eighty-minute sessions are held three times a week for both the lower- and middle-school boys. About once a week all year long, the lower school takes a one-hour adventure walk as their field sport. Two or three times a week in autumn and spring, the boys take aerobic runs of between a half-mile and a mile before sports activities. Each field sports session includes relaxation, stretching, strengthening, and aerobics. In most cases two classrooms of between thirty and thirty-six boys go to the field together with three instructors. The boys are then divided into three groups for sports play.

First-graders are introduced to sports play in a relaxed, non-structured way. In the fall they play soccer, kickball, and other skill games. Twice a week during the winter they walk to a nearby indoor skating rink for skating instruction; they also learn a little ice hockey, using plastic sticks. Once a week in winter, they go out for a walk in the park. In the spring, they play softball and baseball.

Second- and third-graders learn more advanced fundamentals in twice-a-week gym sessions; they also play a semi-structured game once a week.

Second- and third-graders are mixed and teams are evenly matched by the skill of each player. In the autumn, they play soccer and also learn to throw and catch a nerf football. During the winter, the boys skate twice a week and play some ice hockey. Once a week in the winter they go for a walk, weather permitting. Third-graders only ice-skate for six weeks (half the semester). The other six weeks they go swimming twice a week. The first two-thirds of each swim class is instruction. The final one-third is for fitness swimming. During the spring, the third-graders play softball and baseball.

Middle-school boys at Allen-Stevenson have two practice sessions a week at field sports and one game day. In each of the three academic-year semesters, the teachers divide the boys into five groups of about eighteen boys each. For each semester, they rotate the activities every two or three weeks. The boys are placed on permanent teams and the games are mostly structured. In the autumn they play baseball (hardball, with the coaches pitching), flag football, soccer scrimmage, soccer fundamentals, and "hoc-cer"—a combination of soccer and team handball. The soccer and hoccer sessions include plenty of aerobic activity.

In the winter, the middle-school boys have some very interesting options. They take about three-and-a-half weeks of basketball, then swimming, then wrestling. In swimming they are encouraged to swim laps and are awarded a patch if they reach a total of one hundred laps during their short season. As an option, for an additional fee, the boys can play a half-season or twelve-week full season of ice hockey or squash, both excellent aerobic sports. In the spring, these boys take on baseball, softball, and three aerobic activities: soccer scrimmage, lacrosse, or track.

Team sports are used in the middle school to introduce the boys to inter-school competition. In the autumn, winter, and spring, the fifth- and sixth-grade boys compete against a rival school, both at home and away, in soccer, flag football, basketball, softball, and lacrosse.

The upper-school boys must choose a sports team to play on in each semester—a highly unusual requirement. Fall sports include football, soccer, and cross-country running. Winter sports are basketball, wrestling, and swimming, and in the spring the school competes in baseball, track, and lacrosse. The school's administrators feel that team play is an essential part of a boy's education and that excellence in the classroom carries over to excellence on the playing fields. Three sports are offered each semester, an unusual number for a small school. By contrast, the athletic program at my high school in Dansville, New York, had only two sports each semester for about sixty boys in each grade. Allen-Stevenson offers three sports for thirty-five boys in each grade.

The three-sports philosophy offers the boys more selection and spreads the better athletes around. That makes it difficult to develop winning teams, but it also gives each boy, whatever his skill level, a chance to play and develop. "I wouldn't have it any other way," says Pat Lappin. "We believe that by having more teams, more boys get an opportunity to participate, and to excel. We might win more games if we specialized in the basic sports of football, basketball, and baseball, but we would lose valuable diversity in our overall physical education program."

There is another important part to the Allen-Stevenson program: no boy is cut from a team. Each selects the sport he wants that semester and plays. In the popular sports—soccer, basketball, and baseball—both A and B teams compete against local schools. The B team serves as a developmental team for those boys not yet ready for varsity competition and for those whose enthusiasm exceeds their talents. Cross-country, wrestling, and swimming offer exhibition matches for boys not on the starting team. Thus, no boy falls through the cracks and is left off a team.

Each team has two to three weeks of conditioning before starting its season. The coaches and the boys meet three times a week for an hour and forty minutes for fitness exercises and sports practice. These sessions start with relaxation, stretching, and strengthening exercises, plus aerobic activity. They play one game a week.

All sports teams run aerobically during their pre-season conditioning period. Sports that do not require aerobic training, such as baseball and football, include aerobic running as part of each practice session for the entire season. This way, the players on every team maintain a high level of aerobic fitness.

If you look at the pattern of Allen-Stevenson's gym and field sports classes, you can see that they first teach fundamentals and then gradually move into competitive sports. At the heart of the program, from first grade through ninth, is aerobic fitness in every season, along with the sports competition.

One other thing. Recognition is a valuable part of any sports fitness program. An awards ceremony for athletes and their families is held each semester for the sports teams. Varsity letters are awarded based on participation and are worn proudly on school jackets. Three coaches awards are presented for each sport for outstanding contributions to a team. "Honorable mention" school blazer patches are presented to the boys "who worked very hard, not necessarily the best athletes."

Field Days. The school holds Field Day each spring. The events are spirited occasions when the boys can demonstrate their new and improved skills to their parents.

Lower-school boys rotate among four stations: fitness games, soccer, balloon relays, and kickball. Then they play softball with their parents. The middle-school boys play "hoccer," softball, flag football, and soccer. Then they take on the parents in a softball game. The upper school's field days consist of the low-key event of relays with one special addition: they bring in students from a local girls' school to participate in sports with them.

FITNESS TESTING

Twice a year, the P.E. instructors at Allen-Stevenson give all the boys the AAHPERD's Health-Related Physical Fitness Test. The evaluation is then mailed to each boy's parents. The overall fitness test results are carefully analyzed grade by grade and compared to national standards. This helps the P.E. instructors determine the effectiveness of the school's fitness program. If there are deficiencies, the program is adjusted to improve those areas. Not surprisingly, the Allen-Stevenson boys score very high compared to national fitness norms.

At the end of each semester, each boy and his parents receive a school report on all his subjects, plus his physical education. The P.E. report (see the sample below) includes a review of the fitness test results plus a report on the boys' progress in motor skills, cooperation, and effort.

WELLNESS EDUCATION IN THE CLASSROOM AND LUNCHROOM

Starting with the first grade, wellness education is also part of the physical education and academic classes. It is part of the weekly fitness classes and the adventure walks for the lower-school boys. With exercise physiology, wellness topics are re-emphasized during the pre-conditioning periods for each of the upper school's sports teams. By "wellness education," the faculty at Allen-Stevenson means a wide range of health-related topics. These include the following:

Exercise physiology. The study of how the body works and the effect on the body of physical exercise. This is taught in the lower school and covered in depth throughout the middle and upper schools.

Drug education. Starting with the first grade and continuing through the sixth, the boys take Project Charlie, which is an education program about drug use and abuse. Grades six through nine get the Freedom from Chemical Dependence program, which brings former substance abusers into the school during a week of seminars with students and an evening meeting with parents. The students are also made aware of the dangers of tobacco and alcohol abuse, and these discussions generally carry over into the academic classes, particularly the science and health programs.

In addition, since this is New York City, there are discussions and classes about street safety, AIDS, and other safety and health problems that plague cities. As part of this program, police officers visit grades three through

THE ALLEN-STEVENSON SCHOOL

Physical Education Comment

Name: _____ Date: _____

Class: _____ Season: _____

		Excellent	Good	Satisfactory	Needs Improvement
Fitness	Aerobic Endurance				
	Flexibility				
	Muscular Strength and Endurance upper body				
	abdominal				
	Body Composition				
Skill	Agility				
	Balance				
	Eye-Hand Coordination				
	Speed				
Cooperation	Willingness to Accept Instruction & Criticism				
	Positive Attitude				
	Team Play				
	Sportsmanship Competitive & Fair				
	Responsibility				

Comments: _____

Effort: _____ Teacher:

Effort 1 = Exceptional effort; enthusiastic, conscientious, highly motivated
Effort 2 = Consistent participant; eager to improve; generally interested
Effort 3 = Inconsistent participant; cooperates, but interest and motivation vary
Effort 4 = Generally uncooperative; lacks motivation and desire to improve

nine and the school's physician discusses such problems with grades seven through nine.

Relaxation exercises. Being a student these days can be stressful. The Allen-Stevenson boys also learn relaxation exercises as part of their physical education classes. Introduced to first-graders and continued every year, they are designed to help the boys control stress and tension. As I have mentioned, they are part of the P.E. program for all nine grades and part of team sports fitness exercises. The goal is to help the boys learn to deal with the stresses of sports competition, school work, and urban life.

Nutrition. Perhaps because Christopher is growing so fast, Virginia and I believe this is one of the most important wellness concepts. We emphasize good nutrition at home, and we are delighted (and relieved) to see it emphasized in his school.

Nutrition as a subject is introduced to first-graders in the classroom. I don't think schools can over-emphasize this issue. The boys learn what good foods are, where they come from, how to plan a nutritious menu, and how to develop good eating habits. In the third grade, the boys learn about the four basic food groups and how to count calories in various foods, and they study the digestive system. In science, they test various foods for starch and fat content. They also tie in what they learn about nutrition with other academic subjects. In English class, they invent a nutritious food and develop a marketing plan for it. In computer science class, they design a logo to promote their new product.

Nutritious lunch. The school's real lessons in nutrition are imparted through its nutritious lunch program, directed by Monica Matthew. She uses her extensive training in nutrition in the preparation of the food she serves and in her enthusiastic communication to the boys about the value of eating a balanced diet. (Guidelines on nutrition for your family can be found in Chapter 29.)

A balanced and nutritious lunch at Allen-Stevenson includes:

- Hot protein dish: chicken, meat, fish, or cheese.
- Salad bar (as an option to the hot dish or as a supplement): choice of raw salad, protein salad (chicken or egg), or broccoli and roast beef salad.
- Starch: potatoes, pasta, rice, or beans.
- Hot vegetables: carrots, zucchini, broccoli, peas.
- Grains: variety of breads (emphasis away from white processed breads).
- Dairy product: cottage cheese, yogurt.
- Beverage: milk (2 percent low-fat or skim), fruit juice.
- Dessert: fruit salad, yogurt, fresh fruit, pudding, cake, ice cream.

The desserts are sometimes a compromise to induce the boys to eat a healthy lunch. At home, for example, Christopher cannot have dessert until he finishes his vegetables (sound familiar?). Parents who insist on it may instruct their boys to select yogurt or fruit for dessert. The back-up meal for the boys who hate the main dish for the day or pick at the salad bar is the old stand-by: the peanut butter and jelly sandwich on whole-wheat bread—a favorite of Christopher's and mine.

Teachers eat with the boys at each table and encourage them to try some of each type of food offered that day to get a balanced meal. Monica Matthew works with the lower-school teachers to help the young boys understand what foods are best for them. The goal is for lessons learned in school to carry over to meals at home.

To involve the lower-school boys in meal planning and enable them to take advantage of the school's nutritious lunch program, each boy is asked to plan a balanced lunch menu choosing a selection from each food group. "This I have to see," I told Virginia. Without warning, I asked Christopher to write a menu for this book. "That's easy," he replied, and dashed off the following menu.

Christopher Glover's Nutritious Lunch Menu

- Meat: turkey
- Dairy: milk and yogurt
- Grain: bread
- Fruit: apple
- Vegetable: broccoli

As a treat for his hard work in producing this list, however, he asked that we go out for a pizza. Monica tells me that pizza is not such a bad food: it has a protein (cheese), a vegetable (tomato sauce), and a grain (crust). It does have a high sodium level, however.

PARENTAL INVOLVEMENT

Parents are invited to participate in and ask questions about all aspects of the Allen-Stevenson school day: academics, P.E. courses, and evening forums. They join the field days and reservoir run, attend all team sport games and award dinners, and participate in fitness walks with the lower- and middle-school boys. I have organized trips for Christopher's first-grade classmates and their families to attend a New York Knicks basketball game, a New York Rangers hockey game, and a Harlem Globetrotters show. A group of seventy-two boys, parents, and faculty went out to a New York Mets baseball game and cheered as "Welcome, the Allen-Stevenson

School" was flashed on the Met's scoreboard. Such things build school spirit, enhance family relationships, and get kids excited about sports and exercise.

But beyond that, participation by parents in their kids' school has another benefit. If the parents thoroughly understand what the boys are learning at school, they will be more likely to follow that up at home. This is especially important in terms of the focus of this book: sound exercise and nutritional habits. In that regard, the school's P.E. department conducts parent-orientation sessions for the purpose of educating parents about youth fitness and the school's sports programs. The Parents Association is also expanding efforts to educate parents about the wellness programs. Headmaster Cole's frequent letters to parents often discuss drug abuse, mental fitness, stress management, competition, and physical fitness.

Any school that is proud of what it does will welcome parents of its students or prospective students. And it is essential to your child's physical and academic growth that you participate in what he or she does.

Other Innovative School Programs

Daily physical exercise for your child is the ideal. But, as we both know, that's not what goes on in most schools. Many schools turn physical education over to homeroom teachers, who let the kids loose in the gym or schoolyard for 30 minutes of "recess" after lunch. It's a mob scene with large masses of kids of all ages standing, swinging, and chasing, but not learning what fitness is or how important it is to them and their future. It certainly isn't exercise.

The ideal of the daily P.E. classes and the model program at the Allen-Stevenson school can be put into place, to some extent, in almost any school. What I am suggesting is that, at the minimum, schools begin to offer basic fitness education to our children starting in kindergarten or grade one.

There is no reason why they cannot do this. There are many examples of success stories in our public schools across the country, from the poorest ghetto school to the most affluent suburban school with its elegant, sweeping campus and architecturally perfect buildings. The following stories tell about how good teachers, sometimes backed by impoverished but supportive administrations, can make a difference. Here are some examples of what other schools (most of them public) are doing.

SOUTHSIDE ELEMENTARY SCHOOL, JOHNSON CITY, TENNESSEE

This is an example of a corporate-sponsored program for a local public school system. The Paty Company, a regional chain of retail building materials stores, with headquarters in Piney Flats, Tennessee, near Johnson City, sponsors a school wellness program for children.

This story began when John Seward, Jr., company president, trained for his first marathon under a program I directed in connection with the New York City Marathon. Inspired, he had his company sponsor a local race to promote fitness in the community. In 1987, I was John's guest as a pre-race lecturer and suggested that he add a "peewee run" for the kids. It was a huge success, and during a run together in the hills of eastern Tennessee, I suggested that if John really wanted to help promote fitness in his community—and I knew he did—that he start with the kids, including his own.

The result is the Fit Kids program, developed with Paty Company financial and marketing resources and the fitness expertise of East Tennessee State University's Quality of Life Wellness Center. Here, then, is a unique combination of private industry and local university working together in the public schools to improve the health of children.

Southside Elementary School in Johnson City, with about 340 students in kindergarten through the sixth grade, was selected as the pilot school for the 1987–1988 school year. The results of the re-tests of the children showed remarkable improvements in all health fitness areas and as a result the program was expanded in 1988–1989 to include all the elementary schools in Johnson City.

In the autumn, children are tested for all the key fitness components (using the AAHPERD health-related test). They are tested again at the end of the year. After the first test, each student gets a consultation and a plan for improving fitness skills.

The situation at Southside Elementary is not ideal. But the school is doing its best with what it's got. Homeroom teachers are responsible for physical education in their classes three days a week. They were given guide books developed by exercise physiologists to help them lead fitness activities, so that each child can achieve and maintain a high level of fitness. Previously, the classroom teachers were on their own without professional direction. They filled the time as best they could. The Fit Kids program assures that P.E. time is well spent.

After the spring test, students and parents are presented with a fitness profile to measure the child's improvement.

The program emphasizes fun and supplements the school system's existing physical education program. Behind the slogan "It's Hip to be Fit," the program involves parents, teachers, and kids from kindergarten through the sixth grade in a variety of wellness and fitness programs.

The parents of each child are encouraged to join the Fit Club and participate with their child in a home exercise program. The parents get a log to record their family fitness activities. There is an incentive system. After the first fitness test of their child in the fall, parents get a "Hip to be Fit" T-shirt and bumper stickers. All children receive T-shirts, hats, and logo buttons. In the classroom, kids are rewarded not only for reaching certain fitness levels, but also for most improved, good team player, willing to help others, best effort, and family participation.

The program culminates with a "Fit Kid Olympics" at the end of the year. This is a one-day event that allows the children to demonstrate improvement in fitness conditioning and skills rather than competition. At the end of the olympics, the parents, teachers, and kids have a picnic, with awards for various achievements and participation.

"People can make a difference," says John Seward, "when they care about their community and how children grow up."

SOUTH HUNTINGTON SCHOOL DISTRICT, HUNTINGTON STATION, NEW YORK

Here is a case where one teacher makes a difference.

Harvey Pachter has been a physical education teacher in the South Huntington School District since the 1950s. He taught P.E. during the Kennedy era when enthusiasm brought funds, and then during the lean Reagan years when funds were cut. Pachter doesn't give up.

He is able to teach the fifth- and sixth-graders for only forty minutes twice a week. The South Huntington kids start running one to three minutes twice a week from first grade P.E. classes on. That pattern continues until they reach his fifth- and sixth-grade classes. He uses four to five minutes of that class for transitional conditioning to improve flexibility, muscular strength, and endurance. Then the kids do five to six minutes of nonstop aerobic running. The remaining twenty minutes are used to improve motor skills, introduce team sports, or provide other fitness offerings. And as if that weren't enough, Pachter works in nutrition, weight management, stress management, and so forth as part of a two- to five-minute daily discussion with his students following their cool-down period.

But his basic objective, he says, "is to make sure the kids get no less than ten minutes of continuous *vigorous* activity in each class. Our goal is to establish a healthy attitude about fitness for all the kids." Twenty minutes of vigorous activity should be a school's goal, but Pachter is forced to do the best he can with limited time and a New York State curriculum that is not always in tune with scheduled time frames, available facilities, number of personnel, and equipment allocation.

Sixth-graders and the MiniThon. Pachter's program for sixth-graders is worth noting in detail. In September, when the school year begins, he encourages the sixth-graders to strive for five levels of fitness. The program focuses on the excitement of the New York City Marathon, and culminates at the end of the school year in June with a MiniThon—a one-and-a-half–mile fun and fitness event in which the students predict their own times.

To begin the year, the students run laps indoors or run a half-mile course outdoors. They run for five to six minutes and record their laps. Laps are translated into miles and each student charts his or her miles on a large map of the 26-mile, 385-yard New York City Marathon course. These kids see themselves, in their daily workouts, inching along the marathon route. For sixth-graders, 786 laps completed equals the full NYC Marathon. Usually, this is reached by the end of February.

More than this, as they run they study the history of the various neighborhoods along the marathon route, how to train for a marathon, nutrition, and so forth. The marathon becomes a teaching tool, and at least thirty topics are addressed and discussed as the students chart their mileage. They also learn all they can about the marathon in order to "visualize" their route and participation.

That's just Level I. When each of the two hundred students completes the New York City Marathon, he or she moves on to Level II: one thousand laps, or twenty actual miles of running. Level III is fifteen hundred laps, or thirty miles. "Honor rolls" depict their progress and certificates are awarded as each level is attained.

Level IV separates the fit from the followers. At this level, the students must complete a thirty-minute run nonstop. They work out for ten sessions to prepare for this effort. During May, on a voluntary basis, the students use their thirty-minute lunch period to attempt to reach this goal. Parents volunteer to help monitor the run. Almost every student—about 98 percent of them—attempts this level and takes on the thirty-minute nonstop run. Not all of them make it, however, although as many as forty-two—almost half the class—have done so in some years.

Level V, the ultimate level of fitness in Pachter's classes, is the Presidential Fitness Award. The student achieves this by scoring above the eighty-fifth percentile in all of the test items.

The program reaches its climax at the end of the school year in June. This event was started with the help of a South Huntington resident and parent, Nina Kuscsik. Yes, *that* Nina Kuscsik—women's division winner of both the New York City Marathon and the Boston Marathon. She is also the mother of three kids. For the South Huntington MiniThon, each student predicts his or her own time. Students from three other schools in the district also participate; this makes more than four hundred sixth-graders running (and over five thousand since its inception in 1978). Race numbers, water stops, and other special effects line the course to simulate the NYC Marathon experience. The event is played on local cable television, reported in the local papers, and the town supervisor proclaims "Fitness Week" in honor of the graduating sixth-grade fitness enthusiasts. After the event, the boy and the girl from each school who most closely predicted their times get trophies.

This is a fitness run, not a race. The kids can walk as much as they want. The goal is simply to complete the one-and-a-half-mile distance. Afterwards, the students return to their schools for an award ceremony and a "pasta party" organized by the P.T.A.—similar to the parties following the NYC Marathon. All participants receive T-shirts and all finishers get a certificate. In addition, each school sponsors a MiniThon poster contest allowing each child to creatively depict their attitude toward the MiniThon and fitness.

Harvey Pachter feels the tide may be turning his way, with more support for physical education, maybe even a return to the glory years. He proudly notes that the South Huntington school board, with the endorsement of his P.T.A., recently approved ten thousand dollars for fitness equipment for his school, and he is going to use it to fashion a "challenge" obstacle course that will help increase upper body strength and agility. As a result of Pachter's programs, the secondary level has experienced a boom in track and field and cross-country participation, and significant improvement in endurance activities has become widespread.

LEAL ELEMENTARY SCHOOL, URBANA, ILLINOIS

Like Harvey Pachter, Judith Gaston Fisher found a way to motivate her young students. Moreover, the physical education program had been cut in Urbana, and Fisher did a lot with very little. According to *Instructor Magazine*, when Fisher read an article to her thirty-one third-graders about how embarrassingly out of shape American schoolchildren are, they decided to do something about it. They developed an eight-week physical fitness unit and turned their classroom at Leal Elementary School into a health club.

The kids developed a motto: "Mind and Body Fitness." Science and health periods were devoted to discussions of how our bodies work and how exercise and diet affect us. Using the Amateur Athletic Union's physical fitness testing program as a guide, Fisher and her students made fitness booklets for each student. The booklets included:

- A list of six basic exercises to do, including sit-ups, push-ups, standing long jump, endurance run, pull-ups, and shuttle run.
- A space to record initial scores for all six activities and scores at the end of the eight-week unit.
- A page to record height, weight, and measurements.
- A page titled "Personal Goals" to help teach the kids goal-setting. Among the resolutions: no more chips after dinner; only two television programs each night; and twenty-seven sit-ups in one minute.
- Charts for keeping track of TV watching—hours spent and shows watched—with a goal of cutting back.
- A datebook with grids for monitoring eating habits. The kids record all meals and snacks eaten every day during the eight weeks.

Recess and free time were spent exercising. Despite occupying a very small classroom, Fisher's third-graders exercised there. They used the playground and hallway to practice their standing long jumps. Although the P.E. program in Urbana had been cut—despite the proximity of the University of Illinois, with its outstanding P.E. department—the chinning bars remained in the gym and could be used for pull-ups. Shuttle runs, using blackboard erasers for the agility drill, and half-mile endurance runs were done during recess outdoors. The kids learned how many laps around the school building equaled one mile.

Classroom teachers can make a difference in the fitness of their students. All thirty-one of Fisher's third-graders earned certificates from the AAU at the completion of their program. They felt like winners—and they were, in more ways than one.

"Although I have no hard data to prove it," said Fisher, "I'm convinced that the students worked harder in all areas. Furthermore, children who were poor academic achievers excelled in the workouts. Kids who didn't associate with one another previously now work together."

BLACK ELEMENTARY SCHOOL, STERLING HEIGHTS, MICHIGAN

Not every class has to run. Here is an example of a walking program that worked too.

Diane Hoeft-Varisto was shocked when her fifth- and sixth-graders did poorly on a standard fitness test. But what could she expect? Her school, Black Elementary School in Sterling Heights, Michigan, offers only one gym class a week for only half an hour—a level mandated by the school district. That's not enough to even discuss fitness, let alone get the kids into shape.

But Hoeft-Varisto and her students decided to do something about this. They started a walking club. According to an article in *The Walking Magazine*, teacher and students walked a mile at recess. They liked it so much, they voted to add another half-mile to their regimen. Now, the kids plot their miles walked on maps of Michigan—not unlike Harvey Pachter's students and the New York City Marathon—and chart an imaginary journey across their home state.

Both teacher and students are also encouraging each other to walk at home, on weekends, and even during the school vacations. Now, although they may not have the advantages of a regular school P.E. program, the students who pass through Diane Hoeft-Varisto's class will emerge more physically fit and better able to face the challenges of their lives at school and home.

P.S. 118, QUEENS, NEW YORK

During a ten-kilometer race in 1986, Linda Figgers, a fourth-grade teacher at Public School 118 in Queens, a borough of New York City, came up with a brilliant idea. As she ran, Figgers thought about her students and the prevalence of drugs and crime in their neighborhood. What could she do, as a teacher and a runner, to combat those negative influences? Then the idea struck: *Why not use running to provide a positive outlet for my female students?* she thought. Running could boost their morale and give them an incentive to set and accomplish personal goals.

Back at P.S. 118, Figgers challenged her girls: Practice running with me now, and earn the chance to compete in the L'eggs Mini Marathon, a ten-kilometer (6.2 miles) race for women only in New York's Central Park. More than thirty-five girls accepted Figgers's challenge and started training and running in the playground during their lunch hour. These workouts soon continued after school in a nearby park. Then, the girls began running together on weekends.

In May 1987, Figgers brought forty girls to Central Park to run the L'eggs Mini Marathon. They ran as a team and every one of them finished. The next May, on Mother's Day, eighty-two girls showed up from P.S. 118, along with Figgers, assistant principal Marlene Pannell, some other teachers, and several mothers, to run in a five-kilometer tune-up run. Then on June 4, 101 girls from the school joined a field of more than nine thousand women to run the seventeenth L'eggs Mini Marathon.

The girls' running program even motivated the boys at P.S. 118, who wrote a rap song about them and hung banners around the school building.

"Besides greatly improving fitness levels," says Figgers, "the teachers at P.S. 118 have noticed that running has helped bolster the girls' study habits, self-esteem, and overall motivation."

SOUTH BRONX HIGH SCHOOL, BRONX, NEW YORK

At sunrise in the bleak and dangerous Melrose neighborhood of the South Bronx, when the streets are dark and deserted, more than 130 teenagers make their way into the South Bronx High School gym. There, to the beat of rock music and the instructions of Lou Schlanger, they begin an hour of fitness conditioning.

This is no ordinary P.E. class. For one thing, South Bronx High is a tough school in the tough "Fort Apache" neighborhood. Its students are predominantly Hispanic and predominantly poor. The dropout rate for freshmen is 25 percent. Schlanger's P.E. class starts at 6:45 A.M., an hour before school opens. It has an absentee rate of just 10 percent. Schlanger hopes that luring the students into school early will help keep them there. "If they learn to discipline their bodies," he told the New York Times, "maybe they'll learn to discipline their minds."

Some of the kids have to take two buses to reach the school, which draws from the entire Bronx. But Schlanger's class is such a hit that some mornings, up to two hundred teenagers pack the gym. They stretch, then do vigorous aerobics, push-ups, sit-ups, shuttle runs, and broad jumps.

Sharmagne Solis, a seventeen-year-old senior, sets her alarm for 5:30 A.M. in order to reach Schlanger's class on time. "I've learned to push myself physically," she said, "and when you know how to push yourself to do sixty push-ups, you know how to push yourself to do your homework."

Faculty members believe that most of the students who get up and get to the class stay for the rest of the school day. "If we've reached them enough to get them here at an ungodly hour," Schlanger says, "they become the type of kids who stay."

Solis told the New York Times: "I used to go to school because I had to, and I was bored and I cut a lot. But last year, I had perfect attendance because I didn't want to miss the fitness class, and then I began not wanting to miss school."

Schlanger's forty-five-minute workout begins with stretching. On different days the class emphasizes different parts of the body. As the students get into shape, they add a three-mile run to and from Yankee Stadium. On Fridays, Schlanger tests the students, and those who accumulate high scores (based on improvement as well as conditioning) get to compete in a national fitness meet sponsored annually by the Marine Corps. In the 1987 nationals at Camp Pendleton, California, the South Bronx boys' team finished fifth in the country, the girls' team ninth.

The class, says Schlanger, carries over into the rest of the students' lives. "Instead of lowering the standards, we want them to set the standards and feel there's nothing they can't do."

The rewards go far beyond getting in shape and winning national track meets. "I like the idea of doing hard, solid work," says Robert Perez, a senior who has taken the class for four years. When he first started, he was overweight. Now he looks slim and fit.

"This is no Jack LaLanne fairy tale," he says, "and I'm no Sylvester Stallone. But I'm not Fat Albert either anymore."

P.S. 20, BROOKLYN, NEW YORK

Early-morning workouts are also the norm at P.S. 20 in Brooklyn. By 8 A.M., the school's dingy basement gym has filled with fifty fourth- and fifth-graders—80 percent of them black, 15 percent Hispanic, inner-city kids—all ready for P.E. teacher Michael Marcus. But this is no usual P.E. class.

For example, one month Marcus will have the kids working out in a circus theme. He starts a scratchy recording of the Pointer Sisters' "Jump (For My Love)" and off they go! The kids become jugglers who toss frayed green tennis balls, rings (the tops of five-gallon plastic containers), clubs (plastic seltzer bottles with taped-on sticks), and bean bags. The juggling routine goes on until the music stops. Winded, the kids pause.

According to an article in Runner's World, Marcus has been teaching P.E. at P.S. 20 for over twenty years. At first it was traditional sports—basketball, baseball, volleyball, and football. But the kids took winning and losing too seriously, sometimes getting into fights over who won, and Marcus changed the curriculum to "movement education" that features constant movement. Piles of plastic pails, boxes of assorted balls, cardboard musical instruments, and tin-can walking stilts cover one end of the gym floor.

In addition, Marcus instills confidence in his young students. A "Mr. Confidence" poster adorns one of the walls. An "I did it at P.S. 20" banner hangs over the door to his office. At the end of a morning class with kindergarten kids, he sits on the floor and tells them: "I had a wonderful, enjoyable time with you this morning. You are one of my best, best classes, and in the circus you are going to be the stars."

He sends a sixth-grade class into blurs of aerobic movement with a vigorous game of "Simon Says" followed by relaxation exercises. "Sit down, cross your legs, straighten your back, close your eyes, and imagine you've traveled to some beautiful peaceful place," he tells them.

Is Michael Marcus crazy? His classes celebrated the international Olympic games with a Greek breakfast and relay races. During the winter games, he opened the windows and led his kids through rapid ski movements as the frigid air blew in on them.

His classes run around dribbling a basketball with both hands. Sometimes they run around the block.

"I don't herd the kids into the gym and tell them to run thirty laps," says Marcus. "I achieve the same thing with a disguised activity. You have to make the experience worthwhile. So we skip, leap, and juggle, or run like a snake. I get their hearts pumping up to about one hundred sixty."

Marcus intergrates his gym classes with the math and science curricula, to teach the kids about fitness and the cardiovascular system. All of this seems to work: although the grade-schoolers at P.S. 20 have only one P.E. class a week, they are scoring in the sixtieth to seventy-fifth percentiles in the Presidential Fitness Test.

THE HORIZON SCHOOL, PHOENIX, ARIZONA

The Horizon School also offers workouts for its students before school begins. The classes were started because the Glendale Elementary School District could offer only two P.E. classes of twenty-five minutes each during the school week. Now, Danny Knack, the P.E. instructor at Horizon School, has more than two hundred kids showing up to stretch and work out aerobically before their school day begins.

Knack and the students have formed the Horizon School Running Club. They run for half an hour every morning before school on a 440-yard grass track. The school cafeteria serves breakfast and the kids have time to eat before classes start. A large wall chart keeps track of each participant's mileage. Awards are given for mileage accumulation.

"Kids enjoy running," says Knack, "and they can see their progress when they do it on a regular basis." Like some of the other programs mentioned above, the combination of running, setting goals, and keeping a record of accomplishments is a valuable lesson for the kids at Horizon School.

ELKTON ELEMENTARY SCHOOL, ELKTON, VIRGINIA

John Kiser, a P.E. teacher at Elkton Elementary School, uses innovative awards clubs to help motivate his students during gym classes. It has worked so well the kids exercise before and after school.

First, the kids started running, and everyone in each class jogged together. They put up a map of the United States and plotted their mileage. Only laps completed by the entire class counted. In one four-month period, the class logged 4,556 running miles—enough to get them from Elkton to San Francisco and back!

Kiser and his kids also started clubs to encourage the development of upper-arm strength. Students who hang from a horizontal bar or ladder for ten seconds or more get a Monkey Club award. Those who hand-walk across the ladder progress to the Gorilla Club, and those neo-primates who hand-walk forward and backward become members of the King Kong Club.

Before Kiser's imaginative programs started, the elementary school students in Elkton scored in the twentieth percentile in national fitness tests. Now they range in the sixtieth to ninetieth percentiles. Maybe they ought to think about a President's club!

BEVERLY HILLS SCHOOL DISTRICT, BEVERLY HILLS, CALIFORNIA

When school districts cannot or will not fund programs, there are other ways to get fitness activities into the schools. Since 1982, the Beverly Hills, California, school district has offered the Know Your Body program (see Appendix). The program, funded by a local family, involves the entire school staff, and even uses the school cafeterias as nutritional learning centers.

First-grade students learn both wellness techniques and exercise. They are encouraged to give blood samples every year and monitor their own cholesterol levels. They calculate their own training heart rates during exercise by taking their own pulses and recording them.

"Our philosophy is that nobody takes better care of your body than you," says Carolyn McCary, the program coordinator. "We teach the students that by making informed choices they will be better able to control what happens to their bodies."

As we have seen, controlling one's own body often leads to controlling one's own life. From the South Bronx to Beverly Hills, teachers and students are working together to get in shape, plan exercise goals, learn about their bodies, and lead better lives.

Part 4

GETTING FIT

Getting Fit: Exercise Principles

First, we need to ask—and answer—some of the basic questions concerning exercise programs. One is: What kind of exercise is best for my child and me? Next there are three questions equally important for adults and children: How far? How fast? How often? I am asked those three questions more than any others, and the answers now form the basis of my exercise programs.

First we need to understand some exercise principles and to know what fitness is. Obviously, exercise and its effect on the body will be different for an adult than for a child. What is a well-balanced exercise program for an adult and for a child? Understanding the basic physiology of exercise helps in selecting levels of exercise of maximum benefit to you and your child.

Four basic types of exercise are used to achieve health-related fitness: aerobic (for cardio-respiratory endurance and body composition), stretching and relaxation (for flexibility), and strengthening (for muscular strength and endurance). They will be discussed in the next two chapters. Improving your body composition relates to both exercise and diet and is discussed fully in Chapter 30.

To get started, I review ten principles of exercise for you and your child. Then I detail the "1-2-3 Method" of exercise and follow that with a sample total fitness workout.

EXERCISE PRINCIPLES

Principle 1: Overload—the FIT Training Method

To improve your level of fitness, you must increase the amount of work your cardio-respiratory and musculo-skeletal systems have to do. This is sometimes translated by coaches—even kids' coaches—as "no pain, no gain." I don't believe in pain. If you are exercising or playing a sport in pain, you are risking serious injury. I believe in exercise as fun.

But I do understand that both adults and children will need to increase their exercise levels as they gain in fitness. This means that during aerobic exercise, you will need to work your hearts and lungs harder by increasing pace or distance—but not necessarily both. During strength training, you will increase the resistance or the number of repetitions performed; that is, you may need to do more push-ups. For flexibility exercises, you gently increase—over time—the amount of stretch placed on your muscles and connective tissues.

The acronym *FIT* sums up the three key components of increased exercise training: Frequency (how often), Intensity (how hard), and Time (how long).

Principle 2: Progressive Stress—Train, Don't Strain

The body is a remarkable organism and will surprise you in its ability to get stronger. But it can also surprise you by breaking down if you overstress it. Younger bodies break down just as easily as older bodies— perhaps more easily. For both adults and children the workout load should not be too light or too heavy. The body and mind gradually adapt to increasing levels of exercise stress. But that level must be delicately balanced to be intense enough and regular enough to promote adaption to a higher level of fitness—the "training effect."

On the other hand, if the stress is too much (overtraining), you overtax the adaption system and cause fatigue, poor performance, or, worse, injury. "Train, don't strain" is my rule, not "no pain, no gain." That's "no fun." You should train hard enough to improve your fitness level. In the case of children and youth, train to gain. Neither adults nor children should train to the point of strain, which defeats improvement. More—harder and longer—exercise is not always better.

Slow, steady progression will result in increased fitness. As your fitness improves, you will be able to handle a greater training load with the same effort. You may wish to gradually increase the frequency, intensity, and duration of your exercise program. A good rule of thumb is to never increase how much you exercise by more than 10 percent from one week to the next, or one month to the next. Also, do not increase all of the training variables—frequency, intensity, and time—simultaneously. This will increase your risk of injury. Instead, increase one variable at a time.

Principle 3: Recovery—The Hard-Easy Method

It is essential to alternate your stress and recovery periods, what I call the "hard-easy method." In your day-to-day schedule, you and your children should alternate hard exercise days and easy ones. The human body responds best to stressful exercise if it is allowed to recover. Stress applied on top of stress equals breakdown. Stress followed by recovery equals progress. Exercisers at all levels can recover from strenuous exercise with a day off or with "active rest" the following day. This could be an exercise such as walking or swimming that is gentle to the musculo-skeletal system. I believe it should also be fun.

For beginner exercisers, and those adolescents and adults not training for competitive sports, the ideal program alternates an exercise day with a day off or a very easy day to allow for recovery. This can be done best if you exercise three or four times a week. For more advanced exercisers or those adults training for competitive sports, hard workout days should be followed by easier days. The day after a speed workout, race, or long run, a runner should do a short, easy run or no workout at all. Varsity high-school or college teams in track, soccer, cross-country skiing, or swimming—sports with high aerobic workout levels—should have low-level training days and days off before meets or games. A well-conditioned high-school or college soccer or lacrosse team that plays on Wednesdays and Saturdays, for example, should practice on Mondays and Thursdays only—resting on days before games—and those workouts should generally consist of light scrimmages and conditioning running.

The basic rule here is *listen to your body* and recognize its warning signs—sore muscles, aches and pains, and fatigue. Take off a few days when your body complains. (Equally important: You should *not* be exercising so much that your body hurts.) Follow this simple formula: Vigorous exercise plus rest equals improved fitness.

Principle 4: Regularity

To maintain basic levels of fitness, you and your children should work out at least three times a week, year-round. If you take too much time off between workouts, you will lose some of the fitness you have worked so hard to gain. In general, your body builds fitness slowly and loses it rapidly: it takes three times as long to gain fitness endurance as it does to lose it. With complete inactivity, cardio-respiratory fitness declines almost 10 percent per week. Strength and flexibility decline more slowly—but you will lose fitness over time.

John Quincy Adams, our sixth president and an avid exerciser, maintained that there were three rules to living well: (1) Regularity, (2) Regularity, and (3) Regularity. We can still learn from his example. Adams got up every morning at five o'clock and either went for a swim in the Potomac River (wearing only goggles and bathing cap) or for a vigorous walk of between four and six miles at a pace that, according to his diaries, raised a sweat. Nothing stopped him—not even the winters he spent as the first U.S. ambassador in Russia!

Regularity is the key to fitness. But it requires discipline. You and your family should try to schedule your exercise for the same time every day. Make an appointment with yourself—and keep it. Of course, take time off when you are injured or ill. If the exercise gets boring, change your pattern or take a day off. Be regular, but not compulsive. By planning your fitness routine, and following it, you will come to understand John Quincy Adams's basic rule and why it is essential for living well.

Principle 5: Specificity

You have to do specific exercises to get specific fitness benefits. Different exercises might particularly benefit different sets of muscles, such as sit-ups for the abdominals or push-ups for the upper-body muscles. These exercises may improve your overall exercise program. But they will not improve your aerobic fitness. The next chapter includes a balanced program of exercises that will improve your cardio-respiratory endurance as well as your flexibility and muscular strength and endurance.

Principle 6: Variation

Despite John Quincy Adams's emphasis on regularity, also remember that variety will spice up your exercise life. You should vary the exercises you do, the places where you exercise, and the people exercising with you. If you play sports, vary that, too. When I was a kid, I ran cross-country in the fall (with some football), played basketball in the winter (and some volleyball), ran track in the spring, and played baseball all summer.

I encourage Christopher to vary his weekly exercise regimen. He'll run one day, go for an adventure walk on another, then play baseball on the next. Kids especially need variety in their physical activity, and they should be encouraged to continue that variety as they grow up. This not only makes exercising fun, but it also teaches them different ways to get that exercise. These lessons—regularity and variety—will help them find exercises they enjoy and set patterns of exercise behavior that will last a lifetime.

Principle 7: Adaptability

All exercise must be flexible and adapted to the needs of the individual. Find out what exercise routines work best for you. Luckily, not everyone enjoys the same exercises; otherwise our roads would be impassable or our swimming pools overflowing. Some of us enjoy endurance exercises, others prefer strength. As long as you exercise aerobically, you should choose whatever activities are best for you.

Your exercise may also vary by season or by interest. In fact, it is wise to enjoy several different kinds of aerobic exercises (biking and swimming, let's say), in case injury or illness makes you temporarily unable to perform one of them.

Weather conditions, available facilities and equipment, your health, family obligations, and level of boredom may all determine what exercises you do. This will be true of your children, too. Alter your training to fit your needs and moods. Be adaptable, not stubborn. On the other hand, do not switch back and forth so much that you lose regularity and training benefits.

Principle 8: Being Patient

Fitness will not come overnight. But then, you didn't get out of shape overnight either. Success in reaching your fitness goals should be measured in weeks and months, not days. Generally, an adult needs eight to ten weeks to get into fairly good shape after being sedentary. Children and adolescents may take less time. If you are training for sports, success will be measured in years, not months. Runners, for example, "put miles in the bank" day by day and thereby build endurance that will make them stronger year after year.

Whatever your form of exercise, take your time and be patient. You are only competing against the old, out-of-shape you. Every day that you exercise means that you are moving one more day away from the old you and toward a newer and better-fit you. In fitness, the tortoise beats the hare. Regularity, adaptability, and patience pay off. Take your time, enjoy exercise and life, and steadily get into better shape.

Principle 9: Moderation

Too much of anything—food, drink, work, homework, or exercise—isn't good. You need to be moderate in your approach to life. Balancing the major stresses—work, school, family, and friends—with exercise is as important as balancing the individual parts of your exercise program.

Don't overdo your exercise program. As Principle 8 indicates, you will get fit only gradually over a long period of time. Enjoy that time. Put exercise into your life, balance it with the other important things you enjoy, and get on with healthy living. You will be surprised to look up in a year and realize that you are fit, exercising regularly, and enjoying life more. So will your family.

Principle 10: Share the Flowers

A year from now, when you can feel and see the difference in yourself and, if you are exercising with them, your family, pause. Remember the eighty-five-year-old woman who said that if she had her life to live over, she would take the time to smell more flowers and walk barefoot earlier in the spring. Take that time. In addition, look around and find someone else—child, friend, or acquaintance—who is not exercising and might benefit from it. Gently bring that person into your circle and your exercise routine. Share the flowers.

THE 1-2-3 METHOD

Each of the four basic components of exercise—aerobic endurance, relaxation, flexibility, and strength—should follow the "1-2-3 approach": warm-up, peak work (aerobic and/or strength training), and cool-down. This will help you avoid injury and increase your training level.

1. The Warm-up

Warm-ups let our bodies gradually adjust to exercise. This phase is extremely important, but unfortunately is often ignored. This may result in fatigue or injury. The proper warm-up consists of three steps: relaxation, stretching, and cardio-respiratory buildup.

Begin with a few minutes of relaxation exercises to loosen up muscles that are tense and difficult to stretch. These exercises should help ease the tension out of your mind and body. Five to ten minutes of gentle limbering up and stretching will prepare your muscles and tendons for exercise and guard against injury. A few minutes of biking or walking may be added to the routine before stretching. This will warm up your muscles and make them easier to stretch. (Chapter 11 has detailed guidelines on relaxation and stretching exercises.)

Before starting your aerobic workout, you should always spend at least five minutes in cardio-respiratory warm-up—walking briskly, biking easily, jogging slowly, etc.—to gradually increase your resting heart rate toward your target aerobic heart rate. (Chapter 12 details how your heart responds to exercise.) During the warm-up routine, your heart pumps faster, blood flow and respiration rates increase, body temperature rises, causing you to perspire, and your muscles heat up and become more limber; you prepare, gradually, for vigorous exercise.

2. Peak Work

Warm-up routines prepare you for both types of exercise, aerobic and strength training. The sample total fitness routine that follows includes some calisthenic exercises for strength building that can be done after the stretching routine and before the cardio-respiratory warm-up. To prepare for strength training sessions not integrated with an aerobic workout—such as weight training—do the relaxation and stretching exercises suggested below followed by a five-minute (or longer) cardio-respiratory warm-up such as biking or walking. Then do your strength training program. Be sure to end with a proper cool-down.

3. The Cool-down

This is the warm-up in reverse and is equally important. Stopping an activity abruptly may cause injury, the pooling of blood in your extremities, and the slowing of waste product removal in your system. It may also cause cramps, soreness, dizziness, or an abnormal strain on your heart. The majority of exercise-related heart abnormalities among adults occur not during the aerobic phase but following exercise. These may be avoided by gradually cooling down your body, including your heart rate. Never sit down immediately or enter a warm shower or steam room without cooling down properly first.

The purpose of the cool-down is to help your body return to its pre-exercise level. Cooling down helps your breathing return to normal and keeps your muscles from becoming sore and stiff. Why do you think they walk prize race horses after workouts and races?

After your workout, keep moving at a slow pace for at least five minutes. This will allow your heart rate and breathing to gradually return to near your pre-exercise level. Walking slowly is usually the best cool-down. The important thing is to keep moving around so that blood is pumped from your extremities, especially your legs—where it supplied the energy to exercise—back into the central circulatory system. Before moving on to your stretching exercises, you should be breathing normally and you should feel relaxed. If not, walk around some more until you have properly recovered from the workout.

Your stretching routine should last five to ten minutes. You may repeat the same exercises that you do during the warm-up, or add others. It is important to stretch all major joint and muscle groups, in particular those that you used during the workout. This is a good time to work on your flexibility, since it is easier to stretch warm muscles. Thus, you can do more advanced stretches than you did during your warm-up, or if you do the same stretches you may try to comfortably stretch your muscles a little farther.

End your cool-down with relaxation exercises. Properly done, they should leave you feeling very relaxed and energized instead of fatigued. You should no longer be sweating. Your heart rate should be close to normal and your muscles fully relaxed.

A SAMPLE TOTAL FITNESS WORKOUT

The next two chapters will give you details about how to exercise to improve your flexibility, muscular strength and endurance, and cardio-respiratory endurance. The sample total fitness routine below is designed to be well balanced and non-stressful, yet produce increasing fitness levels. All exercises are detailed in the following chapter. The sample adult routine can be completed in forty to sixty minutes. More imaginative exercise routines for young children are detailed in Chapter 13.

1. Warm-up (ten to fifteen minutes)

Relaxation exercises
a. Belly breathing
b. Head roll
c. Shoulder shrug

Stretching exercises (*Do these, if not the whole list.)
a. Swivels
b. Thigh stretch
c. Wall push-ups*
d. Cat back*
e. Pectoral stretch
f. Ankle rolls
g. Groin stretch*
h. Hip stretcher
i. Sitting stretch*

Strengthening exercises
a. Push-ups
b. Sit-ups

Cardiovascular warm-up: Brisk five-minute walk

2. Peak Work (a minimum of twenty to thirty minutes of continuous aerobic activity)

3. Cool-down (ten to fifteen minutes)

Cardio-respiratory cool-down: Slow five-minute walk

Stretching exercises
Repeat warm-up stretches or add new ones for similar muscle groups.

Relaxation exercises
Repeat warm-up relaxation exercises or try the following routine to promote a more complete relaxation.

Progressive relaxation routine: Lie on your back, flex your knees into a bent position, feet flat on the floor. Let one leg slide slowly forward and drop to the floor. Raise the leg ten inches off the floor and tighten. Hold for ten seconds. Drop the leg, relax, return the leg to its flexed position. Repeat with your other leg.

Next, push the small of your back into the floor. Hold for ten seconds, then let go. Raise one arm high into the air and tighten the fist. Hold for ten seconds and then relax. Repeat with your other arm and fist.

Then, tighten the muscles of your face. Really make a contortion. Hold for ten seconds, then relax.

Take a few deep breaths, feeling your belly rise as you breathe in. Now, lie with your knees flexed, eyes closed. Allow your body to go limp. Think of something very relaxing, like floating in warm water. Rest, float for thirty seconds to one minute.

Slowly get up, rising to your hands, then knees, then one leg, then both legs but bent over, then slowly erect. You should feel very refreshed.

Keep this basic exercise routine in mind as you read the next two chapters. The routines here are applicable to almost any aerobic exercise routine. While the specific exercises, and the aerobic exercise itself, may be changed, the pattern of warm-up, peak work, cool-down remains constant.

Getting Fit: Flexibility and Muscular Strength and Endurance

I combine *flexibility* and *muscular strength and endurance* in this chapter because both are essential to muscular fitness. Flexibility is important so that you develop a full range of motion at your joints. This chapter details flexibility exercises and suggests a simple family relaxation and stretching program.

For good health it is essential that you have the level of muscular strength necessary to perform all daily activities efficiently and have a reserve of strength to handle emergencies. Muscular endurance helps you continue that level of strength over long periods of time. This chapter provides a simple family strength training program. In addition, I have included a weight training program for adolescents and adults.

Most of these exercises can be done by both adults and children. In fact, I encourage adults to work out with children so that you may help them learn the proper form for these exercises, and to make the workouts fun for you both. Chapter 13 details imaginative muscular fitness routines that appeal to young children.

FLEXIBILITY

Most flexibility gains come from a combination of relaxation and stretching exercises. Some strengthening exercises that go through the full range of motion, and some aerobic exercises, such as swimming and biking, also contribute to increased flexibility.

Pre-school children are naturally flexible. Who hasn't envied the little four-year-olds who can, at the slightest whim, simply bend over and touch their toes or even put their palms flat on the floor. As muscles develop, however, we need to stretch them carefully and regularly. Even children as young as elementary school age become inflexible and could benefit from a gentle stretching program. In adulthood, our muscles become shorter and shorter. Older children and adults, therefore, need a regular stretching program to avoid pulled muscles and other injuries.

Very few of us, especially children, enjoy stretching exercises. Kids don't want to warm up; they want to play. Parents and physical education teachers need to make sure that our children understand the importance of stretching and that we make it as balanced, regular, and as much fun as possible.

Learning to relax is the first lesson to increasing flexibility. A few minutes of relaxing and gentle limbering exercise release tension so that muscles can be stretched properly. Stretching should condition the muscles and connecting tissues. A muscle works best when at its maximum length.

You should do *static stretching*. This means slow and rhythmic movements. You stop and hold the stretch for about ten seconds at the point of first mild pulling sensation.

It is important to perform about ten to fifteen minutes of static stretching exercises before all vigorous activities, such as weight lifting, running, biking, vigorous walking, and swimming. The time you spend stretching will minimize your chances of injury and enhance your performance. Remember to do five to ten minutes of relaxation and stretching exercises after vigorous workouts to prevent muscle tightness.

GUIDELINES FOR FLEXIBILITY EXERCISES

- Warm your muscles. A relaxed and warm muscle stretches easily. Start with relaxation and limbering exercises. Save more advanced stretches for after your aerobic workout when your muscles are fully warmed up.
- Easy does it. Do not force your stretching exercises. When a muscle is jerked into extension it tends to "fight back" and shorten. It may pull or even tear. When the muscle is slowly stretched and held, it relaxes and lengthens. Stretch easily to the point of mild sensation, and hold.
- Do not bounce or swing your body freely against a fixed joint—such as forcing a toe-touch with your knees locked.
- Breathe properly. Do belly breathing while stretching. Take a deep

abdominal breath (stomach extends as you breathe in) and let it out slowly as you reach forward with your stretch.

- Avoid overstretching. Too much is worse than too little. You can injure yourself by overstretching.
- Stretch all major joint areas. Include areas most prone to injury: hamstrings, calves, Achilles tendons, and lower back.
- Thoroughly stretch those muscles used in a particular activity—for example, leg muscles for runners, arm and shoulder muscles for a baseball pitcher.
- Take your time. Do the stretching step by step and thoroughly. Use the same basic routine every day so you will know it. Stay with the stretches and introduce new ones gradually.
- Don't stretch injured or very sore muscles. Stick to easy limbering movements until the muscle is healed and ready to be stretched.
- Avoid exercises that aggravate pre-existing conditions—especially knee or back pain—or injuries.
- Don't try advanced stretching exercises too soon. Ease into each stretching routine you do.

A RELAXATION AND STRETCHING PROGRAM FOR THE FAMILY

Here is a simple relaxation and stretching routine that you can do alone or as part of a total family fitness program. Your children might follow these or similar exercises in their school physical education program. Even if they do, I suggest exercising together at least once a week as a family.

Relaxation and stretching exercises should be part of your warm-up and cool-down programs before and after peak strength training and aerobic workouts. These exercises can also be done as single workouts to increase flexibility. They should be done at least three times a week to be effective.

Relaxation Exercises

1. Belly Breathing

Lie on the floor with your knees bent, feet flat on the floor. Close your eyes. Take a deep breath. Concentrate on letting your stomach rise as you breathe in. Breathe out slowly. To be certain you are breathing properly, put your hands on your stomach and feel them rise as you inhale. Repeat two more times.

Or, stand with your knees slightly bent, arms at your sides. Rise on your toes, breathing in slowly and deeply as you raise your hands over your head. Then exhale slowly while bringing your arms and toes back to their starting positions. Do this exercise slowly and smoothly. Repeat two more times.

2. Head Roll

Lie on your back. Roll your head to one side, relax, and go limp. Roll it slowly to the other side, relax, and go limp. Repeat three full side-to-side rolls; count left to right, then right to left, together, as one roll.

Or, start from a sitting or standing position. Slowly let your head fall forward and then relax. Roll your head to the right, and relax. Let your head roll to the back, and relax. Roll your head to the left, and relax. Do two or three complete neck rolls at a slow, smooth pace.

3. Shoulder Shrugs

Lie on your back or sit or stand. Take a deep breath and pull your shoulders up toward your ears. Hold for a few seconds. Exhale, letting your shoulders drop limply to a relaxed position. Repeat two more times.

Stretching Exercises

Standing Stretches

1. Swivels (shoulders, back, abdominals, hamstrings)

Stand with hands on hips. Keeping your back straight, slowly bend forward from the waist as far as you can. Hold for five to ten seconds. Return slowly to your starting upright position. Then bend slowly backward as far as you can. Hold for five to ten seconds. You may want to bring your elbows forward as you bend forward, and back as you bend backward.

Next, place your hands at your sides, palms inward. Slowly slide your left hand down your left leg as you bend leftward. At the same time, raise your right hand overhead, palm inward and arm straight. Turn your head to the right and look at the palm of your right hand. Hold for five to ten seconds. Repeat on the other side. Repeat the entire series for a total of three times.

2. Thigh Stretch (quadriceps)

Lean against a wall or tree using your right hand to support you. Reach behind you with your left hand. Lift your left leg and grasp the toe of your left foot. Gently pull your left heel toward your buttocks. Hold for five to ten seconds. Repeat two times with each leg.

3. Wall Push-ups (calf)

Stand an arm's length from a wall, tree, or lamppost. Place both hands on the wall. Keep your hips and back straight, heels firmly on the ground throughout the exercise. Now, slowly lean your body toward the wall. Drop your forearms toward the wall so that you touch it with your hands and elbows. Hold for five to ten seconds. Straighten your arms and push your body back to the starting position. Repeat two or three times.

Kneeling Stretches
4. Cat Back (abdominals and back)
Kneel, resting on your hands and knees. As you breathe in, arch your back like a cat, tucking your head in, chin to chest. Reverse, bringing your head up, expelling your breath, and forming a U with your spine. Repeat three times.

5. Pectoral Stretch (shoulder, chest, back)
Resting on your hands and knees, slide both hands forward, bringing your elbows to the floor and then your arms. Keep your back and head straight, your thighs perpendicular to the floor, hips up. Return to your starting position. Repeat three times.

Sitting Stretches
6. Ankle Rolls (ankles)
Sit cross-legged. Grasp your right foot with both hands and slowly rotate the ankle. Reverse direction. Repeat with left ankle.

7. Groin Stretch (groin)
Sit cross-legged. Place the soles of your feet together. Push down gently on your knees. Bend your head toward your feet. Hold the position with your head down for five to ten seconds. Sit up. Repeat two more times.

8. Hip Stretcher (hips)
Sit with your legs straight out. Bend your left leg across the right and hug your left knee to your chest. Hold for five to ten seconds. Repeat with your other leg. Repeat twice with each leg.

9. Sitting Stretch (hamstring, back)
Sit with legs straight and spread apart, both hands overhead. Inhale, then exhale slowly. Slide your arms along your left leg toward your left toe, exhaling as you go. (Keep the back of your knee flat against the floor.) Reach as far as you can comfortably, and hold for five to ten seconds. Inhaling, bring your arms back overhead. Sit up straight. Exhale as you reach out toward your right toe.

Remember to stop at the point of a mild pulling sensation and hold.

Don't worry if you can't touch your toes. Go as far as you can without forcing it.

Repeat twice for each leg.

MUSCULAR STRENGTH AND ENDURANCE

Why bother with muscular strength and endurance? The exercises are hard—who among us truly loves push-ups?—and they have the sound (if not the actual smell) of an old gymnasium. But to achieve fitness, a minimum level of muscular strength and endurance, along with muscle flexibility, is highly desired. Both will make your exercise easier, enable you to add a variety of exercises to your program, and give you muscle strength to draw on.

What do I mean by *muscular strength* training? This usually refers to the use of heavy resistance to increase muscular strength: lifting a heavy weight a few times, or doing a few push-ups with a partner applying added weight. This is heavy resistance strength training—and not what I propose here. Heavy resistance strength training is of minimal importance to fitness. Its only advantage may be in athletic competition.

I do not recommend heavy resistance strength training for prepubescent boys or girls, or even for adults who are primarily interested in fitness. Instead, I emphasize strengthening exercises that result in moderate improvement of both muscular strength and endurance. Therefore, when I say *strength training* throughout this book, I mean exercises of light to moderate intensity that result in improved muscular strength and endurance. I do not mean high-intensity weight training, which is used to build bulky, powerful bodies rather than lean, strong, supple bodies.

Strength training will improve muscular endurance. This is something quite different from heavy resistance weight training: muscular endurance is the ability of specific muscular groups to continue working over a long period, such as arm muscles that allow you to continue hitting a tennis ball, or upper arm, shoulder, and leg muscles used during swimming.

Muscular endurance improves with repeated movement: lifting a light weight several times or doing repeat sit-ups or push-ups for one minute. Some sort of muscular strength and endurance improvement is essential to any exercise program. Also, this is the area, as you recall from Chapter 1, in which our children are dangerously deficient. We all—children and adults alike—can benefit from strength training as part of our exercise program.

There are benefits here for youngsters and adults. Properly done, muscle strengthening exercises increase your range of motion and thereby improve your flexibility. The strengthening of muscles and other tissue, particularly around your major joints, provides protection from injury in sports and fitness activities. Muscle strengthening improves posture, giving you a better appearance and protection against back pain and other ailments related to weak postural muscles. There are even psychological benefits: you look better and, therefore, feel better about yourself. But best of all, muscle strengthening will allow you to keep moving briskly during aerobic exercise or improve your performance in organized sports.

A STRENGTH TRAINING PROGRAM FOR THE FAMILY

The most simple and safe way to improve muscular strength and endurance is with calisthenics, which use your own body weight for resistance. The strength training program here should be done three times per week to develop and maintain minimal muscular fitness. Ideally, your children will do these or similar exercise routines in their school physical education program. Even if they do, try to exercise together at least once a week as a family. The following strength training routine can be done by itself, or as part of a total family fitness routine.

Push-ups (Arms, Shoulders, Chest)

Lie on your stomach on the floor. Place your hands palms down on the floor slightly outside your shoulders. Put your toes on the floor. Now, push slowly upward until your arms are fully extended, palms flat on the floor, back straight. Regular, full push-ups require that you keep your legs straight and push up off your toes and hands. Do at least ten to twenty full push-ups for minimal fitness. Or, do two or three sets of ten to twenty push-ups, with a brief rest between sets. If you cannot do at least five with proper form (back and knees straight), use the modified push-up.

For a modified push-up, get down on the floor on your hands and knees, back straight, head in line with your spine. Place your hands slightly outside your shoulders, fingers pointed forward. Slowly lower your chest until it touches the floor. Then push your chest up with your arms (knees still on the floor) until your arms are straight again. Exhale slowly as you push up, breathe in as you go back down. Keep your back straight and don't let your fanny arch up or droop. Do as many as you can with proper form. Build to at least twenty modified push-ups before advancing to full push-ups.

Modified push-ups should be used by young children and adults who are just beginning a training program. These allow you to push up only part of your body weight, making them easier than full push-ups. When my son, Christopher, entered first grade as a six-year-old, he could do only three modified push-ups. His school gym classes include push-ups two or three times a week. At the end of the first-grade year, Christopher could easily do three sets of ten modified push-ups.

Sit-ups/Curls (Abdominals)

Lie on the floor on your back, knees flexed at ninety degrees, feet flat on the floor, heels twelve to eighteen inches from the buttocks. The feet should be held by a partner or hooked under a sofa or other stable object. Place your hands behind your head and roll up into a sitting position with your head close to your knees. Then roll back down slowly. Do not jerk with your arms and head in an attempt to get up. Sit-ups should not be done in a fast or jerky motion. Arching the back or bouncing off the floor for high-speed sit-ups puts a tremendous strain on your back. Don't overstrain in an attempt to "gut out" a few extra sit-ups. Full sit-ups should be done carefully to avoid causing injury. Do as many as you can with good form. Build to ten to twenty sit-ups for minimal fitness.

If you can't do this exercise in proper form, use the safer modified sit-up or the curl.

Modified Sit-ups

For the modified sit-up, use the same starting position as for the regular sit-up: on your back on the floor, knees flexed. Your arms should be on your chest with your hands on the opposite shoulders, and should remain in contact with your chest throughout the exercise. (Another version: Cross your hands on your chest, palms down; maintain this position during the entire exercise.)

Have someone hold your feet, or hook them under a sofa or other stable object. (Another version: Leave your feet unanchored and let your knees flatten somewhat as you curl upward.)

Now, slowly roll your head, shoulders, and upper back off the floor, using your abdominal muscles, until your elbows touch your thighs. If you can't sit up with good form, roll to a half sit-up position raising your back six inches off the ground, and then return.

Breathe out as you roll up and then return to the starting position while breathing in. Rest momentarily when your back and head touch the floor, then repeat. Do as many as you can with proper form. A goal for minimal fitness is twenty to forty modified sit-ups. Or, do two or three sets of fifteen to twenty sit-ups with a brief rest between sets.

When Christopher was six years old, he struggled to do a few modified sit-ups before starting the strengthening program at his elementary school. At the end of his first-grade year he could easily handle three sets of twenty modified sit-ups.

Curls

Curls are a variation on sit-ups. They are done with the same form, but you only lift your upper back off the floor six to ten inches. Hold that position for two seconds, and then return to your starting position. Do ten to twenty repetitions. (Another version: Put your feet and calves on a bed or chair, buttocks and back on the floor. With hands crossed on your chest, lift your head, shoulders, and as much of your back as possible off the floor.)

Head Lifters (Back)

Lie face down on the floor with your feet together and hands clasped behind your head. A partner may be needed to hold your feet. Raise your head and upper body off the floor as far as possible, keeping your hands clasped behind your head and your elbows pointing out to the sides. Hold for three to five seconds and then lower to your starting position. Rest for three to five seconds before repeating.

Half Squats (Quadriceps and Buttocks)

Stand with your feet together, hands on your hips. Extend your arms forward and bend your knees to a half-squat position (thighs parallel to the ground). Hold for two seconds or so, then rise slowly to an upright position. Repeat ten to twenty times.

Pull-ups (Arms and Shoulders)

Hang from a chinning bar (you can easily erect one in a doorway at home) using an overhand grip (palms facing away from your body). Hands should be placed at shoulder width. Your arms and legs should be fully extended. From this hanging position, raise your body using your arms until your chin is positioned over the bar. Lower slowly to the starting position.

Do not kick your legs or swing. If you cannot lift your own body weight for at least two or three pull-ups—and very few children or adults can—use the modified pull-up to increase your strength.

To do a modified pull-up, place the bar at a lower height (about two feet off the floor) and position yourself so that your chest is directly under the bar. Grasp the bar with both hands, palms facing away from your body, and hands about shoulder width apart. Pull your chest up to the bar keeping your body straight from head to toe; heels remain in contact with the floor. Lower to the starting position and repeat as many times as you can using good form.

If you don't have a pull-up pole, you might try a strong pipe or two-by-two between two chairs to serve as a pull-up station. Without a good pole or pipe, you might try partner pull-ups. Lie on your back on the floor with your feet together. Have your partner stand erect astride your body. Clasp your hands with your partner's, palms away from your body, arms extended. The standing partner keeps his or her arms straight. You pull up as far as you can and then return to your position on the floor. Do as many pull-ups as possible with good form.

Leg Raises (Hip)

Lie on your left side on the floor, left arm extended overhead with your head resting on the arm. Rest your right leg on your left leg. Place your right hand on the floor in front of your chest for support. Raise your right (top) leg as far (as high in the air) as possible, then return to its starting position. Both legs should remain straight at all times with the lower leg always in contact with the floor. Do ten to twenty repetitions and then roll over and do the opposite leg.

WEIGHT TRAINING

Youths to Age Sixteen

Should your child lift weights?

It is my opinion that weight training should be limited to boys and girls above the age of thirteen—preferably age sixteen—who demonstrate the maturity to train safely and slowly. Young children should not weight train. Period. The risk of permanent injury, particularly to the bones' growth plates (epiphysis), is too great. Moreover, the discipline and maturity that a good, supervised weight training program requires are difficult to achieve with youngsters. Older boys and girls should train only under a conservative, professional strength instructor.

Pat McInally, author of *Moms & Dads, Kids & Sports*, offers some sound advice:

> The problem is controlling the activity. . . . My concern is that kids will give in and go for big lifts as they gain confidence with lighter weights. This could be particularly dangerous when the calcium and growth plates haven't settled and developed enough . . . I think exercises involving a youngster's own body weight—such as push-ups, chin-ups and sit-ups—are safest and will definitely increase strength and stamina. To risk injury lifting weights without having a substantial potential gain isn't worth it.
>
> I just don't feel the risks, time involved, and effort justify weight lifting for kids. They should be playing sports for fun and learning how to handle responsibility and pressure. To push them beyond these in hopes of perhaps playing a little better is unwarranted. I'd advise waiting until puberty when they can benefit the most with greater safety.

Weight training after age sixteen produces considerable benefits for both boys and girls. But, as Pat McInally warns, weight training for youngsters under that age may carry too great a risk.

Adolescents and Adults

Weight training for boys and girls above the age of sixteen, and for most adults, can be both fun and beneficial. Be careful if you have not lifted weights before or recently. Always take lessons from a professional instructor before starting a weight training program. The following guidelines are from *The Runner's Handbook:*

The Warm-up and Cool-down

First, spend about ten to fifteen minutes doing basic stretching exercises. These exercises will loosen up the muscles connecting tissues and joints, and permit you to work out with little danger of injury from muscle tightness. After your warm-up stretching you should do some warm-up lifting. This would be ten to twelve relaxed repetitions using very light weights. This exercise will allow your muscles to warm up and loosen. The cool-down is the warm-up in reverse.

The Weight Training Workout

To improve both muscular strength and endurance, emphasize light weights and between ten and fifteen repetitions. Variable resistance machines like Nautilus are the easiest and safest weight-training equipment to use. The weights are connected to a main housing, which prevents you from dropping them on the floor or on your toes. Weights are changed quickly and easily by moving small levers or rods.

A set of free weights (barbells or dumbbells) is also good if handled carefully. It can be used at home or in your office and you won't have to go to the gym, health club, or Y.

The following routine can be done with any equipment. Allow about fifteen to twenty minutes twice a week. This is a medium-weight workout to build muscular strength and endurance. Each weight training routine consists of the following steps:

1. Select the exercise and the weight to be lifted.
2. Do the specified number of repetitions (ten to fifteen), exhaling as you lift the weight, inhaling as you release the weight.
3. Rest one minute at the completion of the first set to recover and do some flexibility exercises to keep your muscles and joints loose.
4. Do the second set the same way as the first set.

5. Rest one minute at the completion of the second set, doing flexibility exercises to maintain muscle flexibility.
6. Do the third set (if possible) the same way as the first two sets.
7. Rest one minute at the completion of the third set, do flexibility exercises, and set up your next exercise.
8. Continue with the next exercise following the above seven steps.

The trick to proper weight training is knowing how much weight to use, and when to increase the weight for each particular exercise. Here are two general rules to follow:

Rule One: Start Light. Always start every workout with a very light weight. Allow your body to adapt to the increased resistance. Do only a few repetitions. I think one set of ten to fifteen repetitions is best.

Rule Two: Increase the Weight Gradually. You should increase the weight you lift for a particular exercise only after you can easily repeat three sets of the recommended repetitions. Then increase the weight by only five to ten pounds. Reduce the number of sets to two, and gradually work your way back up to three sets at the recommended number of repetitions.

Here are some general rules for weight training:

- Weight training is progressive. You begin with low weights and gradually increase the weights as you become stronger.
- You should lift twice a week, allowing two or three days between each lifting session to let your muscles rebuild themselves.
- Limit the number of repetitions to ten to fifteen and the number of sets to two or three in order to build muscle strength without building bulk.
- Begin each weight training session by exercising the large muscle groups first and then the smaller muscles. Alternate upper-body lifting with lower-body lifting.
- Be sure to do flexibility exercises before and after each repetition.
- All lifts should be done through a full range of motion to work your muscles completely.
- Lifting is done to a four-count pace: count to four as you lift the weight, and count to four as you release the weight.

SAMPLE WEIGHT TRAINING ROUTINE

The following twenty- to thirty-minute routine can be used in a gym with weight machines or at home with free weights. It is only a sample workout: consult a professional weight training instructor if you are a novice at weight training.

Bench Press (Arms and Upper Body)

Use either a bench press machine or a barbell and a bench with a support for the weight. Lie on your back and grip the bar at shoulder width. Using a minimum weight, start with the bar just above your chest, then press the weight straight up without locking your elbows at full extension. Lower again and repeat. Do two or three sets of ten to fifteen repetitions.

Abdominal Curls (Abdominal Muscles)

Lie on your back with your feet anchored, hands behind your head. Raise your torso using your abdominal muscles. When your shoulders are about six inches off the floor, hold to a count of two and then return to the original position. Do two or three sets of ten to fifteen repetitions. Hold a light weight behind your head as you grow stronger.

Arm Curls (Arms and Upper Body)

Use a minimum weight on either a barbell or weight machine. Hold the bar in front of you with a shoulder-wide, underhand grip. Without swinging the weight or arching your back, bring the bar up to your shoulders using only your lower arms. Slowly return to the starting position. Do two to three sets of ten to fifteen repetitions.

Leg Extensions or Barbell Lunges (Upper Legs)

Using a weight machine for leg extensions, sit on the edge of the bench with your legs under the padded bar. Lift upward with your legs, concentrating on using your quadricep muscles. Slowly return to your starting position. Do two or three sets of ten to fifteen repetitions.

For barbell lunges, hold the barbell with a minimum weight across your shoulders behind your head. Step forward with one foot, kneeling so that the back leg nearly touches the floor and the front leg bends at a forty-five-degree angle. Step back and repeat with the other leg.

To ease the strain on your knees and Achilles, try this variation: Stand with your heels on a two-by-four on the floor so that your heels are lifted. With the bar across your shoulders, legs spread to slightly more than shoulder width, slowly squat down until your thighs are about parallel to the floor. Hold and then return slowly to your original starting position.

Keep your head up and back straight throughout the exercise. Do two to three sets of ten to fifteen repetitions.

Pull-downs or Bent Rows (Upper Back)

For pull-downs, you will need to use a weight machine. Assume a kneeling position or sit in a bench in front of the high-bar station. Holding the bar with a wide-armed grip (beyond shoulder width), pull the bar down in front of your chest, hold, and slowly return to its original position. Then, pull the bar down behind your neck. (Be careful not to strike the back of your head with the bar.) Do two to three sets of ten to fifteen repetitions.

For bent rows, place a pillow on a chair and a barbell in front of the chair. Stand in front of the chair, bend at the waist, and place your forehead on the pillow. Using a shoulder-width grip on the barbell and a minimum weight, raise the barbell to your chest. Return the barbell to the floor and repeat the exercise. Do two to three sets of ten to fifteen repetitions.

Toe Raises (Calf Muscles, Achilles Tendon, Ankle Joints)

Stand, hold the barbell (with minimum weight) behind your neck. Raise yourself up on your toes. Slowly return to the starting position. Do two or three sets of ten to fifteen repetitions.

Lateral Raises (Shoulders)

Stand, hold two dumbbells in front of your thighs. Slowly raise your arms out to either side to shoulder height, then slowly return them to your sides. Be careful not to swing the dumbbells out to the side, and don't let them collapse back to your side. Do two or three sets of ten to fifteen repetitions.

A selection of exercises from this chapter will enhance the muscle fitness part of your fitness routine. Next, we move to the core of the exercise program: aerobic endurance.

12

Getting Fit:
Cardio-respiratory Endurance

"The human body," said Thomas Cureton, Ph.D., a pioneer in the fitness movement, "is the only machine that functions better and more healthfully the more it is put to use." This is generally true for both children and adults. And the engine (your heart) that drives the machine (your musculo-skeletal system) must be kept well tuned. Although flexibility, muscular strength and endurance, and body composition are important to our health, the proper functioning of our hearts and lungs is of paramount importance to living a healthy life.

AEROBIC EXERCISE

The exercise we choose should *stress* our bodies. That is, it should make our bodies work harder than usual.

By stressing our bodies with vigorous exercise, we improve the efficiency of our oxygen-transport system. Our lungs and hearts become stronger; our hearts beat less often but pump with greater strength. The benefits occur almost as a chain reaction: the blood carries more oxygen, blood vessels increase in number, the peripheral circulatory system increases in efficiency, and cells pick up oxygen more easily.

Aerobic exercise is the pulse-rated system of exercise developed by exercise physiologists and supported by the American Heart Association. Its basic principle is that your body must exercise at a rate that demands large amounts of oxygen for a sustained period of at least twenty minutes every other day. (The optimum level would be exercising aerobically for thirty minutes, four to five times a week.) The exercise must include continuous movement at a brisk pace and yet be moderate enough not to overtax your heart and muscles.

Most sports activities are not aerobic. Baseball, basketball, bowling, football, golf—stop-go sports—are generally not aerobic because they encourage bursts of activity but not a sustained aerobic workout. Worse, they create the illusion of exercising.

This still leaves a wide selection of activities—and many are a lot of fun for the whole family. The four simplest and most popular are called the "Big Four" of aerobics: walking, swimming, biking, and running. Other aerobic activities include aerobic dance (aerobics to music), jumping rope, cross-country skiing, roller- and ice-skating, rowing, and vigorous games of racquet sports (singles tennis, racquetball, squash, and handball). Chapter 15 includes specific guidelines for enjoying these aerobic exercises.

I recommend that you select several aerobic activities. This will prevent boredom, provide an opportunity to exercise with other people, and let you switch in case of injury or illness. For example, you may enjoy bicycling twice a week and swimming twice a week. Or, you might want to bike and run in the spring, summer, and fall, and swim indoors and cross-country ski during the winter. Whatever aerobic activities you select, remember John Quincy Adams's rule: regularity. Make sure you exercise weekly and year-round.

Basically, you must exercise nonstop at moderate intensity for at least twenty consecutive minutes. This might include such unusual aerobic conditioners as conducting an orchestra, shoveling snow, raking leaves, vigorous gardening, or swinging a baseball bat every five seconds in batting practice. These exercises involve vigorous use of the arms and upper body, which cause the heart to beat faster. Since the upper body doesn't have the strength and size of the legs, you don't have to work much to promote a training effect.

AEROBIC EXERCISE FOR KIDS

Do children benefit from aerobic exercise?

There is some controversy about the benefits of aerobic activity for young children. Many fitness experts, noting that research on children and aerobic training is still sketchy, suggest that children under the age of sixteen, and especially under the age of ten, may not benefit substantially from aerobic training. In her academic paper,* Christine L. Wells, an exercise physiologist at Arizona State University, reported:

*Christine L. Wells, "The Effects of Physical Activity on Cardiorespiratory Fitness in Children," paper delivered before the American Academy of Physical Education, 1985.

The physical growth and accompanying motor development and cellular maturation that naturally occur as a child grows older may be as great as or greater than the adaptations thought to result from an imposed exercise training program. Therefore, it is difficult to distinguish the effects of physical activity from the normal changes occurring with increasing age and concomitant development and maturation.

But other researchers have found evidence linking exercise with improved fitness and performance. Fitness experts state that the cardio-respiratory system in children responds to regular exercise in much the same way as in adults. That is, a child's heart rate and respiration volume increase directly in proportion to the intensity of exercise. Studies suggest that children do improve cardio-respiratory endurance with training. B. Ekblom in the *Journal of Applied Physiology* (1969) reported that endurance training among boys ten to fifteen years of age resulted in significant increases in aerobic fitness, while C. H. Brown in *Medicine and Science in Sports* (1972) demonstrated similar improvements in aerobic fitness among girls eight to thirteen years of age after twelve weeks of cross-country running.

More recently, in 1984 Charles Kuntzleman, Ph.D., had elementary school children in Jackson County, Michigan, exercise aerobically three to four times a week for thirty minutes. This continued for nine to thirteen weeks. As mentioned in Chapter 1, three significant results occurred: The aerobic exercisers increased the amount of exercise the children could (and would) do over the control group, but their heart rates remained the same, demonstrating a marked improvement in aerobic fitness. The aerobic exercisers also improved their academic grades compared to the control group. And the exercisers showed a dramatic drop in major risk factors for heart disease.

WHAT KINDS OF AEROBIC EXERCISE?

What may be an important factor here is the *type* of exercise you and your child get. Young children may not be motivated enough to engage in aerobic activity—or any single fast-paced activity—for twenty minutes. Repeated endurance activities such as running and swimming laps are not usually seen by children as fun. (Many adults find regular running or swimming not much fun either, but our motivation is higher.)

Two doctors, Kaye Wilkins, MD, and Earl Stanley, MD, at the University of Texas Health Science Center at San Antonio, suggest that the best way to keep young kids in shape is through brief bursts of exercise. That is how kids play—they don't stick to one activity for very long before moving on to another. The doctors argue that too much emphasis is placed on "adult" exercise for kids and that a child's attention span is short, so he or she becomes bored and loses motivation. We risk driving our children away from exercise altogether if we insist that they exercise the way we do. Kids are smart; they will see adult exercise as repetitive and perhaps exhausting.

I believe that children can be turned on to exercise—if it is imaginative. Adventure walks, brisk dancing to music, vigorous games of hide-and-seek or tag, and so forth can be used to make aerobic exercise fun for young children. But first we need to explain why it is worthwhile, and then we need to make it fun. My own experience with young children leads me to several conclusions here.

Pre-schoolers are too young to train aerobically. If necessary, they may be motivated to be active—to engage in walking, swimming, moving to music, and so forth. For the most part, however, pre-schoolers get plenty of exercise crawling or running through their daily lives. I've seen some high-speed toddlers who "exercised" all day long—with exhausted parents in tow!

Around kindergarten (about age six) young children should begin to get ten to twenty minutes of continuous aerobic training, two or three times a week at a vigorous pace. Above the age of six, children can follow similar aerobic training guidelines—although not necessarily the same types of aerobic activity—as adults. This should be well within their limits and be imaginative and fun. It must not be imposed on them, and they must not be forced to do the exercises. Some young children will not have the maturity to exercise aerobically in nonstop activities such as running. These youths should be encouraged to at least participate at a minimal level. There are imaginative games for young kids that promote aerobic fitness. These include "Tom Sawyer Adventure Hike," the "Fitness Freeze Game," and "Safari Aerobics" (see Chapters 13 and 14).

A significant goal for children from kindergarten through about the third grade is to give them a variety of aerobic activities. The goal is simple: to encourage our children to exercise regularly and for a sufficient time, establishing a lifelong habit. Most kids this age should have a wide variety of large-muscle games and activities they enjoy. The activities and their benefits should be described to the children as being important to healthy living, in the same category as a wise diet and good dental health care.

Children at this age should not spend long periods of time running, biking, swimming, or whatever; for one thing, they will soon be bored. Ten to twenty minutes is sufficient. If children perceive the duration of aerobic activity as important, and participate for what they see as an extended period of time, they are likely to continue these exercise habits as they grow older.

For younger children, the ideal activity lasts thirty seconds. To create a continuous, gradually extended exercise session, quickly shift the children from one activity to another. (For examples, see the "Fitness Freeze Game" or the "Animal Fitness March" in Chapter 13 to complete a ten- to twenty-minute aerobic workout.)

From age ten and up, most children enjoy activity if properly motivated. All children this age can, and probably should, receive aerobic training three times a week for twenty to thirty minutes. Children are not adults, however. It is important that we find aerobic activities that they enjoy and that we not force adult programs on them.

Our children will most likely get their aerobic exercise from practicing for team sports (lacrosse, soccer, and ice and field hockey are best). I stress practices because the games are generally less aerobic—players are substituted to maintain a high level of intense competition. Two of the best aerobic sports for kids are swimming and cross-country running. Chapters 24–25 discuss guidelines on how to use sports to improve overall fitness. Reminder: Team sports such as baseball, football, and basketball do little for aerobic fitness.

I was amazed at the development of my own son, Christopher, in terms of aerobic fitness and motivation. He actually ran, rather than walked, his first step at ten months and has been running ever since. But he never knowingly exercised for fitness as a pre-schooler. Even as a five-year-old he didn't have any interest in running—other than short bursts. When he was a first-grader, however, his whole class ran together for fun (and, of course, fitness) and Christopher quickly learned to enjoy it. At age six he ran a mile comfortably in ten minutes, thirty seconds, well under the AAHPERD's fitness standard of twelve minutes. He was proud that he ran nonstop all the way and earned a fitness award.

The aerobic exercise program he follows at home and in school—which forms the basis for this book—has meant more to him than just passing a fitness test, however. Christopher can walk for hours, play for hours, while his less-fit friends tire. He has more energy, which allows him to enjoy his fun-filled life to the fullest. The confidence and self-esteem gained in sports and aerobic training parallel a similar growth in his ability in the classroom. The way I see it, if my little six-year-old could get fit and enjoy it, why can't all children?

THREE KEY VARIABLES TO AEROBIC TRAINING

The three important variables in aerobic training are Frequency, Intensity, and Time—FIT. That is, to achieve and maintain aerobic fitness, you need to exercise often enough, at an approriate pace, and for a minimum time. This is why, in the previous chapters, I have emphasized the frequency and duration of the exercise that I have described. The aerobic training summary chart (box) highlights the guidelines detailed in this chapter.

Caution: Before starting, if you have been inactive for any length of time you should check with your doctor. You may be advised to take an EKG-monitored stress exercise test. Be sure to discuss any limitations you may have—asthma, orthopedic problems, or any concerns with your doctor.

Also, check with your family doctor or pediatrician before starting your child on a vigorous exercise program. Discuss with your doctor any limitations your child might have and your concerns, if any, about your child's exercise program.

AEROBIC TRAINING SUMMARY
The FIT (Frequency, Intensity, Time) Method

Category	Frequency	Intensity	Time
Pre-school	3 per week	Fun movement	5–10 minutes if motivated
Age 6–9	3–4 per week	Vigorous activity at approx. 140–180 heart rate/talk test intensity	10–20 continuous minutes
Age 10–18	3–5 per week	same as above	minimally 20 continuous minutes
Adults	minimally 3, optimally 5 per week	Vigorous activity within training HR range/talk test intensity	minimally 20 continuous minutes, optimally 30+ minutes

Let's take a closer look at FIT.

Frequency

How often should I exercise? I hear this question almost daily from members of my fitness classes. To achieve cardio-respiratory fitness, you need to exercise aerobically at least three times a week for at least eight to ten weeks. To maintain minimal fitness, you must continue to exercise aerobically at least three times a week. To improve your fitness level, you must increase the frequency and duration of your exercise. In other words, improvement comes by exercising aerobically more often and for longer periods of time. The gains, however, are not proportionately as large as the first ten weeks once you reach minimal fitness.

Ideally, adults who reach a minimal level of fitness should exercise four or five times a week. Unless you are training at a high skill level for competitive sports, it is not advisable to work out aerobically every day.

Your body needs time to rest and recover. Spread your exercise sessions out over the entire week; this usually means exercising every other day. Beware of the "weekend athlete" syndrome in which some men and women exercise only on weekends and overdo it. Follow the hard-easy program: if you exercise hard one day, follow it with a day off or at least a light exercise day.

Don't push your kids. It is enough of an achievement to get youths to exercise aerobically three times per week. Attempts to get them to exercise more frequently may result in them getting turned off to aerobic training. If they enjoy aerobic exercise, let them exercise more, but not every day. It's the regularity that counts most here—and the fun.

Time

As I have said repeatedly, aerobic exercise must last for at least twenty continuous minutes to give you any cardio-respiratory benefit. But you will not simply step out of your house—or your child will not simply get up from his or her school desk—and go out and exercise aerobically for twenty minutes every other day. You both will have to build up to this with a gradual program—for example, walking and running.

For children under age ten, Dr. Kenneth Cooper's Institute for Aerobics Research recommends fifteen minutes of continuous aerobic training. The American Health and Fitness Foundation's Fit Youth Today program recommends twelve to fifteen minutes as the aerobic exercise minimum for youngsters in kindergarten to the third grade. My recommended range is ten to twenty minutes under age ten, twenty to thirty minutes beyond age ten. For adults, Dr. Cooper recommends an optimal goal of thirty consecutive minutes. Any exercise beyond that limit, he says, is done for reasons other than fitness (such as improving racing times).

Stop-and-go activities like baseball, golf, or doubles tennis are not continuous. You may play them for an hour or more and benefit only slightly in terms of aerobic conditioning. Neither is walking beneficial if you don't keep up a brisk pace. On the other hand, if you run too fast and have to stop to walk slowly, or sit down, you are not gaining from aerobic exercise.

But you should start out by walking briskly and alternating this with running at a slow pace. The entire workout—walk-run—is continuous. You and your child can build from this base by gradually—over several weeks—replacing the walking with running until you reach a continuous twenty minutes. Even when you reach the continuous twenty-minute level, you might alternate exercises. For example, you might ride a stationary bike for ten minutes, quickly move to a treadmill for a brisk walk-run for ten minutes, and then quickly move to the rowing machine for ten minutes. Moving quickly from one brisk movement activity to another is a good way to make continuous aerobic exercise fun for adult and child.

You may prefer to keep count of your exercise in terms of mileage rather than time. Dr. Cooper recommends these *minimum* weekly mileage goals, which are roughly equivalent to exercising aerobically three times a week for twenty minutes each time:

Running: six miles (two miles each session).

Walking: fifteen miles (five miles each session).

Swimming: one and a half miles (one-half mile each session).

Biking: thirty miles (ten miles each session).

Intensity

How fast (vigorously) should I exercise? The answer to this question is easy: not too fast, but not too slow.

Most people—adults and children—start out training too fast. They get injured or exhausted, and quit. Slow down! How fast you exercise should not be measured by speed, but by how your heart and lungs respond to exercise. You want to exercise fast enough to gain fitness, but slow enough to be comfortable.

Three simple checks—training heart rate, talk test, perceived exertion—can be employed to monitor the intensity of your aerobic workout. Use them individually or in combination. Your body basically knows what level of exercise is good for it. If you listen to it—following the talk test or perceived exertion—you will probably be exercising at the appropriate intensity. I only measure my training heart rate a few times a year, mostly to satisfy my curiosity.

1. The Training Heart Rate

This is a good check for anyone starting an exercise program. (It is also a good way to introduce children to their bodies, especially their hearts, heart rates, and even care of their hearts and lungs.) The training heart rate check uses your own heart rate to see whether you are training within, above, or below your aerobic level.

Your heart rate (pulse) is the number of times your heart beats per minute. The faster it beats during exercise, the harder you are working out. The slower it beats when you are under stress, the better shape you are in. For example, before you become well conditioned, your heart rate may go up to 140 beats per minute when you run at a pace of ten minutes per mile. After perhaps two months of training, it may rise to only 120 beats per minute at the same speed.

You can measure your heartbeat at several places on your body, including the left side of your chest or about the middle of your upturned wrist. Use your fingers to take this measure, not your thumb, which has its own pulse. The most common place to count your heartbeats is your carotid artery, which is found just in front of the large vertical muscle along the sides of your neck beneath your jaw. Gently feel for a pulse there with the tips of your first two fingers. Don't press too hard.

When you feel a pulse—and everyone who exercises has a pulse!—count the number for ten seconds and multiply by six. That will give you your heart rate per minute. (For example, if you count twelve beats in ten seconds and multiply by six, that will give you an approximate heart rate of seventy-two beats per minute.) This easily enables you to determine your resting heart rate.

It may be more difficult to count your exercise heart rate. Take your pulse a few times during your aerobic workout and again at the end. For most aerobic activities, you will need to stop very briefly to take your pulse. You should count the pulse immediately after stopping or your heart rate will drop too quickly to give you an accurate measure. Calculate your exercise heart rate and use it to determine whether or not you are exercising at a level to give you aerobic benefit. If you are, then resume your workout at the same level; if not, increase or decrease your workout level depending on your exercise heart rate. At first, you may want to monitor your heart rate three or four times during a workout. Later, when you develop a feel for your pace, you may choose to monitor your heart rate halfway through your workout and at the end.

Should children follow the training heart rate system? Yes and no. For children below the age of ten, the training heart rate system should be used infrequently and largely as an educational tool. They can learn something about the heart's function, and be taught to report whether or not their hearts are beating slow, medium, or fast. With a little experience, they will get a feel for their pulse and learn a system that can be used throughout their lifetime. But these youngsters should train simply according to how they feel. At fourth grade or so, children can calculate their training heart rates themselves and begin to undertake a more formal aerobic fitness program based on the heart rate check.

Four types of heart rates are important in developing a safe aerobic training program: the resting, maximum, training, and recovery heart rates.

Resting heart rate (base pulse). This is your heart rate when you are at rest—either when you wake up in the morning or when you are very relaxed during the day. The average resting heart rate for men is sixty to eighty beats per minute; for women, seventy to ninety. A well-conditioned adult's heart rate may be around sixty or below. Serious endurance athletes often have resting heart rates in the forty to fifty beats per minute range. When I was marathon training at one hundred miles a week, my resting heart rate was forty-two beats per minute.

You should not rush your resting heart rate up to your training heart rate—that would be like starting your car engine on a cold day and then taking off down the highway at a fast speed. You should warm up your engine by walking briskly, biking, jogging, or swimming slowly for five to ten minutes before increasing your pace.

Parents, teachers, and coaches should know that young children have higher resting heart rates than adults. At age six, for example, boys have an average resting heart rate of about eighty-six beats per minute; girls average about eighty-eight beats. There is a steady decrease, generally, among children to about thirteen years of age. Then boys average about sixty-six beats per minute and girls about seventy.

Maximum heart rate. This is at or near your level of exhaustion, where your heart "peaks out" and cannot meet your body's demand for oxygen or beat much faster. You should *estimate* your maximum heart rate—never try to reach it—by subtracting your age from 220. *This is not a goal.* It is merely a figure from which you can obtain your training heart rate range. (See the aerobic chart below.)

In general, the maximum heart rate for a child age five is about 210–220 beats per minute. This has fallen to about 200–210 by age fifteen or so. By age twenty, it has dropped further to about 200, and by age forty to about 180.

Training (exercise) heart rate. There are two heart rates between which we should train to achieve sufficient and safe cardio-respiratory conditioning. This training range falls between two numbers: the *target* of 70 percent of your maximum heart rate and the *cutoff* figure of 85 percent of your maximum heart rate.*

Exercising at a heart rate more than a few beats below the target heart rate will not provide sufficient aerobic conditioning. Exercising at a heart rate above the cutoff will cause you to spend a great deal of extra effort (and agony) and risk injury, with little additional fitness value.

To find your approximate training heart rate, subtract your age from 220 and multiply the answer by 70 percent. Some fitness experts use 60 percent as an acceptable lower limit for aerobic training. Your maximum (slow-down) rate is 85 percent, but this is not a training goal. It is an upper limit.

Youngsters under age nineteen can follow approximately the same formula. In general, youngsters train at between 140 and 180 beats per minute, but they must be able to talk comfortably while doing so.

To save you all the math, the following is a chart showing the target aerobic training heart rate for adults:

---

*The 85 percent figure is the approximate border between aerobic and anaerobic conditions, where it becomes difficult to breathe and talk.

AGE	TARGET HR (70%)	CUTOFF HR (85%)
20–25	140	167
26–30	134	163
31–35	131	159
36–40	127	155
41–45	124	150
46–50	120	146
51–55	117	142
56–60	113	138
61–65	110	133
66–70	106	129

The key here is to keep your heart rate in the target area—between 70 and 85 percent of your maximum heart rate—during twenty to thirty minutes of continuous exercise. At the 70 percent figure, your body will handle the workout easily and gain aerobic conditioning. Your heart rate will increase as you go uphill, increase your speed, exercise in heat or high humidity, or grow tired. At this point, you should slow down or walk briskly to keep your heart rate near your target goal.

Note: The pulse rates are based on a predicted maximum and thus some error is possible. You may find that you can exceed your cutoff without breathing hard. Or, you may be tired at a lower level of exertion. This is a general training target based on averages of many men and women. Don't be a slave to it. Let your body tell you what is best. When in doubt, rely on the talk-test system described below.

Recovery heart rate. A proper cool-down is essential following all exercise. A slow five-minute walk after aerobic exercise should generally bring your heart rate below 120 beats per minute; below 110 for men and women over age fifty. That's your goal. Continue your cool-down with stretching and relaxation exercises until your heart rate is below 100 beats per minute, or within 20 beats of your pre–warm-up resting heart rate. If it takes a long time for your heart rate to drop, you may be exercising too hard or you haven't cooled down properly.

The Talk Test

Instead of taking your pulse, here you *listen to your body*. This simply means that you exercise according to how you feel. You should be able to carry on a conversation as you exercise, or hum if you exercise alone. If you cannot do this, you are exercising too hard. (Most likely you are exercising above your cutoff heart rate.)

Listen to your body. If it yells that you are getting breathless, tiring, or feeling overheated or uncomfortable, slow down and even walk briskly until you feel ready to exercise again at a more moderate pace. There is no shame in walking—in fact, I recommend it as an excellent form of aerobic exercise.

Generally, when you are perspiring and breathing fairly hard, you have reached your target heart rate. To check whether or not your children are exercising too hard, ask them to make animal noises or yell out a team or school cheer.

This system frees you from the trouble of monitoring your pulse or your children's pulses. Yet, it is best used in conjunction with the pulse test. It is a good idea to use the training heart rate (pulse) system while getting into aerobic shape. This will teach you what your body feels like when you exercise within your target range. Then, *listen to your body* and periodically check your pulse to confirm your training level.

Perceived Exertion

This is similar to the Talk-Test method. But it involves a rating scale designed by Swedish scientists, who devised a way to exercise at the appropriate level by monitoring something called "perceived exertion." They created a measuring device, called the Borg Scale. The scale runs from six to twenty. At six, you are at rest. At twenty, you are at total exhaustion.

On the Borg Scale, you adjust your training intensity to reach a perceived exertion of between twelve and fifteen ("somewhat hard" to "hard"). This is a simple idea. You perceive how you are reacting to your training intensity, and you try to maintain it between the "somewhat hard" and "hard" range. Below are the six to twenty ratings of perceived exertion.

BORG SCALE	PERCEIVED EXERTION
6	at rest
7	very, very light
8	
9	very light
10	
11	fairly light
12	
13	somewhat hard
14	
15	hard
16	
17	very hard
18	
19	very, very hard
20	total exhaustion

Imaginative Fitness Workouts

Here is a complete fitness workout that you can do with your child or a few of your child's friends. It would be fun for a birthday party or other special occasion, or your child's physical education teacher might use the workout in a fitness class.

The workout uses several imaginative exercises that Christopher and I have enjoyed. It should be such fun that the kids don't know they are participating in a structured fitness workout.

THE WARM-UP

Use your imagination by following all or some of these exercises (or substituting some that your child invents).

Relaxation Exercises

1. *Whale spout.* Pretend to be a whale. Take a deep breath, swallowing all the water in the ocean, then slowly blow it out like a whale through its spout. Repeat two more times. Concentrate on the belly slowly filling up with water and then slowly emptying. This simulates the belly breathing exercises for adults.

2. *Giraffe neck roll.* Roll your long giraffe neck forward, to the right, back, and to the left in a sweeping circle. Repeat for three circles, then reverse direction.

3. *Turtle shrug.* Pretend you are a turtle. Shrug your turtle shoulders up while taking a deep breath, and tuck your head in like a turtle going into its shell. Then, poke your head out, lowering your shoulders and breathing out, and look around to see what you can see. Repeat two more times.

Stretching Exercises

1. *Elephant trunk swing.* Stand up, hold your hands together in front of your body with your arms extended from your nose to make an elephant's trunk. Then swing your "trunk" back and forth.

2. *Ostrich stretch.* Stand up, bend forward at the waist, hands and arms drooping forward, with your knees slightly bent. Bring your head as close to the ground as possible and "bury it in the sand" like an ostrich. Slowly curl back up and repeat two more times.

3. *Rhino hip roll.* Stand up, rotate your hips in a big circle for three complete turns, then reverse direction.

4. *Cat back.* On your hands and knees, arch your back up, tucking your head in as you arch. Then reverse the direction, forming a U with your spine and hissing like an angry cat. Repeat two more times.

5. *Dog stretch.* On your hands and knees, slide both hands forward, bringing your elbows to the floor, then your arms. Keep your back straight, your thighs perpendicular to the floor, hips up. Return to starting position. Repeat two more times.

Strengthening Exercises

1. *Snail slide.* Lie on the floor with your legs straight and drag your legs and body forward using only your arms. This is an alternative to push-ups, which you can do together following guidelines in Chapter 11. Have your child do modified or regular push-ups while you count and then your child can count while you take your turn. Interaction between you and your child in this and other exercises makes it more fun and more likely that the child will continue to exercise regularly.

2. *Baby Bear sit-ups.* Do modified or regular sit-ups. Follow the guidelines in Chapter 11. Hold your child's feet while he or she completes this exercise and count how many sit-ups are completed. Then, your child can count for you while anchoring your feet.

3. *Gorilla pull-ups.* Do partner pull-ups following guidelines in Chapter 11. First, let your child pull-up using your assistance and count how many pull-ups are completed. Then, let your child help you—you may need to fake it a bit for a young child or enlist a stronger child or adult to assist you while your young child counts. Again, the key here is parent-child interaction.

Cardio-respiratory Warm-up

Start walking slowly in a large circle, then pick up the pace briskly. Complete the following movements while still walking in a circle. (By walking in a circle, you obviously stay in one place rather than start out along a road or path. You might try this in a group along a path or through a park.) Use all of these exercises, or substitute some of your own. They will increase your heart rate and warm up your muscles for more vigorous exercise.

- Swing your arms forward and backward.
- Stretch your arms over your head and walk on your toes.
- Flap your arms like a bird.
- "Swim" forward with the crawl stroke.
- Still walking forward, do the backstroke.
- Walk like a pigeon, stretching your head and neck out forward and backward (Christopher's specialty).
- Walk like a duck. (Bend knees and squat as you walk.)
- Walk like a mime, moving every part of your body.
- Walk like an anteater, bending forward to suck in ants as you move along.
- Do the roller-coaster walk—walk slow, walk fast, walk low to the ground, walk high, walk fast, walk slow, walk fast, walk low, walk high, walk fast, and so forth.

SAFARI AEROBICS

Now, everyone is ready to start on what I call *safari aerobics*. Continue walking briskly in a circle. Do each activity for ten to twenty seconds and then move right into the next activity. Keep moving and you and your children will get a good aerobic workout. Use all or some of these exercises, or substitute some of your own.

- Run, and roar, like a *lion*.
- Crawl—bend over and wiggle—like a *snake*.
- Hop like a *bunny*.
- Run like a *gorilla*. (Maybe King Kong chasing Godzilla?)
- Hop like a *frog*.
- Crawl like a *crocodile*.
- Fly—flap your arms as you run—like an *eagle*.
- Gallop like a *wild horse*.
- Fly—and buzz—like a *bumblebee*.
- Hop like a *kangaroo*.
- Walk like a *spider*.
- Run like a *bull*. (Don't forget the horns! Is anyone seeing red?)

FITNESS FREEZE AEROBICS

This is an alternative to safari aerobics. Or, you can do them both if the kids are having fun. While you and the kids are doing these exercises, you or someone else yells "Freeze!" or blows a whistle. Everyone stops and stands still. Then someone yells "Go!" and you walk briskly again until someone gives the next command.

Do the following for ten to twenty seconds each. Keep moving briskly from one activity to the next to keep the workout aerobic. Use all or some of these exercises, or substitute some of your own.

- *Sergeant Slaughter's march.* March like soldiers to the "Hut two-three-four" cadence of the GI Joe Drill Sergeant.
- *Racewalk.* Walking briskly, wiggle your fanny and keep one foot in contact with the ground at all times to keep from actually running.
- Jog slowly.
- Run fast.
- Run backwards.
- Run sideways.
- Skip.
- Hop on both feet.
- Hop on your right foot.
- Hop on your left foot.
- Walk fast.
- Jog slowly.
- Do jumping jacks.
- Run in place with high knee lifts. Slap your thighs as they come up.
- Walk fast.
- Run slowly.
- Pretend to jump rope.

Note: If anyone tires, have them walk until they are ready to resume the activity.

THE COOL-DOWN

Walk slowly for three to five minutes. Too many people who exercise skip this part of the workout. Here is a chance to teach kids the importance of cooling down.

Finish with a few easy stretching exercises.

Imaginative Fitness Games

Kids, like adults, get bored doing the same thing over and over. They thrive on variety. We, as adults, might like to run different routes or alternate running with some other form of exercise. We should give our kids that kind of change too.

Here is a sample of thirty-one different fitness games to help interest your child in physical activity. Some are best played by just parent and child, some in a small family group, some with a group of children, and others in large groups (save those for birthday celebrations). You may want to show these to your school's physical education director or to the teachers who have to put together their own P.E. programs. They are mostly for pre-schoolers and grade schoolers, but some will be fun for older children as well.

Some of these are traditional games. Others, Christopher and I invented. That's the best kind of game between parent and child. Look for ways you and your child can modify these games and make them new to you.

FAST-MOVING ACTION GAMES

Tag

Christopher's favorite game is freeze tag. Moments after arriving at a city playground and yelling "Anybody wanna play freeze tag?" he's got new friends and they have divided into two teams. Each team has two or three members. One team is "it," and chases the other. When touched (by "it" players), those team members must "freeze" and remain stationary until a teammate can sneak up and touch them to "un-freeze" them. (No baby-sitting the "prisoner.") The game ends when a complete team is "frozen" or when you get too exhausted watching and take your child home. Of course, you can join in. The kids will love your participation.

The game is best played in any place with plenty of room and obstacles to hide behind (playground tunnels are great).

With adult supervision, you can make up a fitness tag game in your backyard or the park. You get opponents out by touching them or by throwing soft foam balls or other safe objects and hitting them. To keep the action going, have the person who is "out" get back in by doing some fitness activity: maybe ten push-ups, sit-ups, or jumping jacks.

You can also play "monster tag," or "Ghostbuster tag," or other variations. Just use your imagination or, better, let the kids devise the game. The only rule is: Keep everyone moving so they get plenty of disguised aerobic exercise.

Cops and Robbers

This has been popular for generations. I used to play it two ways: either on foot running all over my old neighborhood, or zooming around town on bikes.

Divide up into two teams of good guys and bad guys; then they try to capture each other, bringing the "prisoner" back to home base. Guard home base, however, because the other team will try to sneak up and release the prisoners.

There are water guns you can get that will squirt colored fluid. This will prove someone is hit and therefore captured. The fluid quickly evaporates without staining clothing. For parents who object to their children using toy guns, the old method of tagging a prisoner and having him or her go to "jail" at home base is probably best. The team that captures the entire other team wins.

You can play if you want to. But you better be quick!

Hide-and-Seek

This old favorite can be played in a number of ways. Traditionally, one child is "it." There is a home base (usually a rock or tree), where the child counts, eyes closed, to, say, fifty while the others hide. Then the child goes to find them. They can race to the base and are "home free" if they can touch it before the "it" person gets there, and taps base saying "tap, tap (name), one, two, three." If called "out" by the "it" person, that child becomes a "prisoner" at home base and must stay there touching it. He or she can only be freed by one of the other hiders racing in ahead of the child who is "it" and freeing them all. It's not as complicated as it sounds. Ask your kid. He or she will tell you how to play it. (Where did *you* spend your childhood, anyway?)

"Sardines" is another variation on hide-and-seek. In this case, the person who is "it" goes off and hides. The others fan out to search for the person who is "it," and when they find "it" they hide with him or her. In this case, since being "it" is such fun, the first person to find the boy or girl who is "it" and hides with him or her is "it" for the next game.

I have a *fartlek* variation on hide-and-seek. *Fartlek* is a Swedish word for speed play, and runners use this method for training. In *fartlek* training you run fast, then slow, according to how you feel. This creates bursts of energy during a workout. Christopher and I play "hide-and-seek *fartlek*" up and down the hills of Central Park. I'm usually "it." I close my eyes—peeking a bit to make sure he's safe—then go searching for him. I pick a home base such as a tree or rock formation at the top of a hill. When I get close to finding him, he takes off running at full speed to get to home base safe. Then we keep on moving, walking briskly, and find another home base in another section of the park. We cover more than three miles while enjoying "hide-and-seek *fartlek.*"

Follow the Leader

This can be played anywhere: in a circle or confined area or in wide open spaces. If you play it in a small area, select a fitness movement, such as hopping on one foot or doing push-ups. The other players follow. Each child gets a chance to lead.

In a more open space, the kids keep moving and the second in line moves to the front as the others follow. For example: The leader runs fast to a tree, then the next child comes to the front and walks on all fours, then the next hops like a bunny.

Keep Away

Use a ball or other easily thrown object. One team of children passes it around while another team of children tries to catch it. When they do, they switch and try to keep it from the other team. Keep every child active and involved. Kids love playing this with their friends or a group that includes friends and parents. You'll get to see who's in better shape.

Or, you can play this with two children. The "it" person is in the middle, and you and the other child try to keep the ball away from him or her. If there is a noticeable difference in ages between children, add the rule that the ball must bounce once before being caught. Try to keep everyone, including yourself, active.

Tug-of-War

Choose up sides. Get a strong rope. (Be aware that clothesline rots and weakens. Test the rope.)

The two teams stand on either side of a line. Both teams grab the rope and on a signal try to pull the other team *entirely* (not just the first two players or so) across the line.

Some outdoor variations include: tug-of-war across a water obstacle instead of a line; tug-of-war in knee-deep water (make sure everyone is a swimmer and accounted for); tug-of-war across a thick mud barrier. Jack Shepherd tells me there are farmyard variations that are played in parts of Vermont and New Hampshire, if not elsewhere.

Tug-of-war is always a big hit at Christopher's birthday parties. The best part is when the kids beat the parents. (No seconds on cake for you, Mom!)

Simon Says

You can lead the kids through this one. The players move only when the leader (you) says, for example, "Simon says jump up and down." If you only say, "Jump up and down," without saying "Simon says," anyone who moves is out. Stop between activities with the command "Simon says stop." After someone is out for a few minutes, let them back in by doing an energy-releasing activity such as ten sit-ups.

Choose lots of fun activities like jumping jacks, hopping on one leg, push-ups, and so forth. You do it with the kids.

Rock and Roll

Turn on the radio, tape deck, or record player and start dancing. Kids love contests to see who wins in different categories such as craziest, fastest, slowest, etc.

You can also play "rock-and-roll freeze." Let the kids dance and then quickly turn off the music. They have to freeze in place holding a crazy position. Then turn on the music again.

Join in on the fun!

Kangaroo Jumping

Pretend everyone is a kangaroo and start jumping. Call out various commands: jump in place, side to side, forward and back, jump and make a half-turn, jump and make a full turn, jump and clap, jump backwards, and then all together jump forward to a finish line.

Parachute Game

Use an old sheet or blanket, or a parachute if you have one around the home. Jack Shepherd tried one of those lightweight nylon tarps that Vermonters use for covering their woodpiles.

Kids and parents hold the edges around a circle. Put a lightweight ball (a beach ball, for example) in the middle. By pulling up and down, working together, you can toss the ball up high and then catch it. Try to see how many times in a row you can throw it up high and then catch it without the ball hitting the ground. Played continuously, this game provides upper body strengthening and aerobic benefits.

Logrolling

Find a grassy hill. Have the kids lie on their sides (get down there with 'em, Dad!) and then "logroll" sideways downhill. Then, everyone walk or run back to the top and do it again. Try it in mid-winter when the snow is fresh and still unpacked.

This is a great way to sneak in a little strengthening workout for the legs along with aerobic training.

Relay Races

Kids love relay races. They'll play this game for a long time if you just keep coming up with different relays to run.

Divide the kids and parents into teams. Have everyone race to a turn-around point (tree, rock, or wall) and back to tag the next person in line, who takes off for the turnaround and repeats the course. The first team to have all its players finish wins. Made sure the teams are evenly divided in terms of speed and coordination.

Here are some relays you can get the kids and parents to use. (Hey, you'll either be the life of the party or sent home early. Try 'em.)

- *Sprint* as fast as you can.
- *Hop* on both feet, or down on one foot and back on the other.
- *Somersault* down and back.
- *Skip.*
- *Run backwards or sideways.*
- *Racewalk.*
- *Run on all fours.*
- *Dribble a ball* with your hands or feet (as in soccer).
- *Hit a balloon or beach ball* in front of you. (No catching or carrying the ball.)
- *Relay a balloon.* Each player has a balloon and when he or she finishes his run he sits on the balloon and breaks it. When it pops, the next teammate goes.

There are a variety of things kids and parents can do as relay partners:

- Passing a ball back and forth every two steps;
- Wheelbarrowing—your child runs on his or her hands and you hold his or her feet, running behind him;

- Running piggyback with a child on your shoulders;
- Running three-legged—one leg tied to one of your child's.

Obstacle Course

The whole family or gym class can design an obstacle course in the backyard, gym, or playground. Pick a variety of obstacles to go over, under, around, and through. If you wish, you can time yourselves and set a goal for each parent and child to reach the next time. Use natural obstacles—trees, stumps—or make up your own. For example:

- Start by sprinting to a landmark and touching it.
- Then hop through a series of plastic hoops, tires, or circles drawn with chalk on the pavement.
- Crawl under a series of obstacles (a sawhorse, bench, or stick balanced between two chairs).
- Climb over a series of obstacles (a mat covering a picnic table; two mattresses).
- Jump over obstacles (a jump rope loosely tied between two chairs, a broomstick balanced between chairs).
- Zig-zag through a maze of cones or other objects.
- Crawl through a tunnel (a sheet held up by several chairs).
- Sprint to the finish line.

Fitness Circuit Training

Some towns have parks with *parcourses*—an exercise course with points along its path where you do various stretching, muscular strength, and endurance activities. You and your kids can design your own parcourse fitness circuit. This is a great way to have fun and get a good workout.

Here is a sample fitness circuit that you can set up in your backyard, playground, or school gym:

First, warm up with some of the stretching exercises in Chapter 11.

- Station #1: "Racewalk" briskly to a landmark and back (fifty to 100 yards).
- Station #2: Do ten to twenty sit-ups. Then run fifty yards to Station #3.
- Station #3: Jump rope for thirty seconds. Then skip fifty yards to Station #4.
- Station #4: Do ten to twenty push-ups. Then hop twenty yards to Station #5.
- Station #5: Do as many pull-ups as you can. Then run to Station #6.

- Station #6: Run-walk aerobically for two to ten minutes in a large circle. Then walk slowly for two to five minutes to cool down.

Finish with a few more stretching exercises.

Dodgeball

Pick two teams; make sure they are evenly balanced for skill levels. Draw a line with one team on either side. Draw or designate boundaries, perhaps a large circle with the line as its diameter. Use soft foam balls for younger children. One team stands on either side of the line. Using a single, soft ball, each team tries to get members of the other team out by hitting them with the ball. To make the game more difficult, require that the thrown ball must hit a player before it hits the ground. The thrower is out if someone catches the ball before it bounces.

If a child gets out, he or she can re-enter by doing ten sit-ups or push-ups or some other designated fitness workout.

I like to find a wall—side of a building, gym, or outdoor paddleball wall—and use two balls, to keep the game lively. I do all the throwing and the kids do all the running, jumping, and diving as I try to get them out. They run the gauntlet from one sideline to the other as I fire the ball at them. If they get hit, they get one point and keep playing. The child with the least points (having been hit the fewest times) at the end of the game (usually when my arm is too sore to throw) wins.

Aerobic Soccer

Use only two to four players on a team. This will keep everyone active. Don't use a goal keeper. Play with a soft ball to make the game safe for all ages. To increase skill levels, try this with a tennis ball.

If your school or town has soccer fields, use one and play on a half field. Goals can be empty half-gallon or gallon milk containers, or plastic cones.

Aerobic Volleyball

Play with two to four people on a team. Use a beachball instead of a volleyball if young kids are playing. Or, let them catch and throw the ball to keep the game moving and keep them involved. Lower the net, too, for young kids.

Instead of keeping score, when playing with young children count how many times you can volley the ball back and forth across the net without it hitting the ground.

Try this in shallow water, at a pool or the beach. In water, when playing with adults and children, do keep your eyes on the little kids.

Frisbee Football

Play with two to four on a team. Use a long field to have lots of room to run. Designate two goal lines. The idea is to try to advance the Frisbee across your opponents' goal line by throwing the Frisbee to a teammate, who catches it and is allowed two controlling steps before throwing to another teammate. If the Frisbee touches the ground, the other team gets possession. Or, the Frisbee may be intercepted or an opponenet holding the Frisbee may be tagged; in either case the other team gets possession.

This is also a good game in a pool or on a beach.

Home Run Aerobics

You can play this with your child, or with up to six kids. Set bases a long distance apart—sixty feet or more. When the ball is hit, the child races off around the bases. You (or another child in the field) must get the ball and run after the batter before he or she can run back to home. Make the chases as dramatic as possible. When playing with more than one child, have them take turns batting and running and fielding and running.

Christopher has played this game with me for more than an hour. This imaginative adaption of baseball is a lot more exercise than just standing and hitting a pitch, or waiting around in the field or on the bench.

Fast-break Basketball

Play this with your child alone or with up to six kids. The ideal place would be an empty gym. But this is tough to find, so use a basketball goal at either end of a small field, tennis court, or racquetball area. Improvise: a wooden peach basket nailed to a pole is fine. Use a whiffleball for a little variation.

Let the kids run to one goal, shoot one to three shots, and then "fast break" to the other. With younger children, don't worry about dribbling. Let 'em run.

If you have only one goal, have the kids fast break out to a marker and then back to the basket.

Aerobic Kite Flying

Find a big field. Get at least two kites. Have contests flying the kites—running as you pull the string—from one end of the field to the other into the wind.

Have contests flying the kites higher. First, run into the wind to launch the kite. Once it is up and away, reel in enough string to take you downwind about fifty yards. Then run into the wind while letting the string out. (A good kite reel helps here, or a foot-long rounded stick.) Try this over and over: sprint upwind, walk briskly downwind. Repeat.

Tom Sawyer Adventure Hikes

You will find imaginative walking games, such as "Tom Sawyer adventure hikes" and "king of the mountain" detailed in Chapter 19 under the section on walking.

These are excellent ways to introduce young kids to the adventure of walking and hiking. Then, you can progress to family outings in a nearby park or to hikes on nearby walking trails. By the time your kids are age ten or so, they will be eager to try their strong legs in state and national parks. Many of these are within an hour's drive of our major cities and well worth the time.

Shuttle Run

Make a line, and add four lines at increasing distances from it. This is best done on a soccer or football field, perhaps at your local high school. Or it can be done in any open space using a line and four obstacles at varying distances from that line.

Stand behind the line and run to the next closest line or obstacle, touch it, and run back. Run again, to the second closest line or obstacle, touch it, and run back. Repeat to another line/obstacle and return. Then run to the farthest point and return.

If playing with more than three or four kids, run in heats with the winners contesting in a "championship"; second-place finishers compete together in a final round, and so forth.

Body Slam

This game, Christopher claims, made him strong.

We wrestle on the bed. I concentrate on keeping his arms "active" by applying resistance. I pick him up and "body slam" him to the mattress, then he lifts me up (with a little faking on my part), and "body slams" me. "OOOOOOF!" I yell.

When Christopher plays this game with his friend David Pena, they take turns lifting and throwing each other down. They play this over and over for up to thirty minutes—developing upper body strength as they play. *Note:* Friends (and fathers and sons) should agree that no one will get hurt, or mad, and that the game ends if anyone does.

Christopher hasn't dared to try this yet with his mother—and neither have I.

Ocean Wave Running

Here's another of Christopher's summer favorites. Run out into the ocean, turn around, and run fast as a big wave comes crashing down behind you.

Running in water applies extra resistance, and you not only get aerobic benefit, but also strengthening of the leg muscles. Children will play this aerobic game for more than the twenty-minute aerobic goal—especially when their parents join in.

WINTER GAMES

When the snow flies, so can you and your kids. Snow creates a whole new fitness environment for imaginative kids and their parents.

Snowball Tag

Running through snow creates lots of resistance and leg strengthening. Try to tag each other with soft snowballs (no ice balls and no hitting in the face). This is a variation on water tag, which can be done in the summer at a beach in thigh-deep water.

Uphill Sledding

After you slide downhill, pull your sled back up while walking as briskly as you can. This is something like hill running: a vigorous workout going uphill, recovery while sledding downhill. Mom and Dad should jump in and share the exercise—don't just watch from the bottom of the hill. Throw in a large, hairy dog and you've got a winter wonderland.

Christopher and I have frolicked nonstop for two hours in this type of fun and exercise. We stopped when I got too cold and wet.

Sled Pulling Races

Line 'em up and take off running. Who can pull his or her sled the fastest and the farthest? Racing back to the top of the hill is a real fitness challenge.

Making Tracks

Fresh snow offers children a great game: making tracks. Scuffle along and make a secret path. Draw your initials with your feet or designs like a heart, dog, or moose. Make the design as large as a field.

This is great for leg strengthening.

Snow Baseball

Christopher and I discovered this game at Grandpa Glover's house in upstate New York. His backyard was filled with almost two feet of snow, which became our white baseball field. Use a plastic bat and plastic ball. Trees and other landmarks are bases. Take off running after a hit and keep going until you are tagged out or reach home. Christopher soon discovered that sliding into bases in the snow was the most fun!

A variation on this is snow football. Same snow, same field—now you leap and dive for passes. Play it with a soft football. Try gentle tackling if the snow is deep and you are bundled up.

Snow Shoveling

Believe it or not, kids can have a lot of fun shoveling snow. (They can also make a lot of money by shoveling other people's sidewalks.) I can hear you saying, "Yea, sure, Bob."

Give them a toy shovel when they're little and a junior one as they get older. Set up a goal, such as shoveling a path from the front porch to the driveway. They can also shovel secret paths in the backyard to a special hiding place, a clump of trees, or a snowhouse or igloo.

If the snow is the right texture, shovel it into one huge pile and tap it down with your shovels. Then, as a reward for shoveling the walk, let the kids tunnel in to make a hideout.

Part 5

LIFETIME AEROBIC FITNESS ACTIVITIES

15

Aerobic Fitness Activities

I believe that the best workout you can get produces an aerobic training effect and promotes muscle fitness, weight control, and a general feeling of well-being. There are activities that do all this and can be enjoyed by an individual, rather than requiring team play, and they are suitable for anyone in the family—from the kids to the grandparents.

I call these *lifetime aerobic fitness activities* because they are things you can do your whole life. They should be taught to children at an early age—ice-skating and cross-country skiing, for example, can be learned almost as soon as a child knows how to walk.

Fitness experts have identified what they call the "Big Four" of aerobic exercise—walking, running, biking, and swimming. These give you an aerobic workout and are simple and fun. I detail them in separate chapters in this section. The Big Four are not the only forms of exercise of benefit to you, however.

The President's Council on Fitness and Sports asked seven fitness experts to rank exercise activities for various fitness and general well-being factors. The seven experts ranked the activities from zero to three, with zero indicating no benefit and three, maximum benefit. The maximum score was twenty-one (the seven experts all giving an activity a three). The top scorers: running, biking, and swimming. Chart A has the results.

Dr. Kenneth Cooper and his colleagues at the Institute of Aerobics Research also ranked the most common physical activities by their "aerobic conditioning potential." They came up with five in this order of importance: cross-country skiing, swimming, running, biking, and walking. Beyond these came roller-skating, and then, of equal value, aerobic dancing, handball, racquetball, squash, and basketball. Lagging behind them was tennis.

Another way of comparing the value of physical activity is in terms of calories burned. Chart B lists approximate caloric expenditure per minute.

Fitness and Well-Being Ranking of Physical Activities

Factors	Running	Bicycling	Swimming	Skating	Handball Squash	Cross-Country Skiing	Basketball	Tennis	Calisthenics	Walking	Golf	Softball	Bowling
PHYSICAL FITNESS													
Cardio-respiratory endurance	21	19	21	18	19	19	19	16	10	13	8	6	5
Muscular endurance	20	18	20	17	18	19	17	16	13	14	8	8	5
Strength	17	16	14	15	15	15	15	14	16	11	9	7	5
Flexibility	9	9	15	13	16	14	13	14	19	7	8	9	7
Balance	17	18	12	20	17	16	16	16	15	8	8	7	6
GENERAL WELL-BEING													
Weight control	21	20	15	17	19	17	19	16	12	13	6	7	5
Muscle definition	14	15	14	14	11	12	13	13	18	11	6	5	5
Digestion	13	12	13	11	13	12	10	12	11	11	7	8	7
Sleep	16	15	16	15	12	15	12	11	12	14	6	7	6
Total	148	142	140	140	140	139	134	128	126	102	66	64	51

Source: President's Council on Physical Fitness and Sports.

CHART B

Estimated Calories Used per Minute for Physical Activities

Activity	Calories per minute
Cross-country skiing	10–15
Running	10–12
Handball/Squash/Racquetball (singles)	8–11
(doubles)	6–8
Canoeing/Rowing	7–11
Swimming (crawl stroke)	8–10
Biking	5–10
Jumping Rope	7–10
Tennis (singles)	7–10
(doubles)	5–7
Ice- and Roller-Skating	5–10
Walking	5–7
Dancing (rock/disco)	4–6
(square, western, polka)	5–8
(aerobic class)	5–8

Actual caloric expenditure will vary by activity depending on your body weight, exercise intensity, skill level, and the weather. I have listed only the activities discussed in this section.

Although the values are listed per minute, remember that you will need at least twenty minutes of continuous exercise to provide aerobic conditioning. Some activities here—tennis, handball, and squash, for example—will vary in intensity as you stop-go during the game.

Cross-country skiing, running, biking, swimming, and walking are all efficient calorie burners and easy to do continuously. Tennis, squash, dancing, rowing, and jumping rope are good calorie burners if done continuously and intensely, but you may find it difficult to do so.

As Charts A and B indicate, there are many beneficial forms of lifetime aerobic fitness activities. I recommend some of them in this chapter: cross-country skiing, ice- and roller-skating, aerobic exercise dancing, rowing, and jumping rope.

There are many forms of physical activity that may interest your children and provide for aerobic fitness benefits. One that surprised me with its value is horseback riding. Kayle Morrison, one of Christopher's classmates, ran a very fast time for the one-mile run as part of our Sports Club program. Yet, his mother claimed he seldom runs. Further questioning revealed that he vigorously rides horses on weekends in the country, and ice-skates regularly in the winter. Both activities strengthen his legs and promote aerobic fitness without his realizing that he is exercising.

Other activities that involve stop-go exercise—thus not keeping your heart rate in a constant aerobic training range—can produce aerobic benefits only if you play them vigorously. These include: tennis, handball, racquetball, and squash. Playing doubles in any of these activities sharply reduces their aerobic value. These sports do offer good workouts that can be enjoyed long into adulthood by every family member. But you probably should establish an aerobic base to get in shape for these individuals sports by running, swimming, or biking.

SELECTING YOUR ACTIVITIES

Which activities should you choose? I believe you should select several and try them out. Then, you might want to mix them—for example, running most of the year, mixed with swimming in summer and cross-country skiing in winter.

You can even combine activities for family fun. Roberta Brill, a top masters division marathoner on my team, was concerned that her ten-year-old son, Ben, was gaining weight despite his participation in sports activities. He wasn't getting enough aerobic exercise. She bought new bikes for each of them and they started enjoying long bike rides of fifteen to twenty miles together. Then, fascinated by the concept of the triathlon event, Ben challenged his mother to do one with him. She quickly capitalized on his interest and they began to train for the three portions of the event: swimming, biking, and running. They agreed to work together on the day of the event and record their times so they could set a goal of improving them in the future. First they swam a quarter mile in the lake near Ben's grandmother's house. They emerged from the water and quickly mounted bikes for a four-and-a-half–mile hilly bike ride. Then, they dismounted and ran one and a quarter miles back to the finish line. Not only did this family triathlon program improve their fitness, it strengthened the mother-son relationship and was a lot of fun.

Your child may enjoy a variety of activities. Just be sure to select *lifetime aerobic fitness activities*, and in whatever combination of exercises you choose, work out vigorously for at least twenty to thirty continuous minutes three times a week.

Whatever you select, also be certain to follow the warm-up and cool-down principles and review the FIT aerobic training variables detailed in Chapter 12. These apply to each aerobic activity.

Most important of all, before you start, check with your doctor about exercising and what exercise might be best for you. If you are over age thirty-five, you should get an exercise stress test that searches for any hidden coronary artery disease or heart problems. Be cautious, start slowly, stretch, warm up, and cool down.

CROSS-COUNTRY SKIING

Dr. Cooper ranks cross-country skiing (also called Nordic skiing) as the number one aerobic activity because it involves all the upper and lower body muscles in vigorous activity. The driving action of the legs strengthens those muscles, while the motion of using the ski poles to pull you forward uses your shoulders, arms, and abdominals. The gliding action stretches the muscles in your back and the backs of your legs. In one invigorating workout, you promote all the components of fitness: cardio-respiratory endurance, muscular strength and endurance, flexibility, and body composition. The gliding motion of cross-country skiing makes it a low-injury exercise. Finally, cross-country also burns more calories for effort than any of the other aerobic fitness activities. It is great fun for the entire family. The little ones find plenty of downhills, jumps, and snowball fights to keep them from getting bored.

Equipment. Cross-country skiing is inexpensive. You can—and, for your first winter, should—rent skis, boots, and poles. Most ski touring places and many country inns offer cheap daily, weekend, and weekly rental packages. Try both the bamboo poles and the plastic ones. Try also the wooden or plastic skis that require waxing and the cross-country skis that do not require waxing (so-called waxless skis). Each has a different feel. Jack Shepherd and his wife cross-country ski all winter long in Vermont. Jack has old wooden skis and Kathy has waxless. Jack prefers to study the snow conditions and determine which "wax day" it is: blue, red, green, and so forth. Cross-country skiers have their own language, and you'll hear them talking about a "red-wax day" or a "blue-wax day," depending on the temperature, "age" of the snow, and other conditions. Kathy likes the waxless skis: you just step out the door and go. No scraping, waxing, testing, or re-waxing.

Clothing. Cross-country skiing appeals to people like Shepherd and me, who like to run in old, torn, but comfortable clothing. On sunny January-February days in Vermont, Jack and Kathy put on knickers, ski socks (add gaiters, if you have them, to keep your legs dry), undershirt, wool shirt, wool sweater, and down vest. Before too long, they unzip the vest. Bring along a hat and mittens to protect against frostbite.

Sometimes, one of them carries a light day-pack with chocolate and a snack. You might also pack a lightweight portable one-burner stove, de-hydrated soup or hot chocolate, cheese, and bread. Melt the snow for water. Do not take wine or other alcohol into the woods with you in winter; it does not keep you warm and may cause you to have an accident or become confused. Also, if you stop, bundle up and keep moving to stay warm.

Where to ski. If you ski along a groomed trail you can easily cover ten miles in an afternoon. Or you can strike off on your own across farmland and meadows. In deep snow, almost all obstacles are covered, and it's easy to cross stone walls and roads. But fresh, unpacked snow is a serious obstacle, and new cross-country skiers should stay on groomed cross-country trails, ski-mobile tracks, or snow-covered dirt roads. Shepherd and his family prefer trails that follow ski-mobile tracks. The snow is compacted and yet the path is narrow; if you want to get off it into the unpacked snow you can.

How to ski. Cross-country skiing is also a great sport for groups of friends or a family. Anyone can learn to ski in less than half an hour, and young kids seem to be born to it. Lessons would be helpful. Be sure to warm up before setting forth. Stretch both your leg muscles and your upper body, arms, and hips. Ease into the skiing, even if you are an experienced skier.

Until you've mastered reasonably good technique, you may have difficulty reaching your training heart rate range. If you ski too much too soon, you could find yourself very sore the next day, as I found out the hard way. Try to limit yourself to thirty minutes of skiing the first few days and gradually build up to an hour or more once you get in shape. Remember, keep moving in order to keep your heart rate in your training range. Family members may need to pair off with those of similar skill and fitness in order to get the best workout. As with other activities, exercise at your young child's level and put in your personal workout at another time.

The technique is like ice-skating or hill running. You "grab" the snow with the ski poles, alternating your arms in a pumping motion, kick the ski ahead of you, and then glide. It's harder to describe than to do. To go uphill, most skiers simply jog up with the skis in a herringbone pattern. (Ah-ha, says Shepherd, here is where the waxed skis outperform the waxless.) Some also run down hill, but most, like Jack and Kathy, prefer to ski down bent in a crouch. If you get going too fast, all you do is roll into the fresh snow.

Perhaps the best thing about cross-country skiing is the quiet. You ski deep into the meadows or woodlands listening to the wonderful sound of the ski tips cutting through snow—a kind of shush, shush—broken only by the occasional call of a chickadee.

Snowshoeing. This is highly aerobic and lots of fun in deep snow. Kathy and Jack go snowshoeing in the full moon in January and February. Take along one ski pole to help yourself up if you fall. After one enormous New England storm, Shepherd set out on snowshoes down his long driveway. He turned around to wave at his family—warm and snug inside—and fell over. He sank into forty inches of powdery snow, and it took him four or five minutes to turn over, find something solid to push on, and get himself righted again. His kids thought it was hilarious, but he thought it was like drowning in cotton flakes. Now he and Kathy each take a ski pole when they snowshoe.

Remember: Stretch and warm up for this aerobic activity. It's hard work—and fun.

ROLLER-SKATING AND ICE-SKATING

Dr. Cooper's research indicates that skating at a speed of ten miles per hour (six-minute miles) is the aerobic equivalent of running at five miles per hour (twelve-minute miles). In other words, you need to skate twice as fast as you run to benefit aerobically. Further, you need to keep skating continuously with your arms and legs in motion. It's too easy to coast along and thus lose fitness benefits. Roller skating is fun for young kids, but probably not a good fitness activity for them since they tend to coast so much.

Keeping fit by roller-skating can be fun. I'm always amazed by the roller skaters in Central Park who zip up and down the hills or dance to music for what seems like hours. They are in great shape and their legs look very strong.

Also, Shepherd tells me that roller *skiers* abound in the hills of Vermont and New Hampshire during the warm months. This involves wearing a pair of high-top shoes that look like roller skates or ice skates, but they have a straight row of small wheels along the bottom. You skate with them on the paved roads, using your ski poles—a great way to extend cross-country skiing to all four seasons, or to keep in shape for the snow. Shepherd tells me that the good roller skiers can stop on a dime, even going down steep hills. But he also says he'd never try it!

Ice-skating is a good fitness activity. Christopher learned to ice-skate at school and goes skating regularly with his mother. He could zoom around the rink faster and for a longer period of time as a six-year-old than most of the adults. He loves the music and the companionship of all the other kids he meets on the ice. My brother roller-skates with his boys and they all enjoy the exercise and fun.

Skating slowly is a gentle way to ease into aerobic workouts. First, build up to skating twenty to thirty minutes nonstop. Then increase the intensity so that you reach your training range.

It's important to get some lessons and a good pair of skates. Poorly fitting skates and lots of falls will discourage the most ardent youngsters. Spend money on equipment, not on expensive clothing to wear while working out.

TENNIS, HANDBALL, RACQUETBALL, AND SQUASH

These activities are excellent for developing hand-eye coordination, muscular strength and endurance, and flexibility. But they also depend on a series of sprints and bursts of energy rather than continuous lower-level muscle activity.

Therefore, to improve your aerobic fitness, you should combine any of these four sports with an activity such as running, biking, or swimming. In these cases, the sport benefits from your aerobic workouts. I agree that there is a certain satisfaction in playing a hard, competitive game. But these sports often do not benefit your cardio-respiratory system sufficiently, and are therefore incomplete as fitness workouts.

You can increase your fitness benefits by playing singles rather than doubles. Play at as high a level of intensity as you can, with minimal resting between volleys. The better shape you are in, the longer and more intense the volleys. You can also wear down an opponenet by being in better aerobic condition. Reserve doubles time for family fun.

Be sure to warm up properly. Beware of the "weekend tennis warrior" syndrome: only exercising on weekends, and irregularly at that, and then playing too long and too hard. You will be susceptible to muscle aches and pains, and may risk more serious injury or even heart problems. I lost a good friend several years ago because he was out of shape, played a very competitive and intense game of squash, and then sat down in exhaustion without properly cooling down. He died on the court from a heart attack. He was a very skilled player who thought he was in good shape.

Don't start playing these sports to get into shape. Get in shape first, then play the sport. Once you are exercising aerobically for twenty consecutive minutes three times a week you should be safe to play a reasonably controlled game.

These sports are excellent lifetime activities that children should learn. When playing with young chidren, concentrate at first on the skills of the game and the fun of the activity. Fitness benefits should come later when the child is more skilled—perhaps not until he or she is a young adult. As with all fitness and sports activities, play the game the child wants, not the one you want the child to learn. And don't be too competitive too soon. There's time for that. And be sure to balance your child's sports activities with other exercise that will gradually provide more aerobic training.

CANOEING AND ROWING

Both of these sports are good aerobic exercise. But they require a high degree of skill—and the ability to swim—before you can enjoy them and use them as workouts.

Of course, you can always use a rowing machine on dry land; here, too, you should work up gradually to rowing for twenty to thirty minutes. A quality machine has several choices of arm resistance, a sliding seat that allows for proper leg movement, and sturdy oars. The best—which costs about two thousand dollars—is a simple bicycle wheel with chains; rowers say it duplicates the feeling of water almost exactly. But you can buy good machines for under two hundred dollars if you shop carefully. I suggest renting one (or any other exercise machine) for a while to see if you like this kind of workout. There are a lot of rowing machines and stationary bicycles that stay in closets. (For that reason, look for a second-hand machine when you decide to buy.)

Shepherd bought a rowing machine three years ago—after renting a bicycling machine that he hated—for winter workouts when the roads were too slippery for running. He always warmed up and cooled down, and rowed for only five minutes the first week. He paid special attention to stretching his lower back, which stationary machines seem to aggravate. Then he built up to thirty minutes over a six-week period. Now, he just snaps a tape in his headset, and rows for one side of a tape, about thirty-five to forty minutes.

Canoeing and rowing on water are somewhat different than on machines. Canoeing works the upper body more than the legs. Rowing—especially in sculls or boats with sliding seats—works the entire body. It's an excellent workout.

Canoeing can be enjoyed in shallow streams, ponds, and lakes. It's a lot of fun for everyone. Jack and Kathy often take their summer visitors out on the Connecticut River in two canoes, paddle a mile upstream, tie the canoes together, and eat a picnic dinner as they float downstream. Canoe trips can be fun adventure for the entire family.

Canoeing is harder to learn than rowing, however. You should master several different strokes to move the canoe in a straight line, sideways, and backwards, and to turn it quickly in an emergency. You also need to canoe kneeling—don't sit on the seats, since your center of gravity is too high—and learn how to move about in a canoe and get into and out of the water in a canoe.

Rowing a rowboat is easy to do, and can be an aerobic workout. If you want to row as an exercise, you should have access to a rowing club or sculls and a long, smooth body of water. This can be a wonderful exercise. But get some lessons. Remember that a scull (the narrow, wooden boat with a sliding seat and fixed oars that is rowed alone, by two people, or by eight) tips over very easily. Your instruction should include safety and how to right the boat.

Whether you are canoeing, rowing, or using a rowing machine, be sure to warm up and cool down, and don't overdo the workout. Gradually move up to your desired exercise level.

JUMPING ROPE

Kids love to jump rope. Some get very good at it and learn elaborate double jumping and team jumping. Like other exercises in this section, it's both fun and, when done vigorously for a period of time, aerobic.

Properly stretch before jumping rope, and wear well-cushioned shoes. It is also wise to jump on some surface that has some give, such as a gym floor or carpeted area, rather than a street. You might want to jump rope for a few minutes, do sit-ups, push-ups, or other brisk exercises, and then return to rope jumping as part of a circuit training program. Kids enjoy this kind of routine. You can buy fancy ropes with ball bearings in the handles or inexpensive ones, or you can make your own out of clothesline.

Length of rope. This is determined by your size. Stand on the rope with your feet together. The handles should reach to your armpits. Here's a guide for rope length: Kindergarten through third grade, about seven to eight feet; grades four through six, about eight to nine feet; grades seven through nine, about eight to ten feet; grades ten through twelve and adults, about nine to ten feet.

Jumping rope takes coordination and a high ceiling. After warming up, try these tips:

- Hold the rope loosely, using your thumb and index finger for control.
- Keep your elbows in at waist level with your arms extended sideways at about ninety-degree angles.
- Hold your back straight and your head erect; your body should be erect but flexible. Relax.
- Use a circular wrist motion to turn the rope forward or—after you master the technique—backwards.
- Jump on the balls of your feet and land softly. Start with a two-foot landing and then advance to one-foot landings or a gentle sort of running in place.

- Hop just enough to allow the rope to clear beneath your feet. Bend your knees slightly as you land.
- Alternate from foot to foot as you skip at the rate of about seventy to eighty jumps a minute. You may jump slower at first and then increase the pace as you become more skilled.

The goal is not that you skip rope fast, but that you get your heart rate up into your aerobic exercise range. If you get tired too quickly, you may be jumping too high or turning the rope too vigorously—using your arms rather than your wrists.

Beginners should start by counting how many jumps they can make in a row. Then stop, pause, and start again. As you get better, you will forget about counting and jump rope for a period of time. Build slowly for three- to five-minute intervals, with brisk walking in between for one to two minutes. Your goal is twenty minutes of continuous rope jumping. Do not try this right away, but build up to it.

You can make the rope jumping interesting by adding crossovers, heel kicks, one-foot hops, and other variations. If you want a real workout, stop at any playground and try to copy the kids! "Double Dutch" is a tough variation where two long ropes are turned simultaneously by partners as the jumper(s) enter, jump, and exit without touching the rope.

The American Heart Association (AHA) and the AAHPERD have together developed the "Jump Rope for Heart" program. This promotes rope jumping for physical fitness and raises money for heart disease research. The event is held in March every year, and school kids, teachers, and parents may participate. For more information and their guide book "Jump for the Health of It," contact your local AHA. You might want to encourage your school to become part of this program and use rope jumping to promote fitness and motor skills.

DANCING

Dancing can be fun and a fitness workout. The more skilled you are and the more vigorously you dance, the better the fitness benefits. Traditional ethnic dances—polkas, rumbas—are fun that the whole family can enjoy. Christopher loves square dancing with his mother—although at age seven he refuses to dance with other "girls." Any type of dance that involves body movement is fun and good for the kids, including disco and rock dancing. The key is to keep it continuous. Play record after record, song after song to keep everyone moving for at least ten minutes, if not twenty.

When you go dancing, make it a workout, too. Try to dance nonstop for the complete set that the band or D.J. plays. Your rest comes when they take a break.

With young kids, it is more important that they dance for fun than for fitness. Anything that can get them to enjoy moving their body is a step in the right direction—so to speak.

AEROBIC DANCE EXERCISE

This is choreographed exercise to music. It might be an "aerobics class" at a fitness studio, or a workout at home to a tape on your TV set. Aerobic dance is indeed an effective way to gain aerobic conditioning as long as you do it properly. More and more men are also joining these classes—even top athletes. The 1988 college basketball championship finalists—the high-scoring, fast-breaking University of Oklahoma Sooners—were in much better shape than their opponents all season. Why? Their pre-season conditioning program included high-intensity aerobics dance classes.

What should you look for in an aerobics class? Here's a checklist:

Instructor. This person should be enthusiastic and take the time for individual help to make sure you and each student exercise safely and aerobically. Instructors should have a degree in exercise science and/or be certified by a reputable organization like the American College of Sports Medicine, the Aerobics and Fitness Association of America, or the International Dance-Exercise Association.

Periodic pulse checks. Class members should take periodic pulse checks to make sure that they exercise safely within their training heart range. Each class member responds differently to various exercise movements. You should listen to your body rather than attempt to keep up with those around you.

Warm-up, cool-down. Your class should include a thorough warm-up and cool-down as well as at least twenty to thirty minutes of continuous aerobic work. The exercises should be smooth and continuous, not jerky.

Classes. They must be challenging, progressive, but not exhausting. Classes should be divided by skill levels—beginner, intermediate, and advanced—rather than lumping everyone together in one class. This will make the workouts too difficult for some and too easy for others.

Floor. The floor you dance on should provide some cushioning. The harder the floor, the greater your chance of injury.

A good forty-five-minute class will improve both aerobic and muscle fitness while burning calories—all as you are having fun dancing to music. Make sure that you have well-cushioned shoes, which will decrease you chances of injury while increasing your enjoyment.

In an effort to minimize injuries, "low-impact" aerobics classes have become popular. These classes minimize the jumping and replace it with lots of upper body movements to keep your heart rate up.

Video tapes. Be cautious when exercising to tapes. Without an instructor to monitor you, you may exercise too intensely—or not hard enough. You may also miss the fun of a class—there is something reassuring in seeing others puff and sweat along with you.

AEROBICS FOR KIDS

What about your kids? The older ones should take the classes right along with you. There are a lot of classes for kids, too, some called Huff-N-Puff, Funky Dancer, or Jump for Joy. These are good for kids age ten and up as long as they enjoy them and the instructors are well qualified to not only teach exercise, but specifically to teach children. Programs for young children should be directed more toward fun than fitness. If the kids like them, good. But don't force it.

Many schools, including Christopher's, are starting aerobic dance classes as part of their physical education programs. It is an excellent way to get kids to exercise—all kids like to have fun to the beat of music.

Many Y's and fitness clubs offer co-ed aerobics classes for the entire family. Family aerobics can be fun. Each member can adjust his or her intensity to the best maximum training effect. Even the pre-schoolers can get involved—jumping, twisting, and twirling whenever the mood strikes them.

16

Biking

By now, more than ninety million Americans are bike riders. We are buying more than thirteen million bikes a year. But biking has changed. More of us are biking for fun, fitness, and competition; we're taking biking vacations and tours, commuting to work on bikes, and training for bike races and triathlons. Best of all, we are biking for family fitness. *Sports, Inc.* magazine reports that "baby boomers and their children are financing cycling's rise."

Biking is a good, total fitness workout that can be done indoors or outdoors. It provides aerobic benefit, strengthens your leg muscles (especially the quadriceps along the top of your thighs), hip, lower back, and abdominal muscles, and increases the flexibility of your hip and knee joints. Also, as a non–weight-bearing exercise, biking is good for the overweight or older person.

Outdoor biking gives you a wide variety of training—hills, flats, rolling countryside. You can bike to and from work—an exercise that saves you gas and makes a good impression on your children and out-of-shape neighbors. Your kids may be able to bike to school, friends' houses, and other activities. You should encourage them to bike or walk to these activities instead of asking for a ride in the family car. Better yet, whenever you can, bike with them to their activities.

Dr. Irvine H. Page, former president of the American Heart Association, said: "We ought to replace the automobile with bicycles. . . . It would be better for the coronaries, our dispositions, and certainly our finances." Indeed, in many countries—China, for example—bikes far outnumber cars.

So what's wrong with biking? One disadvantage is bad weather; you cannot ride a bike when it snows or when the roads are slippery. Also, bikes can be dangerous: about six hundred children and adolescents die from bicycle injuries every year in the United States; over three hundred thousand are injured badly enough to require emergency care.

Let's discuss some safety guidelines and various types of bikes for you and your family.

SAFETY GUIDELINES FOR BIKING

There are more serious injuries to adults and children from biking accidents than from any other aerobic sport. I see at least one bike accident for every six-mile loop I run in Central Park. Out in the country, Jack Shepherd sees kids who get careless, hit loose gravel, and skid off the country road into the woods; he's taken several of these to the emergency room. One day, a family was riding the wrong way in Central Park and the father's bike clipped my foot, sending me flying and causing his child to fall out of the small rear seat. Everyone was all right, except me: I was so bruised I couldn't run the New York City Marathon two weeks later after three months of one-hundred-mile training weeks. If you are a runner, watch out for bicyclists. If you are a bicyclist, keep alert for everyone else.

In *Around Town Cycling*, Donald Prudden offers four tips for survival on a bike in the world of the automobile and truck: Be aware; Be defensive; Be predictable; Be visible. Other tips:

- Ride with traffic; you are considered a vehicle. Commuters should select their routes with care, and watch for turning cars, car/truck doors suddenly opening, and jaywalking pedestrians.
- Obey all traffic laws.
- Make eye contact with everyone you pass who might get in your way: runners, pedestrians, drivers.
- Wear bright and reflective clothes—a bright, lightweight hunting vest is excellent and inexpensive—and have reflector material taped onto your bike. Include the spokes so you will be seen from the side.
- Wear a hardshell biking helmet, sometimes called a "mushroom." This is essential for every bicyclist of whatever age. Start your kids wearing them even before they are riding tricycles. Anyone can suffer serious injury falling from a speeding bike. Protect yourself and them.

BIKES FOR KIDS

Most kids start on plastic bikes they push with their feet, and progress to tricycles, small bikes with outrigger training wheels, youth-sized bikes without the training wheels, and on to adult bikes. Here are some general rules:

Young children cannot use hand brakes. Your child's first bike should have coaster brakes that he or she can operate simply by reverse pedaling.

Training wheels are controversial. Some specialists believe children shouldn't use them, but should start on a grassy slope coasting downhill without pedaling to get a feel for the balance. Others recommend training wheels to get the child off and pedaling, steering, and stopping the bike before worrying about balance.

Choose what works best for your child. Don't rush him or her. Christopher didn't take off his training wheels until he was seven years old. Instead, he learned how to handle his bike with confidence.

Do not buy a bike your child can "grow into." Bikes are not like shoes. They should fit the child and not be a few sizes too big to last longer as your child grows. Get a bike that allows your child to touch the ground with the balls of his or her feet when seated on the bike. If the bike is too big, your child will not be able to control or stop it, or get off quickly in case of danger. The Bicycle Federation of America recommends not allowing a child to have a ten-speed bike until at least age eleven or twelve. Single or three-speed bikes are recommended until skills and maturity develop.

Get a bike with regular upright handlebars at shoulder width. Do not get a bike for your child that has fancy racing handlebars. The regular ones are easier to control—and for all young riders, control is the key element.

Equip your child's bike with a horn or loud bell to warn others.

Trail bikes (BMX, or bike motocross) have been a problem for some parents and kids. These are a cross between all-terrain bikes and motorcycles. They are one-speed with rugged twenty-inch knobby tires, a strong frame, and padded crossbar. Christopher's cousins in Buffalo, New York, ride them over dirt trails; they are fun for exploring Class Four (unpaved, unrepaired) roads in the country. They can also cause a lot of environmental damage to hiking trails, and therefore should be used only on roads. Inspect the area your children will be riding and insist that they wear helmets, long pants, and shirts or jackets to minimize scratches when they fall—and they will fall.

SAFETY FOR CHILDREN

All safety tips also apply to children. But there are some other points to add especially for them.

The Physician and Sports Medicine magazine lists a consensus from four major cycling organizations about bicycle safety for children. They include:

Helmet. As stated above, your child should not be on a bike with you until eight months or older. Whenever you start him or her on the bike seat, always make this simple rule: Everyone wears a helmet.

You and your child should wear a tough helmet that meets the standards of the American National Standards Institute or the Snell Memorial Foundation. Sadly, less than 2 percent of children and adolescents who ride bikes bother to wear helmets. The American Academy of Pediatrics has said that most parents are unaware of the risks of head injury while bicycle riding. Invest in a good helmet for your child and for yourself.

Bike. Your child's bike should be in good shape and its brakes, handlebars, and reflectors should be checked. The bike should not have any sharp, exposed parts.

Training. Your child should know how to stop quickly by using the bike's brakes (not by dragging a foot or jumping off the seat), how to look for traffic and pedestrians, how to signal turns, how to ride a straight line, and how to stop and dismount without falling.

Your child should also obey all traffic signals, ride with traffic (not against it), avoid busy streets, and not show off on the bike.

In *Woman's Day,* Jim Fremont, education director for the Bicycle Federation of America, a national, non-profit organization that promotes the safe use of bicycles for transportation and recreation, suggested safety guidelines for children:

- Children age six and under should always bicycle with an adult, even on sidewalks. "Drivers of cars entering and leaving driveways may not look for bikes," says Fremont, "so riders must look for and stop for cars crossing sidewalks."
- Seven- and eight-year-olds may ride alone. But they should not ride on the street. They may not understand such traffic laws as right-of-way and they may have difficulty judging the speed of oncoming cars. Children this age assume that adults will get out of the way of bicycles.
- Kids nine and older may, with proper training (above), ride on their own. You may want to restrict them to safe streets and dependable routes. You should also teach your child traffic rules necessary for safe bike riding, such as riding with the flow of traffic, stopping at all stop signs and red lights, and waiting for oncoming traffic before making a left turn. Go over these things repeatedly with your child, before and after every outing.
- Don't let your child ride his or her bike after dark. Also, make sure that your child's bike has a light and a noisemaking device. Horns and bells attached to the bike are favorites. Adults sometimes wear

police whistles around their necks, and blow them repeatedly while riding through heavy traffic.

Also, don't allow children to ride in heavily congested areas (like Central Park), since they aren't very adept at avoiding speeding bikes and pedestrians that may suddenly swerve into their path.

ADULT BIKES

Bikes for adolescents and adults should be chosen carefully too. How do you plan to use the bike? Regular old-fashioned single-speed bikes—the only kind I've ever used—are fine for easy riding on flat roads. These have pedal brakes (not hand brakes), upright handlebars, and wide, padded seats. They are good for short distances and are an excellent workout bike. They also require few repairs and little maintenance.

If you plan to ride in hilly country, and want to make biking a fitness workout, you may want a three-speed bike. These are also recommended for older children as they move up to more complicated (and expensive) bikes. Three-speed bikes have narrower tires than the single-speeders, but come with hand brakes. Your child will have to practice using these before getting out on the road.

If you will be riding long distances, climbing steep hills, racing, or want a good bike for steady fitness workouts, you may move up to a ten-speed. These bikes have more low gears, which make biking uphill easier. They are expensive, lighter, and less sturdy, and require more repairs and upkeep. They have dropped handlebars and narrow seats designed to let you use your muscles more efficiently on long rides. The additional gears are unnecessary for fitness biking, however.

Whatever bike you like, it should have a seat and handlebars that are adjustable. Raise the seat until you can reach the handlebars and pedals easily. When you are sitting on the seat with the ball of your foot pushing one of the pedals all the way down, your leg should be just slightly bent. You should be able to touch the ground with your toes. Toe clips on the pedals will allow you to exercise the muscles in the front of your leg and give you more power as you ride.

Here again, I recommend renting bikes first to see what you like—both in terms of numbers of speeds and brand—and then look for good used bikes to buy. You can get some outstanding bargains at garage sales, school fund-raisers, and from friends. You should not have to pay top dollar for any fitness equipment.

BIKING THE RIGHT WAY

If you have regular, upright handlebars, just lean forward slightly as you ride and rest your hands on the handgrips or the bars.

If you have lower racing bike handlebars, you will gain speed and control by holding the grips and bending the body forward. This is often tiring for new riders and you may need some stretching and rests before you become comfortable with it. Sitting upright is also tiring over a long ride and creates greater wind resistance. A comfortable forward lean distributes your weight more evenly on the seat, handlebars, and pedals.

Riding style is less important for short fitness rides of up to thirty minutes. But it does become important as your ride gets longer. You can create more power in pedaling by "ankling." Using toe clips, drop your heel when the pedal is at the top of its circle and push forward and downward with your ankle to add power to the motion. Drop your toe at the bottom of the pedal action to allow a backward and then upward pull.

How fast should you pedal? You should shift gears on your bike to create a smooth and steady pedaling pace. Don't pedal slowly uphill and fast downhill. A beginner will bike at about sixty to seventy pedal revolutions per minute and work up to ninety to a hundred with increased fitness and skill. A common mistake for beginners is to pedal too slowly in too high a gear. This is not only inefficient, it also places a lot of stress on your knees.

Find the pedaling rate that is most comfortable for you, at your present level of fitness, and yet allows you to achieve an aerobic benefit. Gear down on the uphills to save your tired thighs, change gears on the downhills to allow you to keep pedaling rather than coast. Safely control your speed.

On long rides, stand on the pedals and stretch every ten minutes or so. By getting up from your seat you can stretch your lower back and leg muscles and give your fanny a rest. Roll your head from shoulder to shoulder to relieve any neck tension. Change your hand position every few miles to relieve hand and arm tension.

GETTING FIT WITH BIKING

First, review the exercise principles and warm-up and cool-down routines in Chapter 10. Look over the FIT aerobic training variables in Chapter 12.

Start your biking program with a slow five- to ten-minute warm-up ride, followed by riding for about twenty minutes at a steady rate of pedaling. Ride at a pace that allows you to talk with someone and keeps you within your training heart rate range. If you find that your heart rate or breathing speeds up too quickly, slow down. If necessary, alternate pedaling briskly for two minutes with pedaling slowly for two minutes until you can pedal steadily and briskly for twenty continuous minutes. Conclude by biking slowly for five minutes. Then get off the bike and walk around for another five minutes to cool down properly.

For the first few weeks, ride every other day. After reaching the point where you can ride for twenty minutes within your training heart rate range, increase your mileage slowly until you are riding a minimum of thirty minutes per workout. Don't ride for more than an hour at once until your legs, buttocks, and upper body have adjusted to the new strains and stresses. You may find that your legs will tire, and your upper body, hands, and neck—along with your fanny—will become uncomfortable long before your heart and lungs give out. Try to work up to thirty miles a week.

Avoid steep and long hills until you are in good shape and have practiced climbing moderate hills. As your fitness improves, don't fool yourself and coast. It's easy to coast, and thus cheat on your workouts. If you are biking for fitness, rather than fun, you will need to keep pushing. Speeds less than ten miles an hour produce limited fitness benefits. Speeds above twenty miles an hour are racing speeds. Slow biking requires very little effort and produces very little fitness benefit. The more fit you are the harder you need to pedal. As with all fitness activities, training within your target heart rate range is far more important than distance or speed.

COMPETING

After you have mastered all the fancy gears and the technique of riding—and you have a good fitness base—you may enjoy competing. This is similar to runners who reach a certain point in their fitness, and then start building races into their workouts. You might want to do that with biking.

Contact your local bike club. This may be located through your bike shop. Most of the good clubs have programs to introduce beginner bikers to the sport.

TOURING

Your local bike club will also introduce you and your family to bike touring, in which local groups sponsor day trips or week-long rides. This is a great way to see the countryside. In some parts of the country—New England, the Pacific Northwest—you can bike from country inn to country inn. Your luggage is transported ahead by van.

In many areas, local bike clubs sponsor bike festivals that can be fun for the entire biking family. Make sure you and your kids are in good enough condition to enjoy an outing, and that your children understand and know the rules of safe biking mentioned above.

Citibank and the American Youth Hostels sponsor a thirty-six–mile, five-borough tour of New York City which attracts more than fifteen thousand bikers, including a lot of families. Christopher is already getting in shape to participate in this fitness parade of bikes.

FAMILY BIKING

When should your family start biking together? Bring them along for the ride as infants so they'll grow up in an exercise environment. The Bicycle Federation of America suggests that your child be at least eight months old before you take him or her along on a seat securely attached over the rear wheel of your bike or in a bicycle trailer towed behind you.

Child seats: Your child's neck must be strong enough to support his or her head wearing a helmet. A quality helmet is *essential*. This is not a place to save money.

Make certain that your child's seat has a high back for support, a sturdy seat belt and shoulder harness, and guards to prevent his or her feet from becoming entangled in the wheel. As with the helmet, this is essential equipment and not the place to save a few bucks. Buy quality.

Remember: Be extra careful with your child riding behind you. Avoid heavy traffic—cars, bikers, crowds—and ride slower, smoother, and with control. Also be aware that your bicycle won't maneuver as easily with the added weight of your child.

By introducing your child to biking around age one—in a bike seat, wearing a helmet—your child should grow up knowing that bicycling can be fun and safe. Eventually you will find the little rascal standing up back there. It's time for her own bike. As I detailed above, there is a somewhat set order for children and bikes. I leave the age to start and to switch bikes up to you. This will depend on the child's size, skill, desire, and the safety of your biking routes. I do suggest that age ten to twelve is generally safe for your kids to bike along with you more or less on their own.

Your local bike shop will know about bike paths where your family can ride without fear of car traffic. Start with short biking trips together, perhaps to the grocery and back. Work up to extended trips of several hours if your kids enjoy this. (Be sure to bring along beverages and perhaps some light, healthy snacks.) Make the biking goal very clear—"We are going to the store," or, "We are going to do a loop of the park." Kids understand short-term goals better than aimless riding around.

As with any family activity, be sure to adjust the speed of the workout to the fitness level of the slowest member of the group. You may need to sacrifice your fitness workout to the cause of family fun and the fitness of your children.

Let your children help you plan your bike trips: where you go, what to bring, what to eat and drink. Use this experience to teach a little fitness, health, and nutrition to them. What drinks best replenish lost fluids? What foods are good to eat while exercising? Make sure that the distance of the trip is well within your and your child's fitness capacities.

Be prepared to make unplanned stops if the kids see something interesting. You might later organize day trips around a theme—counting wildlife (or cows, horses, sheep) or spotting birds. Many clubs and schools sponsor family bike trips.

For fun, you might want to rent a bicycle-built-for-two. Christopher loves to rent a bicycle carriage in Central Park. The bicycle carriage comes with four wheels, a bench seat, a steering wheel, and an overhead umbrella to shield you from sun and rain. Up to four people can fit in it, and you pump away on pedals located on either side of the steering wheel in a team effort to move along. It's great fun and exercise.

CLOTHING AND ACCESSORIES

Unless you plan to race, keep your clothing to the basics. Wear loose clothing, but avoid any garment that might get caught in the gears of wheels. Don't wear clothing that is too tight, which will be uncomfortable and may cause chafing. You can purchase fancy biker's seamless shorts or tights. The modern, skin-hugging Spandex outfits are expensive, but also comfortable. Cycling shorts should have a soft chamois crotch to absorb perspiration and buffer you from the seat. The mid-thigh cut of cycling shorts helps prevent chafing and the skin-tight fit improves aerodynamics.

A bright-colored T-shirt is fine for your upper body. If you want a fashionable, high-tech look you might buy a biking jersey. The shirt has extra-long tails to prevent it from coming untucked as you ride. It should also have pockets for keys, money, and so forth; cycling shorts do not have pockets.

Finally, a reflector vest is a good investment. It immediately focuses the attention of drivers on you. The easiest to see are those bright orange ones with the yellow horizontal stripes that hunters wear. Any sporting goods shop carries them.

Whatever you choose to wear, in cold weather make sure that it is in layers so you can peel off or replace clothing as your temperature changes. Dress warmly with the inside layer designed to wick off perspiration from your skin. Make sure your head, ears, and hands are protected and that no body parts are exposed to the wind. If you ride in very cold weather, be aware that the wind created by your speed increases the wind-chill factor.

There are other accessories you might consider. Padded, fingerless gloves improve your grip and absorb shock on long trips. Biking shoes have flexible soles to keep your feet from flexing and overworking. Toe clips, as mentioned, hold your feet on the pedals and give you more power through the full range of pushing and pulling. They also increase the work of your quadricep muscles and the muscles in the front of your shins.

Sunglasses or tinted goggles will keep the sun—and bugs—out of your eyes. A basket, saddlebags, or bike rack can be attached to your bike for carrying items on trips or when running errands. If you want to wear a small day pack on your back, try it out first. It may shift your center of gravity and make pedaling trickier. For your long trips, you may want to bring along a patch kit, spare inner tube, a tool kit, and a pump that attaches to the frame of the bike. You may never need them, but if you do, it's nice to have them along. A water bottle attached to the bike will help you keep hydrated on hot days. Finally, you may want to invest in an extra-wide, padded seat if the narrow seat is uncomfortable.

STATIONARY BIKES

If getting out on a bike is difficult, you might want to try an indoor stationary bike. You can regulate your exercise and your heart rate better simply by adjusting the speed and resistance of the pedaling. Modern, high-tech computerized bikes flash your heart rate on a small screen in front of you; they can be programmed to vary the speed and resistance you encounter. Other bikes require you to pump with your arms as you ride, which gives a better aerobic workout, as well as upper-body training.

With an indoor bike, you don't have to slow down for curves or watch out for traffic. You don't have steep uphills, which dramatically increase your pulse, or long downhills which allow your pulse to drop. You are also free from environmental conditions: no wind, heat, sun, rain, or snow. You also avoid dogs. I also advise all of the women runners I coach to get a stationary bike so they can train on days when it's too late to go out and run safely. An added advantage: you can exercise at home while keeping in touch with your family. Christopher plays next to me while I ride.

But indoor biking can be boring: there's no passing scenery and no other cyclists to admire or secretly compete against. You can enliven things a bit by watching television, reading (with a special reading stand), or listening to music. You might program in some interval training: after warming up with five to ten minutes of steady biking, do a series of fast rides for thirty seconds to two minutes, separated by one or two minutes of steady riding.

As I mentioned earlier, rent before you buy. Jack Shepherd rented a stationary bike one winter; he found it boring, too easy, and hard on his back. He switched to a rowing machine and ended up buying it. If you do buy a stationary bicycle, choose one that is stable, strong, with adjustable tension control, a good chain drive, and a flywheel.

If you prefer, you can ride your own outdoor bike inside by getting a wind-load trainer. You remove the front wheel of your outdoor bike and attach the front fork to an upright bar on a wind-load trainer. The real wheel of your bike then rides on a free-moving cylinder connected to bladed fans on each side. As you pedal, the fans are cranked, causing resistance. The faster you pedal, the greater the "wind" created and the harder your workout.

Whatever you decide to do, you will find bicycling a lot of fun, both as a fitness exercise and as a family outing.

Running

17

Running is an extension of walking, a natural movement for adults and kids. To run, however, adults usually have to plan the activity. Kids, especially my kid, seem to be running all the time. Youngsters run as part of play. You would think, therefore, that running would be something we did naturally from childhood until old age.

Running, like walking, is one of the best aerobic activities. You just do your warm-ups and head out the door. You don't need special equipment (like a bike) or facilities (like a pool). Running also requires very little skill compared to swimming or cross-country skiing or ice-skating. Running also burns more calories—about 650 an hour—than any of the other Big Four aerobic activities.

I'm often asked, What's the difference between running and jogging? My answer: They're spelled differently. Some people who run slowly and avoid competition like to call themselves joggers. That's fine with me, as long as they exercise aerobically. Other runners would never call themselves joggers. I call everybody a runner no matter how fast or slow they run.

RUNNING AND CHILDREN

I like to see children exposed to running at an early age, but not forced into it. After all, running is a natural extension of play for them.

Christopher's first race as a runner was a peewee event. He was five years old. I helped organize the New York Road Runners Peewee running program, and he could have participated at age two. He didn't want to, and I didn't force him. In fact, I played down running as an exercise option for him, partly because I was a running author and coach. Still, he went to races with me and enjoyed watching. But I never suggested that he enter.

Finally, one day Christopher asked me if he could run in a race so he could try to win a finisher's ribbon. He did, and loved it. I gave him and all his classmates who ran their first race together one of my old trophies with the new inscription: "Chrissy's First Race." It still occupies a cherished spot in his room.

I told you the story about Christopher training for and running the one-and-a-half-mile loop of the reservoir. He generally prefers running with his classmates and learned to enjoy the one-mile youth runs with the Road Runners. With me he usually only wants to run sprints. He will, however, run races of two to three miles with me because he enjoys the race day excitement. The point is that he prefers running with his classmates. He goes on adventure walks and plays aerobic baseball with me. That's fine. We cannot and must not force our kids to run with us. But we must encourage them to run.

It's also important that kids enjoy running. Otherwise, they will quit this form of exercise. To keep them motivated, parents and teachers need to think like children. That may be my greatest advantage when working with kids. I'm always being told that I act like a seven-year-old (sometimes a two-year-old)! I try to break the boredom of running for kids with their limited attention spans with walking, skipping, hopping, and other fitness games. For very young pre-schoolers, brisk walks and a few dashes let their enthusiasm erupt.

The trick for any age—adults and kids—is to make running fun. This may mean running with one's peers, as Christopher prefers, or as a family group. If you run with kids, follow their lead, and when they want, chase them through fields, pick flowers, and play games along the way. Older children, like adults, enjoy talking during the run to pass the time. A good thirty-minute conversation is a great way to find out what your child is doing and thinking—and both of you will be surprised how fast the run will go.

Baby-carriage running. When Christopher was born, Virginia and I let our exercise drop to almost zero. We spent our time living for the baby. Then we discovered baby-carriage running. We could be together, although Chrissy often slept through the four-mile loop of Central Park. Cameras clicked, and people said: "Look at that family running together!" We were a novelty back then; now I see baby-carriage runners every day in the park.

If you have a baby, don't give up running. Put the little nipper in a baby carriage, and push him or her around your favorite running route. Baby-carriage running is a great way for beginner runners to start out or for mothers who stopped running temporarily to get back into the activity. Start with brisk walking while pushing the carriage. The resistance of the carriage will push up your heart rate. Then, alternate slow jogging with walking until you can run pushing the carriage for twenty minutes without stopping.

Run at the same heart rate you would maintain if you weren't pushing a carriage. You can also do some speed work while pushing the baby and carriage uphill. You'll find that the increased weight will make you work a lot harder.

Here are some tips:

- Use only a well-made carriage with good shock absorption. Do not use lightweight, collapsible strollers. The front wheels may catch in a crack and catapult both baby and running parent. Strap your baby in with a full harness. Specially designed carriages are available for running with your baby, such as the Baby Jogger we used (Racing Strollers, Inc., P.O. Box 9681, Yakima, Washington, 98909).
- Run at a slow, comfortable pace. Walk down steep hills and stop if there is any danger.
- Adjust the carriage handles to fit your height. Increase baby's comfort by shifting the child to different positions during the run.
- Be sure to bring extra clothing with you to keep you both comfortable, and include a supply of diapers.
- The best time to run is right before baby's nap. When baby wakes, perhaps during the run, talk to him or her and point out interesting objects along the way. If you wish, pause and let baby out for a crawl. By the time Christopher was a year old, we often had to stop and let him out for his own run.
- DO NOT run in races pushing your child in a carriage. Show him or her off before or after your race, but don't endanger the safety of your child or other runners by competing for attention rather than concentrating on your performance. I've even seen fathers finish the New York City Marathon while pushing a stroller. The crowd thought it was cute. I thought it was irresponsible. Most race directors around the country have outlawed this practice in the interest of safety.

STARTING THE KIDS RUNNING

Let the child decide—like mine did, and still does—when and how often he or she wants to run. Don't push them. Make the early experience positive, successful, and fun. They might want to run for several days and then move on to other activities, returning on and off to running. As long as they are exercising and happy, you should be satisfied. Focus the running on your child's needs, not yours.

The best way for parents to introduce children to running is to make it a natural part of their play. Let them run after you while playing baseball or going up and down hills while playing hide-and-seek in the park. Take running breaks while walking briskly to the playground or home from school. Very few young children will enjoy running for distance, so don't force them. Use your imagination to integrate running into your child's play.

Pre-school Running Tips

For kids two to five, most running is just playtime activity. And it should be. Even at this age parents can get too involved and push their kids to compete against their peers. Let the kids exercise for themselves, not you.

I remember two experiences that illustrate the lack of competitive instinct in pre-schoolers. In 1973, I directed a youth track program in Rome, New York, and we had more than three hundred kids participating in a big meet under the lights at the high-school stadium before a large crowd. About twenty little kids lined up for the "Peewee 440." They really didn't understand what all the commotion was about, but they liked the excitement. When the race started, many parents ran along cheering madly for their little ones. Less than a hundred yards into the race, however, the lead runners discovered the long-jump pit along the edge of the track and naturally assumed it was a sandbox. That was the end of the race; all the kids stopped to play in the sand.

As a five-year-old, Christopher bolted off the starting line for one of the peewee events in Central Park. He was in second place and I was biting my tongue when he suddenly stopped and looked back. Over half the runners went by while he searched for and then waved to his little friend David Pena, who was running his first race. They held hands all the way to the finish line. When I asked Christopher why he had stopped, he replied: "I was worried that David would get lost and anyway it was more fun running with my friend."

If the kids want to run, encourage pre-schoolers to sprint short distances—maybe a few yards on a track to a sandbox. Four- and five-year-olds may enjoy running around the block or the local track. Praise them for trying, no matter how fast or slow they run, or how many times they stop. Run against them, letting them beat you to boost their self-esteem. The goal is to establish in their minds that running and exercise are good for them and fun for the whole family. Sometimes a good book helps. A wonderful book that Christopher loved as a pre-schooler and still reads is *The Adventures of Albert the Running Bear* by Barbara Isenberg and Susan Wolf. I won't give the plot away, but Albert gets fat on junk food, escapes from the zoo when his supply is cut off, and gets caught up in the excitement of the New York City Marathon. Then . . .

The New York Road Runners Club's Peewee running program was born with Christopher in 1981. In fact, he "ran" our first event at age one month—in the baby carriage with his father and grandfather on Father's Day. No, I'm not contradicting my earlier statement on this subject. We walked briskly and ran slowly as a fun run with other parents pushing carriages.

Our peewee program is designed to develop an awareness and joy of running for pre-schoolers. The program has attracted as many as 300 peewee runners to the dozen events the NYRRC hosts each year, usually before adult races. We divide the kids into three groups: age two and under run fifty to one hundred yards; ages three and four run two hundred yards; ages five and six run three hundred yards. The shorter the distance the better, since the object is not fitness but developing a feeling that running is fun and something that adults encourage. Parents cheer (and some run along with the youngest kids). At the finish line everyone is a winner; each kid gets a ribbon (a different color for each event to make their collection brighter!).

As this book was being completed, Christopher and I served as spokespersons for the Post Raisin Bran Peewee Run in Central Park. We led three hundred kids through some of the exercises described in Chapter 13 and then walked them to the starting line imitating the California Raisins. The experience was a happy one as the youngsters were made aware that running is fun. It was so successful that a half dozen of these events were scheduled to be sponsored for 1989.

See Chapter 20 for further fitness tips for pre-schoolers.

Elementary School Age Tips

Attitudes about fitness and exercise are established primarily in this age group. Fitness running should be emphasized for most kids of this age, and controlled competition can be introduced for some at around age ten. My preference for this age is to limit their fitness runs to one to four miles. Again, let your child make the choices here.

Here's a tip for running with young children: Keep talking to them to keep their minds off when it is time to stop running. Play games you make up on the run, discuss their favorite toys, vacation plans, etc. Encourage these children to participate in activities with a lot of running (but don't tell them that's why they should do these things): soccer, lacrosse, even singles tennis. They should be encouraged to try other aerobic activities, such as ice-skating, cross-country skiing, biking, and swimming.

I'll tell you a secret here. Christopher completed both a two-mile and

five-kilometer fun run with me without doing any formal running during
his summer vacation. How? First of all he had built up a good running
fitness level during the school year having fun running in his P.E. classes
with his friends. The summer was so hot that he didn't want to go
"running." No problem. He ran and walked briskly so much in his daily
play—including running for hours under the sprinkler in the park—that
he easily maintained the running fitness established in his school program.

As the peewees in our New York Road Runners Club program, including
Christopher and his buddies, outgrew our age-six-and-under program, we
looked for a low-key fitness challenge to condition them aerobically. In
1988, a series of one-mile youth fitness runs was developed and tested.
Christopher's response to his first race beyond the peewee distances:
"Great!" These runs were so successful that Post Raisin Bran now sponsors
them six times a year for youth ages six to eighteen. These, too, are held
prior to adult events, thus gathering a large and enthusiastic audience. This
is a non-competitive event with all finishers receiving the same ribbon.
Children may stop at the half-mile turnaround point and receive a participant's ribbon for that distance if they don't feel ready to complete the full
mile. Most of the kids are motivated to keep going. We encourage them
to take as many walk breaks as they like in order to finish and earn the
one-mile finisher's ribbon. A digital clock at the finish line lets the kids
compare (if they wish) their times to the health-related fitness standards
described in Chapter 4. In our first trial event we had seventy-five kids
complete the mile, including twenty-five physically disabled "runners"
from the Achilles Track Club. We have over three hundred disabled youths
of this age in that NYRRC program, which is conducted with the New York
City public schools.

Tips for Teenage Runners

Teenagers vary greatly in size and growth rates. The simple point is
this: Kids in this age group change physically and emotionally almost
week by week, and this will affect every aspect of their lives, including
their running.

Teenagers at every athletic level should get plenty of praise and encouragement. They have fragile egos, and, as mentioned above, they can
grow and change, and anyone who makes a judgment about them last
month may look foolish next month.

Running is an excellent form of exercise for teenagers. It helps them
learn to set and attain goals, and it helps develop them physically.

Training for Elementary Age and Teenagers

Teenagers who start running for fitness can follow the same program described for adults in this chapter. Elementary age children may also be able to do the ten-week beginner's program described.

To be effective, a parent or teacher must keep the program interesting and the kids focused and disciplined. It is my experience that youngsters are better motivated if they run for distance, not time. Tangible goals are necessary for these kids. Children in kindergarten through the third grade should build gradually to ten minutes of running—about one mile. Kids in grades four through six should build to twenty minutes of running, or about two miles.

To start them training, have the kids run half-laps on a 440-yard track, or about 220 yards if you don't have access to a track. Let them walk/run and repeat the lap again. They should keep moving until they have completed a half-mile of running and walking. This should give them a sense of accomplishment.

After two weeks, have the children run three-quarters of a mile (again, taking walk breaks as needed). A week or two after that, have them try a full mile on the track. Next, work to extend the run to twenty minutes if they are interested.

If you can get the kids to enjoy running a half-mile to a mile regularly, even if they don't last twenty minutes, then you are achieving fitness gains and helping them to learn a lifetime exercise option. Two good minimal goals for kids are: running for twenty minutes nonstop; and, meeting the AAHPERD's one-mile run health fitness standards for the various age groups. (See charts in Chapter 4.)

Where to Run

Kids, and perhaps especially teenagers, may not want to run where neighbors and friends might see them. Your local park may be best, or a nearby track. Parents have told me stories of taking their young children to a nearby high-school track, and letting them play in the middle while the parents ran. Before long, the children joined them to copy Mom and Dad.

Kids seem to like ovals small enough to see around. They may feel secure knowing exactly how far they will be running. Also, on a track, each family member can work out at various paces and yet be together— see each other—and encourage one another as they pass back and forth. With young kids, of course, one parent (or two, alternating) may have to spend time with an easily bored young child/runner.

On the road, I would avoid running where my child has to compete with traffic. As you and your child get better (and older), you may run at different times and places. If your youngster wants to run outside the safety of a track, you might accompany him or her on your bike if you can't keep up running. Also, I've seen parents running in the park with their kids alongside riding bikes.

How Fast?

One rule you should always follow: Run at the pace of the slowest runner. A sure way to discourage family members is to run off and leave them or to keep pushing them to a pace beyond their training. Run a step or two behind the slowest runner in the group. You should also always exercise at a conversational pace and that includes the slowest member of your group (faster runners can get their aerobic workout later). The goal of family running is fun and unity.

Parental Competition

The worst thing that can happen between parent and child is competitiveness. Sometimes, your child may sense that he or she is good enough to compete against you during your training runs together. End this immediately. We all run only against ourselves.

Even now, I have to hold back to stay at Christopher's pace and not force him into running too fast. I let him get about a half-step ahead so he has a sense of controlling the speed. He likes to sprint at the end and beat me. It makes him feel good. As he gets older and faster, and I get older and slower, I'll have to hold off the urge to get competitive with him. Maybe he'll let me run a few paces ahead of him sometimes, to set the pace, and sprint at the end—just to even things off.

Parents who are runners, especially serious competitors, must understand the danger of their role model backfiring—turning off their child from running and exercise. I think it's best to keep your running/training separate from your family and child. Run with them for fun only. Don't suggest that they train with you. Let the kids stretch with you before and after your runs. But that's all.

Also, stop complaining about your training injuries and aches and pains in front of your family. Who wants to hear all that? Serious runners love to complain, and serious kids don't like to hear it! Kids should learn that running at certain levels is injury free and fun.

RUNNING THE RIGHT WAY

Most children naturally run with good form. Adults, however, often have to re-learn how to run properly. Yet teaching running is a little like teaching bike riding. It's easier to do than to describe.

Basically, you run the way you walk, using a heel-to-toe motion. You gently land on your heel and roll forward to the ball of the foot before pushing off. You should not land and bounce on your toes. That places too much stress on your lower legs. Nor should you land hard on your heels. That will put too much stress on your back.

Your lead foot, after it has stretched forward and started to swing back, should strike the ground more or less directly under your hip. Push with the rear foot, don't reach with the front one. Don't overstride (take too long a stride). That is inefficient and may cause injury. You'll get the best results when you concentrate on lifting your knee just enough to allow your leg to swing forward naturally. Combined with a gentle heel landing, this will give you an economical yet productive stride.

Allow your body to move as freely as possible. Hold your head high, your eyes focused directly ahead, and keep your back straight. By "tucking in" your buttocks, you can run in an erect, comfortable position. Leaning too far forward or leaning too far back is inefficient and may cause injury. It will also, over time, be uncomfortable. Your shoulders should hang loose, parallel to the ground. Don't stick your chest forward or throw back your shoulders. Try to make the position and movement as natural as you can, so that after a while you simply forget about all of these things; you just do them.

The arms balance a runner. The left arm moving downward balances the right leg lifting forward; the right arm moving downward balances the left leg lifting forward. If you carry your arms too high or too low or move them across your body, you will lose good forward movement and efficiency.

The best arm position is fairly low. Your hands should be somewhere between your waistline and chest. At the midpoint of your stride, your forearms, wrists, and hands should be parallel to the ground. During the forward swing, your forearm moves slightly upward and inward; during the backward swing it moves slightly downward and outward.

The fingers of your hands should be cupped loosely, your wrist firm but not locked, your palms turned slightly upward, thumbs resting comfortably on the fingers. Some runners make a small circle with their thumbs and first two fingers. Others let the thumb gently touch the edge of their first finger. Again, try out different ways of holding your hands until one way feels natural.

Breathing properly helps you run better. When you run, you should get as much air into your lungs as possible. The best method to use is "belly breathing," which is nothing more than breathing so your stomach expands outward with each inhaled breath. Take air in any way you can—through the mouth and nose. Belly breathing is important, because it helps stretch muscles that cause the dreaded runner's side stitch.

Having read all of this, forget it! The most important thing to do is to run relaxed. If you feel comfortable when you run, then you are running correctly. More detailed information on running form is available in *The Runner's Handbook*. For a quick lesson, watch a child run—most of them have almost perfect form. Somehow, we adults unlearn this gift.

EQUIPMENT

All you need is a good pair of running shoes. The best shoes provide cushioning, flexibility, and comfort for your feet. Your best bet is to go to a store that specializes in running shoes or athletic equipment.

Children do not need special running shoes if they are just running in short bursts of energy during play. If they start running more than a mile, they should have running shoes to cushion the impact of feet striking a hard surface; all runners hit the ground with about three times the force of their body weight.

When you or your child run in cold weather, be sure to wear layers of clothing and cover your head and hands. Most cold weather runners wear a ski cap and woolen mittens, and then take them off when they get warmed up. In summer, dress in light, bright clothing that will reflect the sun and that is loose-fitting. Be alert to the heat; you may want to change the time of day that you run to take advantage of cooler early morning or late evening temperatures. Stay in the shade, avoid the hottest part of the day, drink plenty of fluids (hydrate yourself) during and after your runs, slow your pace and walk if you get fatigued or overheated. If it's too hot, you may want to switch to a less demanding or cooler workout, such as walking or biking or swimming, or use an indoor stationary bike, rowing machine, or treadmill.

INJURY PREVENTION

Runners, including children, get injured. Chapter 26 gives you the basic guidelines for preventing and treating injuries and *The Runner's Handbook* includes extensive details on this subject.

Generally, you can minimize injuries as a runner by stretching, warming up, and cooling down properly. Well-cushioned shoes also help prevent injury. Be sure to keep your running shoes in good repair, especially the heels, which tend to wear down. Also, do not try to do too much too soon. Sometimes it is important to slow down, or not to run at all for a day or so. Your cardio-respiratory system can generally handle more than your musculo-skeletal system. So be conservative in your training.

GETTING FIT WITH RUNNING

First, review the exercise principles and warm-up and cool-down routines in Chapter 10 and the FIT aerobic training variables detailed in Chapter 12. These apply to all aerobic activities.

Next, check with your doctor and get his or her approval before you set out. Men over age thirty-five may want to have an exercise stress test to be certain there is no hidden coronary artery or heart disease. Have your doctor also check your child before he or she starts a running program.

Then, get yourselves a good pair of running shoes purchased from a specialty store.

Now, make a commitment to give yourself two months to get into shape and follow one of the training programs described here, which are taken from *The Runner's Handbook*. You may want to add variety to your training by using other aerobic activities. But to improve as a runner you will need to work up to running at least three times a week. Because of the pounding, you probably should run every other day as a beginner, and take it easy on the off day.

My running programs for beginners are for teenagers and adults who have not been physically active and want to ease into running. Some children between the ages of six and twelve may also benefit from these programs if they can follow the guidelines and have strong support from their parents, or the programs are taught in school by a qualified physical fitness instructor.

Start with Walking

Anyone who is elderly, overweight, has joint problems, or has been inactive should start with a walking program before running. Think of this as a pre-conditioning program. Once you can walk for at least thirty minutes at a brisk pace three to five times a week, you are ready to start a gentle running program.

BEGINNER RUNNER

Who is a beginner runner? You are if you cannot run nonstop for twenty consecutive minutes—smiling and talking all the way. Admit it, and get started on your running program.

I use three conservative, progressive methods for starting beginner runners. The first two methods allow you to select how far you run before taking a walk break and give you more flexibility for increasing your run-walk ratio. The third method is for runners who need the discipline and motivation of a precise, structured program. I suggest the third method for most beginner runners.

Method 1: The Twenty-Minute Run-Easy Program

Warm up properly, then walk for five to ten minutes and then alternate walking with running for another twenty minutes. Start your running slowly, taking walk breaks at a fast pace whenever you need to slow down. The signal for this may be shortness of breath, weakness in your legs, and so forth.

Be conservative. Take several walk breaks during your twenty-minute run and resume running only when your body is ready. Don't stop moving. The goal is to alternate brisk walking with slow running (but running with your heart rate in your training range). Walking too slowly may lower your heart rate out of your aerobic training range, in which case you'll get fewer fitness benefits.

Over a period of several weeks, shift the walk-run ratio so you are progressively running more and walking less. Your goal is to run for the full twenty minutes nonstop and at a conversation pace.

Don't try to run a specific distance at first (like a mile) or see how far you can run. This puts too much pressure on you and may cause injury. Since you are exercising within a time measurement—twenty minutes— it doesn't matter how far you run. Your goal is to keep your heart rate within your training range for twenty minutes. You do this by walking-running, and over several weeks you shift your training from mostly walking to mostly running, and then to nonstop running.

How many minutes you can run at one time and how long it takes you to build to that twenty nonstop minutes depend on many factors: your age, previous athletic experience, body weight, weather conditions, and so forth. Most beginner runners take eight to ten weeks to run twenty continuous minutes. Be patient.

Method 2: The One-and-a-Half–Mile Run-Easy Program

This method is the same as the previous one, with a minor difference. Instead of alternating running and walking for *time* you alternate running and walking for *distance*. In this method, that distance approximates twenty to thirty minutes in time.

I use this method for people who "see" distance better than time. (This is especially true for kids.) For example, the one-and-a-half–mile loop of the reservoir in New York's Central Park is an excellent goal for beginner runners. The day they complete the loop nonstop, you can hear whoops of joy throughout the park. If you prefer distance to time, here are some suggestions:

- Walk and run a measured loop in a local park.
- Or, walk/run from your house to a friend's house.
- Walk/run a specific number of laps at a local high-school or college track.
- Walk/run a measured loop or an out-back course in your neighborhood.

Caution: Do not combine time with distance yet. That's racing. Either run for twenty to thirty minutes, or a distance that approximates that time (perhaps one-and-a-half to two miles). If you start timing your runs each day to see how fast you are running, you will be racing yourself. This may pressure you to run faster than a conversational pace or run too long before taking walk breaks.

Method 3: The New York Road Runners Club Run-Easy Program

This is a structured program I developed for my New York Road Runners Club classes. It's ridiculously easy. We start out running only one minute at a time! It has not only been effective for adults, but also for a number of nine- to twelve-year-olds and teens who have taken the class with their parents.

True, most of you can run more than that at first. But we start running for just one minute. Very gradually, we increase that amount to twenty minutes of continuous running—a level that comes after ten weeks.

By taking it easy, we cut to almost zero the chances of being hurt—or discouraged. Each week you improve, and you discover that less is more: by running less than you can each week, you make it easier to run more week after week.

The following schedule should be run at least three times a week. All running should be done at a conversational pace, and all walking should be done briskly. Of course, warm up and cool down properly.

You can even fall a little behind and still get back on schedule easily. Once you reach the halfway mark, however, you will find it difficult to keep up unless you run faithfully at least three and preferably five times a week. If you cannot keep up, or lose time because of illness or injury, don't panic. Stay at the level you can handle (or go back a level) until you are ready to move up. You may take twelve to fifteen weeks to reach twenty nonstop minutes of running. So what! Just remember how many years it took you to get out of shape. Now, take your time getting back into it.

If you find the program too easy, adjust by moving up to a level that is more difficult for you, and continue from there. Don't try to go too far too fast. Your goal is running for twenty minutes nonstop—smiling and talking all the way.

TEN-WEEK BEGINNER'S RUNNING PROGRAM

Week #	Run-Walk Ratio (20-Minute Total)	Total Run Time
1	Run 1 minute, walk 2 minutes—do 6 sets, followed by running 1 minute	7 min
2	Run 1 minute, walk 1 minute—do 10 sets	10 min
3	Run 2 minutes, walk 1 minute—do 6 sets, followed by running 2 minutes	14 min
4	Run 3 minutes, walk 1 minute—do 5 sets	15 min
5	Run 4 minutes, walk 1 minute—do 4 sets	16 min
6	Run 5 minutes, walk 1 minute—do 3 sets, followed by running 2 minutes	17 min
7	Run 6 minutes, walk 1 minute—do 3 sets	18 min
8	Run 8 minutes, walk 1 minute—do 2 sets, followed by running 2 minutes	18 min
9	Run 10 minutes, walk 1 minute—do 2 sets	20 min
10	Run 20 minutes nonstop	20 min

ADVANCED BEGINNER

You are an advanced beginner when you can run twenty minutes nonstop—and finish smiling.

After you can run nonstop for twenty minutes, stay at this level. Run for twenty minutes each time, three to five times a week, for three to four weeks. You are putting minutes (miles) in the bank, as runners say.

You may have started in the beginner program, and progressed to this level. Or you may have been doing some running, or other aerobic exercise, and feel comfortable starting at this level. Don't push it. I cannot stress too much: Do not start at this level to inflate your ego. You will deflate all too soon—and probably quit.

For increased fitness, you may wish to progress to thirty minutes nonstop running by following this four-week program:

Week	Run
1	22 minutes nonstop, at least three to five times a week
2	25
3	27
4	30

When you reach thirty minutes, three to five times a week, pause. Hold your running at this level for at least three to four weeks, and put more miles in your running bank. What's the point of rushing now, anyway? Why risk fatigue, boredom, or injury?

INTERMEDIATE RUNNER

This is a runner who can run for thirty nonstop minutes at a comfortable pace at least three to five times a week.

If you can do this—and I said comfortable pace!—you might want to start adding a few runs that are longer than thirty minutes. and switch to counting miles instead of minutes.

Go easy here. This is a serious and important transition. Keep your easy days to thirty minutes per run (about two to three miles). Add one or two days a week of longer runs (four to six miles). Here is a typical four-week progression:

Week	Mon.	Tues.	Wed.	Thurs.	Fri.	Sat.	Sun.	Total
1	2	3	2	2	Off	4	2	15
2	2	3	2	3	Off	4	3	17
3	2	4	2	3	Off	5	3	19
4	3	4	3	3	Off	5	3	21

Never increase your mileage by more than 10 percent a week. This is a basic rule for *all* runners at all levels. Alternate long runs, which are stressful, with shorter runs. After reaching fifteen to twenty minutes a week on a regular basis, you may want to prepare for your first race.

Remember: Once you reach the intermediate level, you can run for thirty minutes at least three times a week. You do not need to progress any further. You have achieved the basic level of fitness I have been talking about in this book. Many runners do advance. But at this level, you can run for fun—sightsee in any city you visit, run with friends, join a running club and its workouts, or just enjoy the running experience.

FUN RACING AND COMPETITION

After running for a few months, you might want to enter a race just for fun. Consider it your next fitness challenge. If you can comfortably run for twenty to thirty minutes three to five times a week, you can complete races of 10 kilometers (6.2 miles) or less for adults, five kilometers (3.1 miles) or less for children.

Many people run these races for fun and talk throughout the event. Look for a "family fun run" where the entire family can run the distance together, or split up to each run at your own pace or distance. Be sure to regroup at the finish line and compare notes. The goal of the Post Raisin Bran Family Fitness Festival, which I developed for cities around the country, is to highlight the value of families sharing the experience of fitness running and fun racing. In some cases the kids run first for short distances while the parents cheer them on and then the parents run longer distances while the kids support them. For others, the entire family runs or walks together for two miles. I love watching families run together in these events, talking and laughing. Some wear family "team" uniforms of colorful shirts emblazoned with logos like "The family that runs together, stays together," "Mom," "Dad," and "Kids," their names or funny sayings.

Let me tell you a typical story. Christopher liked his first one-mile youth run with the New York Road Runners Club because, he said, he got to run with lots of other kids and earned a nice ribbon. When I showed him the application for the final one-miler of the season, he said he wanted to run it, too. Then he noticed on the application that there was a two-mile run and he asked if he could run that. I told him that this event was mostly for adults, but that some kids would probably want to run the longer distance with their parents.

"Yeah, that's what I want to do," he said. "Will you run with me, Dad, please?" Remember that he never before wanted to run with me—just his friends. The prospect of running in an event with his dad was very exciting to him.

On race day, we lined up in the back row for the two-mile event. I had a special job: "water boy." I had to run along with the water bottle and pour water on Christopher's head whenever he "dinged me"—a little game he played to keep the run interesting for him. He would sneak up on me and pull on my arm as the secret signal for me to pour water over his head, getting him all wet—kids love to get wet.

I made sure that we were in last place when the race started to make the event less pressured for him. After the start, we talked and talked, laughed and laughed, and ran at a steady ten-minute-per-mile pace. Whenever he got bored, he would signal for another dousing of water. Along the way we passed several families running together and exchanged greetings. We passed the mile in ten minutes—a good effort for a seven-year-old—and I tried to encourage Christopher to take a walk break. He was determined to run nonstop. We continued passing runners—mostly adults—which added to his confidence (the reason I made sure we started last so that we would be passing runners rather than being passed along the way). We passed over three hundred runners. "That was one of the fun parts," Christopher said later.

At the finish, the race announcer called out his name: "Here comes Christopher Glover, age seven, and his dad." The crowd cheered and Christopher smiled proudly as he crossed in 20:10. When asked what he liked best about his first two-miler, he said: "Running with you, Dad." How's that for a family fitness reward!

A month later Christopher and I enjoyed another fun run experience. As part of a Post Raisin Bran Family Fitness event in Central Park, a five-kilometer family run was conducted. To further test the concept of family running for this book, I invited the daughter of one of the top marathon runners I coach (Stephanie Kessler) to participate with Christopher and me. Jaclyn, age six, was accompanied by her grandfather and was very excited about her first race. Christopher, who met her for the first time at the starting line, quickly took a liking to her and as an experienced racer gave her tips on pacing. They both ran the entire 3.1 mile race without stopping, talking all the way. Halfway through the race Jaclyn asked Christopher for a date. Afterward, Christopher said: "Dad, how come we ran three miles and it only seemed like a mile?" They were so busy having fun that the distance went by very quickly.

Adults may want to train to improve their time over a certain race distance, or increase their race distance after enjoying a few fun runs. The goal of improving your race performance can serve as the motivating factor to keep you exercising and in good shape. *The New Competitive Runner's Handbook* contains detailed training programs for all levels of runners from first-time racers to marathon veterans.

COMPETITION FOR KIDS

But what about competition for the kids? The American Academy of Pediatrics recommends that pre-adolescent children not run long-distance races held primarily for adults. I strongly agree. Unless it is a low-key fun run for families (as described above), let the kids run against each other, not adults. Family fun participation in races can extend up to five kilometers—my limit for Christopher—for ages six through nine, and up to ten kilometers for ages ten through twelve, as long as the children are properly trained, well supervised by an adult running with them, and don't attempt to race competitively. Additionally, the adult running with the child should be there to provide support, not attempt to push the child to run faster. Run at the pace which the child chooses—and take as many walk breaks as they wish to make. One additional rule: Participation in the event should be the kid's idea of fun, not just the parent's.

A few running clubs exist for young children. Some are good, some are bad. Don't allow your child to join one unless he or she really loves to run and wants to learn how to compete. Make sure the competition doesn't get out of hand and that the coaches emphasize sportsmanship and self-improvement, not just winning. I have enjoyed coaching youth running teams in the past, and as this book went to press I organized a team of seven- and eight-year-old boys as an informal program through Christopher's school. The boys trained once a week with me as part of our Sports Club program by running a mile, and trained twice a week by running with their regular P.E. classes. The New York Road Runners Club conducts the National Road Runners Club Age Group Cross-Country Championship each fall and we used this event as our program goal. The children are divided into events by two-year age groups, starting with the sub-bantam division for seven- and eight-year-olds who run one-and-a-half miles. The boys enjoyed running as a team under the direction of their school coach. Competing against teams that held regular, serious practices, the Allen-Stevenson School boys won the team title.

It is important to point out that the boys we coached in this program started as fitness runners. We only recruited them for mild competition after they expressed a desire for more of a challenge. I prefer low-key competition for pre-adolescent children to organized running teams. More important in the "long run" are the fun and fitness aspects of running, not competition.

Teenagers may choose to participate on their junior-high or high-school cross-country or track teams and should be encouraged to do so. Others will choose to enjoy a few local road races rather than compete on a team. Teens should be encouraged to learn how to run fast over short distances. They should concentrate on the distances run by their school's team: one hundred yards to two miles. Detailed training guidelines for youth competition for the one-mile track event and cross-country running are included in *The New Competitive Runner's Handbook*. Older teenagers have increased stamina over long distances and may compete on a low-key basis in road races up to 10 kilometers. I do not recommend marathon training and racing until the late teenage years or older, when young men and women are better able to handle the training and race distance physically and mentally. This is why the New York City Marathon extended its minimum age from sixteen to eighteen.

RUNNING-BASED FITNESS PROGRAMS FOR KIDS

The key to successful running-based fitness programs is that they stress fun, fitness, and family participation. This is the formula I used to develop the Post Raisin Bran Family Fitness Program. A key ingredient is the Family Fitness Festival, which showcases the comprehensive fitness and nutrition educational program. Our first event was scheduled to kick off in New York City's Central Park in the Spring of 1989, just as this book was released. The NYRRC-directed event offers something for everyone: peewee runs for pre-schoolers, one-mile fitness runs for children, and a two-mile family run/walk for parents, grandparents, teens, and aerobically fit elementary school kids. All youth participants receive equal prizes for finishing: everyone is a winner. Special certificates are awarded to families with three generations of fitness participants. The feeling of parental pride and youth happiness after an event like this is tremendous. The Post Raisin Bran Family Fitness Program will be expanded to include additional cities around the country. For information, contact the New York Road Runners Club, 9 East 89th Street, New York, New York, 10128 (phone number: 212-860-4455).

The National Road Runners Club of America has also been very active in youth fitness. They can provide a promotional package to help you or your local running club start a youth running program. It includes information on several outstanding programs around the country, including Huntsville, Alabama (as many as 3,000 young people participate in one-mile cross-country runs), Long Beach, California (2,500 kids turned out for a 2.62-kilometer run), and the biggest kids' race of them all—the Junior Bloomsday one- and two-mile runs in Spokane, Washington (do you believe ten thousand kids in one event!). All of these programs include a training program coordinated between the local running club and the area schools. For further information contact: Henley Gibble, President, RRCA, 629 S. Washington Street, Alexandria, Virginia, 22314 (phone: 703-836-0558).

Swimming

Swimming is one of the best aerobic exercises. It uses all of the major muscle groups of your body and provides a total fitness workout. Plus— no sweat! The movement of your arms and legs against the resistance of the water also improves the muscular strength and endurance of your whole body—arms, shoulders, abdominals, hips, legs, and ankles. The long, sinuous movement of swimming improves range of motion and flexibility. Also, swimming burns about six hundred calories an hour—depending on your stroke, speed, and skill as a swimmer—and thus improves body composition.

Swimming is especially beneficial if you are overweight, have orthopedic or other problems that prevent you from doing other forms of aerobic exercise, or are pregnant or getting back in shape after childbirth. Because you are suspended in water, there is no stress on your joints and muscles. For these reasons, swimming is an excellent option if injury prevents you from enjoying weight-bearing exercise such as running.

There are, of course, disadvantages to swimming. First, you need a place to swim. Second, you need to know how to swim. Third, in order to exercise aerobically, you have to take the time to master certain swimming skills. Finally, there is the question of safety. You need to be concerned about yourself and/or your child in the water, be vigilant, and be careful. I will discuss equipment, facilities, and safety guidelines in a moment.

SWIMMING FOR KIDS

Kids know how to have fun in the water. They can run, dive, and spash around for more than an hour in virtual nonstop physical activity. It may not be continuous aerobic action, but their enthusiastic physical activity is vigorous enough to give them a good workout. Certainly the arm and leg action against the resistance of the water contributes to muscle fitness and growth.

How soon should your child start swimming?

From six to fifteen months is a good time to introduce your children to the water. They are uninhibited, yet coordinated enough to enjoy themselves. Keep them in very shallow water—no deeper than six to ten inches—and stay close at hand and hold onto them. Let them kick their feet, splash, fall down, and make a lot of noise, and sit down in the water to "patty-cake" the surface.

Swimming for pre-schoolers? Kids seem to be ready to learn swimming at various ages. Christopher started a local "water babies" class with his mother when he was one year old. We wanted him to start feeling comfortable in the water, but not to swim yet. Most kids are ready for lessons between the ages of three and five. They have the motor skills to learn the leg and arm rhythms, and they know to be cautious. Swimming programs for children under age three are not recommended by the American Academy of Pediatrics or the National YMCA.

Babies in diapers can spread infections in swimming pools; they can also get viruses that cause diarrhea or get water intoxication and convulsions from swallowing too much water.

The Y recommends water fun and water adjustment classes for kids under three years old. For ages three to six, the Y suggests classes where the emphasis is on fun and safety. Pre-schoolers and young children not yet able to swim may use a flotation device when in the water. As a two-year-old, Christopher used a small, padded bubble that tied under his arms and around his chest. He would paddle and kick around shallow water for hours. We kept our eyes on him and one of us stayed close by. But he got the feeling of freedom and movement in the water, which was an important foundation for later swimming lessons. It also enabled him to get a lot of fun exercise.

Don't rush your child into the water or into learning to swim. The old 1960s method of so-called "drown-proofing" kids by getting them into deep water at a very early age has been debunked. Marilyn Segal, Ph.D., director of the Family Center at Nova University in Ft. Lauderdale, Florida, told *Children Magazine:* "The research coming out is showing that the earlier you teach the child to swim, the greater the chances of the child drowning. That's because the child who has been a great little swimmer is going to lose that natural sense of fear. Add to this the fact that his or her parents may not be as vigilant. No child is ever really safe around the water."

Older children as swimmers. Older children, above the age of thirteen, may want to follow the aerobic swimming program in this chapter (above). Most kids, however, will find it boring to swim lap after lap just to stay in shape. Participation in a swim team will give them incentive to swim for conditioning and meets.

At Christopher's school, the grade-schoolers swim twice a week in winter. They get instruction, lap swimming, and free time. They are motivated to swim aerobically by keeping a record of laps completed in order to qualify for the "100 Lap Club." Other swimming clubs and teams chart their laps as miles, and put their mileage on maps of the Atlantic or Pacific oceans. As with any physical activity, use of the imagination can result in both fun and fitness.

As with any aerobic sport, your child's progress should be measured by improved times (and thus fitness) rather than just their competitive place. Properly supervised, school (or community) swimming teams are a great way for older kids to enjoy team sports while establishing a base for lifetime fitness.

COMPETITIVE SWIMMING

Local swimming clubs, Y's, community organizations, and some schools offer competitive swimming teams for children of all ages, and even masters swimming for men and women. Like competitive running, these clubs and events can serve as motivators to keep you or your children working out and in shape. But remember, you need to swim only for twenty to thirty minutes three times a week for fitness—anything beyond that is for performance.

Competitive swimming on junior and senior high-school teams is a great option for your child. He or she can enjoy a team sport while building a base of fitness for life. Competitive swimming for grade-school children is all right, as long as they really want to do it and they aren't overworked by win-at-any-cost coaches.

WATER EXERCISE

Even if you cannot swim a stroke, you can get in shape with aerobic exercising in the water. Classes such as Watercise and Water Aerobics put non-swimmers in shallow water. The classes use movement to music and water resistance to create aerobic conditioning, while also increasing muscle strength and flexibility. *Donna DeVarona's Hydro-Aerobics* details an excellent program you and your children can use in any shallow body of water.

SAFETY GUIDELINES

Water is essential to life, and a threat. Here are some points to remember:

- Don't let young children play in or near water without adult supervision.
- Observe water-depth signs. Don't get in over your head if you aren't a good swimmer.
- Don't be a show-off. Don't let the peer pressure get you in trouble. Stress this to your children—especially teenagers. If you get in over your head running, your body forces you to stop. With swimming, you can drown.
- Don't depend totally on a lifeguard to protect your children; be your own lifeguard and use the "buddy system." Each young swimmer should have a "buddy" in the water or near him or her. Half of all drownings occur when someone swims alone.
- Never drink alcoholic beverages before swimming.
- When swimming in an ocean, lake, or river, know the bottom and don't underestimate your distance from shore. Check with the lifeguard or beach patrol about tides, currents, depths, and natural dangers such as sharks, jellyfish, or other critters.
- When there is a designated roped-off area, always stay within it; it has a purpose (to protect swimmers from motorboats, for example).
- Always look before you dive. Diving into shallow water is very dangerous. Save diving for designated areas. If in doubt, walk into the water, or jump feet first. When floating in a river on a raft, always head downriver feet first so you can see where you are headed.
- Don't swim after dark unless there is a lighted, after-dark swimming area with a lifeguard on duty.
- Don't eat a large meal before swimming. You may get stomach cramps.
- If you are swimming and start to feel very cold—numbness in your fingers and toes—it may be a warning sign of hypothermia. Get out of the water, dry off, and put on warm, dry clothing. Leave the water immediately if you feel anything unusual happening to your body: cramps, nausea, dizziness, chest pains or tightness, or difficulty breathing.
- In case of emergency, notify the lifeguard immediately. Don't try to be a hero and make a rescue yourself, unless you are the lifeguard of last resort. You can help with rescues without swimming by offering a pole, branch, or towel to the person having difficulty in the water. Or you can toss them a life preserver.

You and your family may want to take some water safety courses at your local YMCA or community organization. You might also want to take courses in CPR (cardiopulmonary resuscitation), offered in almost every community.

GETTING FIT WITH SWIMMING

Before diving in, review the FIT aerobic training variables in Chapter 12, and the exercise principles, including the warm-up and cool-down routines, in Chapter 10.

If you already know how to swim, give yourself about two months to get into shape. Check with your doctor, and then follow the training program below. This training program is for adults and teenagers. Some pre-teen kids will benefit from this program if they are mature enough to follow the guidelines and have sufficient parental support, or if the program is offered by a school with supervision from a qualified instructor.

Swim-for-Fitness Training Program for Beginners and Intermediates

You can't just jump in the water and splash around and expect to get fit. As with any aerobic program, swimming workouts have to be well designed and done on a regular basis. You have to become a "lap swimmer." You may find it difficult—and boring—to swim nonstop for the minimum of twenty minutes.

Begin your program by alternating swimming with short breaks—short enough to keep your heart rate in your aerobic target zone—for ten to twenty minutes. For example, swim the length of a twenty-five–meter pool and then take an "active rest" break of fifteen to thirty seconds (or up to a minute) by walking in or out of the water, bobbing, or flutter kicking. Keep moving, swimming a lap or two at a time alternating with these short breaks until twenty minutes have elapsed.

You should try to swim fast enough to get a training effect, but slow enough that you don't become fatigued and unable to complete the workout. Gradually increase the number of laps you can swim nonstop until you can swim continuously for twenty minutes. Don't be in a hurry. Depending on your fitness level and your skill as a swimmer, you may take anywhere from four to twelve weeks—two months is average—to reach the nonstop level.

After that, your next goal will be to maintain that level for two to four weeks. Then gradually build—over a period of four to six weeks—to thirty minutes of continuous swimming.

You may prefer to swim for distance rather than time. To do this, you simply count laps. Down and back in your lane is one lap: in a twenty-five–meter pool a complete lap would be fifty meters; five hundred meters (ten laps) is a good goal to aim at for beginners for a single workout and one thousand meters (twenty laps) is a good goal for intermediate swimmers.

THE WARM-UP AND COOL-DOWN

Although swimming at a leisurely pace gently warms up your muscles, it is wise to do some specific stretching exercises to get ready for this workout, as for any other workouts you do. You can follow the general pre-aerobic training program in Chapter 10 or substitute some of the exercises below, recommended for swimmers—many of which can be done while standing in the water. Take five to ten minutes for a pre-swim exercise warm-up. Be sure to stretch your leg muscles and upper-body muscles, which take the most stress from swimming. Take special care to stretch your lower-back muscles, which are used for kicking and pulling. Here are some recommended stretching exercises:

Shoulder and lower back. Stand an arm's length from a wall. Reach up and put your hands on the wall one foot higher than your head. Lean forward and lower your head somewhat between your arms. Hold for ten seconds. Next, bend your knes slightly and hold that position for twenty seconds. Repeat three times.

Shoulder and upper body. Stand up and put your feet about twelve inches apart. Clasp your hands high over your head, and lean slowly to the left, hold for ten seconds, then lean slowly to the right and hold for ten seconds. Repeat three times.

Hamstring. There are several ways of stretching this important muscle. Sit against a wall, legs straight in front of you, grip your right ankle, and slowly pull it toward your left side. Hold for ten seconds. Release. Repeat three times for the right and left ankles.

Or, while standing, pull your right knee to your chest. Hold for ten seconds and release. Repeat with your left knee, and do each leg three times.

Forward bend. Stand with your back straight. Slowly bend at the waist (knees slightly bent) and try to touch the floor with your fingers. Don't force it. Let your body hang as far as you can. Holding this position, fold your arms across your body, cupping your left elbow with your right hand and right elbow with your left hand. Hold for ten seconds and repeat.

Ankle stretch. Stand erect, hands at side, feet flat on floor. Raise your body on your toes. Stand on your tiptoes and hold for several seconds. Return to the starting position. Repeat three times.

Overhead stretch. Also standing, feet together and flat on the floor, make a fist and raise one arm as high above you as possible. Stretch as far as you can. Return that arm to your side and repeat with the other fist and arm. Do three repetitions with each arm.

Shoulder rolls. Stand, feet about twelve inches apart. Roll both shoulders forward until you feel the muscles across your upper back stretch. Now, with your hands and arms motionless, roll your shoulders in a circle. Repeat three times.

Head turns. Stand, feet apart, hands on hips. Keep shoulders facing forward, and turn your head slowly to the left as far as you can. Turn it slowly to the right as far as you can. Repeat the right-left motion three times.

Next, swim—or walk in shallow water if you are a beginner—at an easy pace for five minutes as part of the cardio-respiratory warm-up.

Now you are ready to start your twenty-minute swim (or swim-walk, depending on your fitness level). After your aerobic swim, be sure to cool down. If you find that you are tight after swimming, you may want to add some other stretching exercises, from Chapter 11.

SWIMMING THE RIGHT WAY

You will need swimming lessons to learn how to swim properly. And then skill is required to make swimming an effective aerobic workout. You must keep moving in the water for twenty to thirty minutes. The better your swimming form, the more enjoyable and safe your swimming workout.

Youngsters and adults can take swimming lessons at your local YMCA or with other community organizations. You might consider this for several reasons: to learn how to swim (if you or your child do not know how), to have access to a pool for workouts and fun, and to improve your swimming techniques to allow for better performance. Here are some basic tips on improving your freestyle (crawl stroke), the most popular of the swimming strokes:

Body position. Jane Katz, author of *Swimming for Total Fitness*, recommends: "Your body should have a long-stretched-out feeling. It should be streamlined along its central axis (your spine), and the water level should come between your eyebrows and your hairline." If your head is held too high, your body drops from the hips down and acts as a drag in the water.

The flutter kick. When doing the flutter kick, move your legs up and down alternately. The power comes with the downward movement. When done properly, kicking will help you maintain your body position and the tempo of your arm stroke. The kick provides only about 20 percent of the power of your freestyle stroke. But done improperly, it can slow you down and create a drag on your arm pull, which provides 80 percent of your power. Donna DeVarona, my friend and Olympic Gold Medalist swimmer, offers some excellent suggestions in her book *Donna DeVarona's Hydro-Aerobics* about the basic swimming kick.

Most swimmers, she says, use only the lower leg for kicking. Experienced swimmers use their entire legs, from the hips to the toes, when swimming the crawl. Check the following:

Knees. Relaxed, not much bend. Hips and thighs should do the work because they have the larger and stronger muscles.

Feet. Slightly arched, toes pointing outward, ankles loose and flexible.

Leg position. Keep your legs close together without touching.

Size of kick. This will probably be twelve to eighteen inches.

The arm stroke. Start with your hands. Your little fingers (pinkies) should enter the water first, your thumb last. Your hands should be angled slightly outward, fingers slightly apart. (DeVarona writes that the "air pockets between the fingers will actually aid in cupping the water.")

Your hands should strike the water almost straight ahead of your shoulders, and about shoulder width apart.

The pull and recovery. As soon as your hand hits the water, pull it down and toward you. Make sure your elbow is bent as you pull. "It's almost as if you're doing a push-up in the water," DeVarona writes, "except that your ultimate strength comes from your back muscles." She also suggests "rolling your shoulder into the water as the elbow enters."

As you complete the movement, your pull should be as strong as possible at your thighs. Recover with your elbow emerging from the water first, followed by the hand as it begins the next pull.

Don't chop at the water. Make long, graceful strokes and try to get as much distance as possible from each one. Pull the water by you and bring your arms in and out with as little splashing as possible.

Coordinating the kick and arm stroke. According to DeVarona, make sure your kick stabilizes your stroke and keeps your body on top of the water. This will help you with your arm pull. Do not worry—as some swimmers do—about counting the number of kicks made during the time both arms make the full pull cycle. Like bike riding and running, the best motion here is a natural one.

Breathing. Swimmers inhale fully and exhale slowly through their mouths and noses in an easy, rhythmic way. The basic key is to get all the air you can. Swimming offers the additional challenge of getting air without getting water in your mouth.

As you get into better shape, you might try interval swimming. Swim fast for twenty-five to fifty yards, then rest ten to fifteen seconds, followed by a lap or two of regular-pace swimming. Then repeat the cycle again. Do five to ten cycles, or so, and end the workout with your usual cool-down swim and stretching.

Rhythmic breathing, writes Jane Katz, "consists of pivoting your face out of the water to inhale, then pivoting it back down into the water to exhale. Pivot your head, don't lift it."

Coordinating the head motion with your arm reach and pull takes some practice. You might want to start with lessons and then progress to holding the edge of a pool or swim board as you pivot your head and breath. To breathe while swimming, turn your head and inhale on one side while your arm on the opposite side extends and enters the water; the arm on your breathing side is completing its stroke near your thigh. Then you blow out the air underwater, turning your head, and inhale on the opposite side as the other arm starts its stroke.

Different strokes. For variety and a more balanced exercise program, you might want to switch your strokes. The most popular ones, after the crawl, or freestyle, are the sidestroke, backstroke, breaststroke, and butterfly. To do these properly, you'll need personal instruction, but here are brief descriptions.

Sidestroke. Lie on your side, move your top leg forward and your bottom leg back. Bring both together quickly in a scissors motion (called a scissors kick). As you do this, your top arm sweeps in a stroke from a little above your shoulder to your waist. The bottom arm points straight ahead.

Backstroke. This is a nice, relaxing stroke. Roll over on your back. Using a flutter kick, reach with one arm from your waist out of the water past your head and into the water and pull back to your waist. Alternate arm strokes.

Breaststroke. On your stomach, push both arms along the surface of the water in a straight line in front of you. When fully extended, pull your arms in a wide circle from your shoulders to your waist. With a "frog kick," then bring both arms together again in front of you and repeat the stroke.

Butterfly. On your stomach, extend both arms ahead of you, and push hard down to your stomach. Bring the arms around and out of the water, extend them in mid-air far in front of you, and repeat the stroke, while maintaining a continuous dolphin kick. This one of the hardest strokes to do over a long period of time, but it does strengthen your upper body.

EQUIPMENT AND FACILITIES

What to wear when you swim? All you really need is a swimsuit—although Shepherd says that in many wooded creeks and rivers of Vermont you can dive in with only your birthday suit on! But for most workouts, you will want a bathing suit. Nylon is inexpensive and dries fast; Lycra and other materials are preferred by competitors who think they are "faster" and look better. A clean pair of running shorts will also do as swimming trunks.

If you swim in an indoor pool, you may want to get a pair of goggles to protect your eyes from the chlorine. Unfortunately, many of our lakes and rivers now have bacteria that may also trouble your eyes. Goggles will help.

A swimming cap will hold long hair in place and keep it out of your eyes.

Ear plugs are advised if you get ear infections easily, and nose plugs will protect your sinuses.

A kickboard offers swimmers variety and improves their leg kicks.

Pools. Olympic-size, or "long course," pools are fifty meters (about fifty-five yards) long. Most communities and schools have a twenty-five–yard, or "short-course," pool or perhaps a twenty-five–meter (twenty-yard) facility. These are fine for fitness swimming and most competitive needs. The small ten-to-fifteen–yard pools are good only for beginner swimmers. The constant turns interfere with the aerobic workout.

Some new homes are being built with long "lap pools" in them. These are only one lane wide by fifty meters or more, and are solely designed for the aerobic workout.

Often during your workouts you will need to swim within a lane at a pool. You may also have to share lanes. If so, you may want to talk with your lane companions before your workout, and stagger your entrances into the water to give each of you maximum room. Generally, you swim counter-clockwise within the lane, staying to your right.

Outdoor aerobic swimming is more difficult. Added to the rigors of your workout are factors of nature: currents, hazards, wildlife, and weather.

Don't let any of these obstacles deter you or your children from this excellent aerobic exercise. But be safe.

Walking

Walking is an excellent fitness exercise. In fact, it is my preferred start-up exercise routine. Like running, it requires no special skills, little equipment, and can be done almost anywhere. Best of all, walking is easily done by children, parents, and grandparents. Christopher enjoys brisk three-generation walks with me and my father (who can reallly step!). According to the U.S. Bureau of the Census, more than one hundred million Americans now walk for fitness and pleasure.

Walking is also very good for you. It exercises most muscle groups, especially if you swing your arms vigorously or use hand weights to aid in muscle development. When asked his advice on staying sharp into ripe old age, Harry Truman said, on his eightieth birthday: "Take a two-mile walk every morning before breakfast." My uncle Louie Snyder walked several brisk miles a day past his one hundredth birthday. According to research at Harvard University, a brisk two-mile walk every day can cut one's risk of a heart attack by 28 percent. Hippocrates knew this twenty-four hundred years ago when he said, "Walking is man's best medicine." It is a safe form of aerobic exercise, even if you are under medical care for heart disease, high blood pressure, obesity, or osteoporosis.

We are now learning that walking—like other forms of vigorous exercise—is also good for relieving stress. Because it is slower and takes longer, walking teaches patience. Slowing down, taking your time, is often the best therapy for dealing with severe stress.

In a survey of more than one thousand people participating in a "Walk for Wellness" program in Owensboro, Kentucky, 81 percent strongly agreed that walking helps them relieve tension and stress. Walking can also aid sleep. Late night walks, at an easy pace, can help drain off tension and worries from your system. A short walk of five to fifteen minutes will relieve muscle tension and help you sleep better. It also facilitates conversation between family members. During my walks with Christopher he opens up and discusses his greatest joys and biggest fears.

Walking is also a way of slowing down and seeing more. It encourages curiosity about life going on around us. Oliver Wendell Holmes said: "In walking, the will and the muscles are so accustomed to work together and perform their task with so little expenditure of force, that the intellect is left comparatively free."

WALKING FOR KIDS AND FAMILIES

It's tough to get young kids excited about taking a walk. They will hike all over the place if it's play or their idea. But to take a family outing and hike someplace—yuk! Even before suggesting a fitness walk, you must first think like a child and develop an imaginative and flexible plan. Adjust to your children's views of exercise and their environment, and you will enjoy a wide variety of adventurous family walks.

Special Supplies

The first ingredient to successful walking with kids is to be prepared for every small "emergency" that will come up. Here are a few tips:

Pre-schoolers. When wandering far from home with pre-schoolers, take a change of diapers, bottle, pacifier, toys, and other necessities. Walking along pushing a stroller is fine when the child is not walking, but as soon as the infant wants to join in, let him or her in on the action. Then, put him or her back in the stroller after a few minutes and continue.

If you have a very young child in a stroller and some older ones, take occasional breaks to let the little one out to play. As your child gets older, encourage him or her to walk more and ride less. Continue to bring along the stroller even when the child can do a lot of walking—or you may end up having to carry him or her on your back.

Be prepared and be flexible with pre-schoolers. At this age, exposure to walking for fitness and fun is your only goal.

Key goodies. Christopher requires four important supplies for our walks. First, Band-aids. Anytime he gets the slightest cut or scape—and he is so adventuresome on our walks that they are inevitable—a Band-aid is required.

Second, a water bottle and/or juice. Christopher gets hot and thirsty very quickly during walks. Unless you know there are plenty of water fountains along the way, pack a few containers of juice. (Nutrition note: Make sure they are fruit juices, not imitations.) Throughout the summer, Christopher's water bottle is a constant companion. We take a plastic soda bottle and fill it with water. He drinks it and pours it over his head to stay cool.

Third, paper towels. These items do triple duty: wiping runny noses, cleaning cuts and scrapes, and being used as toilet paper if you have to use the woods. Fourth, some small strong bags. These are used to collect things found along your path: rocks, pirate's gold, leaves, bones, and so forth.

We also bring along some sugarless bubblegum. It helps to quench thirst and divert kids who are temporarily bored with walking. Christopher and I have bubble-blowing contests that last at least a mile.

Nutritious snacks like apples, dried fruit, unsalted nuts, raisins, or grapes should also be carried along to feed kids while they walk and again divert them from the fact that they are basically on a fitness walk.

All of this can be easily packed into a small day pack. Be sure to get one with padded shoulder straps and several exterior pockets. Stash goodies in the exterior pockets so the kids can simply come up to you and unzip a pocket and help themselves. You won't have to take the pack on and off a dozen times to find raisins or bubblegum, store a bag containing a squashed salamander, or give them a drink.

Games Along the Way

The attention span of a child varies with the activity. Most very young children may be able to walk for only a few minutes. But by age five or six, the kids should be ready to log at least twenty minutes.

Goals. Kids like to have clear goals on their walks. First, simply get them to walk out the door and around the block. Then you may expand to walking to school or church. Once beyond that, you'll have to be more imaginative and challenging. Here are some goals I've used with Christopher:

- Walking to a friend's or relative's house where he will be greeted with praise for his accomplishment and perhaps a nice reward (apple cider at Grandma's house, with a hug).
- Walking to a landmark. Christopher first walked the one-and-a-half–mile Central Park reservoir, then the six-mile loop around Central Park. He also picked some landmarks to walk to: the Empire State Building and the South Street Seaport.

The Shepherds took their kids overnight camping when they were six and four. Both kids carried little packs that they made and went off like mountain goats. They had the best climb when the kids were shown a lake on a map as their destination. After four hours, the two little hikers went over the crest of a hill and looked down on that same lake—and set off running toward it shouting, "We did it! We did it!"

- Walking to a place that offers a fun activity. Christopher eagerly walks two miles to basketball games in Madison Square Garden, and about a mile to the carousel in Central Park.
- Climbing the highest "mountain." This might be a small hill in your local park or a major mountain in a national park or national forest. When we were visiting Phoenix, Arizona, Christopher spotted Squaw Peak. A popular trail leads to the top of this very high hill. Off we went for more than an hour's climb to the top until Christopher was satisfied that he had conquered his mountain—and could see miles of desert below.
- King of the mountain. This is a favorite of Christopher's. We go for walks where there are plenty of hills, rock formations, and other landmarks to explore. When we get close, I yell: "Who will be king of the mountain?" and Christopher and anyone else with us sprints to the top of the nearest spot. Then we look for the next mountain to climb.
- Getting wet. Kids love to get wet. I haven't met one yet who can walk around a large rain puddle. Christopher will walk and run in the rain having a great time. As long as it isn't cold or there is lightning, we go out and get wet. Look at it this way. On a hot day you pour water over your head to keep cool; when you finish a workout you shower. So why not walk in the rain on a hot day?

  Plan hikes along streams, or to lakes or rivers. Look for waterfalls, fish, frogs, and other wet friends.
- Walking to a mysterious destination. During the summer of 1988, while I wrote this book, Christopher and Virginia vacationed at Point o'Woods, a family community on Fire Island, along the Atlantic shore of Long Island, New York. There are no cars or television sets. The kids have to use their imagination to have fun and their legs for transportation.

  One day, Christopher heard about a mysterious place on Fire Island called the Sunken Forest. He begged his mother to walk him there to check it out. While standing in the breakfast line, Virginia told some other parents about the hike they were going to take, and before long found herself leading a pack of about a dozen kids and four mothers on a one-way walk of about two miles. None of them had ever walked that far before, except Christopher and Virginia.

  Within a quarter mile, several of the out-of-shape ten- and 11-year-olds, and their huffing parents, dropped out. By the half-mile mark, only Virginia, Christopher—the youngest of the original group—and a tired nine-year-old girl remained. When she begged to turn back after a mile, Christopher begged her to finish. He didn't want to miss his goal. She struggled, but made it to the Sunken Forest, where they played in the low and dark woods growing just behind the sand dunes, before walking back. They returned to the community as heroes.

The little girl was proud that she had made it. She told her friends about the wonders of the Sunken Forest and they became determined to walk the distance themselves. The next morning, the dropouts came to get their fitness leader, Christopher. But his mother had other plans for the morning and said he couldn't go. Off the others went, bravely committed to reach their newfound fitness goal and the forest. Christopher cried so hard for so long that his mother finally gave in and changed her plans. They took off running and caught up with the group.

During the hike, Christopher ran ahead of the group and came back to give scouting reports and encouragement that they could make it. They did, and spent hours exploring the dark seaside forest. When they returned, Christopher became known as the "little Pied Piper of fitness." The kids admitted that the hike was a lot of fun. They said they wanted to go for a walk every day. Christopher summed it all up: "I just knew they could all do it. It was so much fun."

Collecting and counting. Kids love to collect things and count objects. Christopher returned from his first adventure walk in school, for example, with a bag full of "Indian arrowheads." Actually, they were rocks that sort of looked like arrowheads if you held them a certain way. His class had pretended they were Indians and gave each other special names. Christopher chose "Chief Gathering Stone." And gather he did, as part of a three-mile fitness walk.

Any walk offers its collectibles: acorns, fall leaves, seashells. Christopher and his friends count "punch buggies"—Volkswagen cars—while they walk along city streets. At Easter he counts Easter bunnies in store windows; at Thanksgiving, turkeys. For Christmas 1987, Christopher and his friend David Pena counted more than two hundred lighted trees and wreaths during a two-hour fitness walk, and they never once complained of being bored or tired.

There are birds to see and animals to look for. You can play "Who will be the first to see?" and look for spiders, a green car, or a moving animal.

Games. You can use games requiring educational skills, like "follow the alphabet": you walk to an object that begins with the letter *a*—apartment or alligator (just kidding!). Then you go on to *b* and work through the whole alphabet. Or you can play the version where you call these objects out as you see them while on your walk.

You might look for a certain number of objects, starting with one and moving up to a set number—such as ten or even one hundred. For example, you might start by finding one singing bird, then two croaking frogs, and on up to ten mooing cows. You can also try to count—as individuals or as a group—how many objects you can sight of a certain color or shape. A variation is to divide up the colors or shapes among your family and have a contest while walking.

Exploring: Tom Sawyer Adventure Walks

Since he was barely able to walk, Christopher and I have gone exploring. We wander around looking for interesting sights to see and things to do. This is the way walking must be for kids. Let them change directions and speeds as often as they wish. Let them pick imaginative distractions.

You can pick obstacles/events to keep them busy: walk up some steep stairs, climb up a hill and roll down, run to a tree and climb it, skip or hop for thirty seconds, race to the corner, hop over cracks in the sidewalk, walk on benches or balance while walking along a wooden beam. Whatever, be prepared for a series of diversions to keep the fitness walk fun, or you will be stuck with a whining kid complaining, "I'm bored. I'm tired."

Try saying "Who wants to go exploring?" instead of "Let's all go out and exercise." Watch how your child's enthusiasm increases when the walk is an exploration.

Christopher's all-time favorite is our "Tom Sawyer adventure hikes." These walks, I believe, have been the key to his advanced level of aerobic fitness. Having done these workouts, he can run two miles nonstop even without "practicing" as a runner.

Christopher loves to have me read Mark Twain's books about two rascals who I tell him are just like him: Tom Sawyer and Huckleberry Finn. For our walks, he picks one character and I take another. If friends come along, we give them names too. We go by these names for the remainder of the adventure.

We enter Central Park with a mission: to search for the treasure hidden by the pirates. We climb up and down "mountains" in our search. Whenever we see signs of pirates—such as a person approaching who is wearing black or a beer can marked with X's, we take off running. We sneak up on suspected pirate ships, castles, and hiding places, and then go scurrying at the first sign of trouble. We look for signs of pirate activity: messages (graffiti) on the sides of rocks, "swords," "cannons," and other objects (actually sticks, pipes, and rocks). Sure signs of the presence of bad guys are discarded whiskey bottles and cigarettes (pirates enjoy things that are bad for you).

When a road race in the park goes by, we take off running because we realize that the pirates have scared these people into a wild stampede. We climb trees and huge rock formations to look out for pirate activity and signs of where treasure might be buried. Once we found a discarded letter and in it was a picture of a boy named Josh. We knew he had been captured by the pirates and we set off to save him.

In order to protect ourselves, we fashion swords out of sticks and carry them along. The game goes on and on as I lure the kids into covering the back woods and trails of Central Park for distances of four to eight miles. After several hours of creative exercise, we all return home exhausted and exhilarated. The kids are full of wild stories to tell parents, teachers, and friends, and Virginia is further convinced that I am a wild man running amok in the park, which, of course, I am. We always finish with a "continuation" plot, so the kids can look forward to the next adventure walk.

GROUPS

Kids love the company of their peers. The best way to ensure a successful fitness walk, whether for a pre-school group or teenagers, is to bring along one or more friends. You can organize a group of parents for a family fitness walk, or take a group like a scout troop.

As mentioned in our model school program (Chapter 8), adventure walks make a great activity for school physical education classes. Regular classroom teachers can use educational walking field trips to promote both fitness and academic skills. *Walking for Little Children*, by Robert Sweetgall and Robert Neeves, includes a chapter of advice on educational walking field trips. Here are a few examples that they suggest for classrooms: nature walks around the schoolyard; neighborhood discovery walks; education walks to other schools; community service walks to a senior center, fire station, or police station; historic walks to a local landmark or museum; agriculture walks on a farm; and "let's stay healthy" walks to the hospital. They give two good tips: Develop experience charts to compare what you expected to see to the actual experience; and keep a class scrapbook of each field trip.

EQUIPMENT

What do you need to go walking? A place to walk and some good walking shoes.

Shoes are as important to walkers as to runners. You probably should invest in a pair of well-cushioned, good-fitting walking or running shoes.

A good walking shoe is well cushioned in the heel, where the foot strikes first, and has a stable heel to keep the foot from rocking sideways. Allow room in the front for your toes to spread as you push off. You might also consider lightweight shoes. As in the case of running shoes, shop at stores that specialize in walking shoes. Try on several pairs, and walk around in them at the store. Make sure they feel comfortable on your feet.

I don't recommend hiking boots for people who want to walk for exercise, aerobic or not. Regular hiking boots are too heavy, and the cleats are large; walking fast in them can cause you to trip. The new, lightweight nylon hiking shoes are better for fast walking. Still, I recommend regular walking or running shoes, unless you are hiking over rugged terrain.

Clothing is easier. In hot weather, wear loose-fitting and light-colored clothing to protect you from the sun and allow air to flow freely around your skin. Keep your shoulders covered with a full, cotton T-shirt (cotton absorbs perspiration and lets excessive moisture evaporate as you walk). Wear a light-colored lightweight hat and sunglasses.

In cold weather, dress in layers so you can remove clothing as you heat up. It is better to overdress than to underdress—you can always peel off layers and tie clothing around your waist. Mittens keep your hands warm. Wear a ski hat to trap body heat off the top of your head.

HOW TO WALK

This is almost ridiculous. Bob Glover is now going to tell you how to do something you've been doing since you were about twelve months old. Why? Because many people walk incorrectly. Others, who walk correctly, get sloppy over long distances. Walking with a relaxed, proper form needs to be learned, and it is safer, faster, and more rewarding than the improper form.

Proper walking starts with good posture. You should not look down at your feet or slump while walking. Look straight ahead, and see the sky, buildings, trees, and faces. Without an erect stance, with your head and body bent slightly over, you will soon be uncomfortable when walking briskly.

The most comfortable walking position is with your weight over your feet, or just slightly ahead of them. Your body should be relaxed, with a slightly forward lean. Your back should be straight, stomach and buttocks pulled in. Hold your head up. If your eyes are looking ahead, not down, they will help keep your head in the proper position. The scenery will improve too. Correct posture will give you a higher center of gravity, which will in turn result in a longer, more efficient stride.

Use the heel-toe foot strike. Point your feet straight ahead, reaching forward with your heel down. Touch the heel of your lead foot to the ground just before pushing off the ball of your other foot. Gary Yanker, author of *Exercisewalking*, writes:

> The back edge of the heel should strike first, with ankle set slightly to the outside. Roll forward on the outer side of the foot. Pull forward with the leading leg, while pushing off with the back leg until toe-off. Don't kick off, as runners do, but push off straight back as your feet roll forward. During the swing phase, toes are pointed in the direction of travel, and the leg is reaching forward—not pushing or pulling—to become the supporting leg once more.

Try walking at a brisk pace with your hands in your pockets. You will see how arm drive makes a big difference in your ability to walk briskly. A strong arm swing is essential to walking for fitness. Not only does it help you keep your body in balance, but the arm movement also increases your heart rate. The result is a better aerobic workout.

Keep your shoulders loose and your arms low. If you carry your arms too high, you will become fatigued and tense in your neck and shoulder muscles. Your arms should swing back and forth from the shoulder like a pendulum, and should balance the opposite leg action: right arm drives downward as left leg drives forward; left arm drives downward as right leg drives forward. Your elbows are relaxed at a ninety-degree angle—this shortens the arm swing and allows a quicker leg motion.

Inhale and exhale using deep, relaxed abdominal breaths. If you are huffing and puffing and can't breathe properly, slow down.

The key is to walk comfortably and smoothly. At the same time, you should put some effort into each strike and arm swing to get an aerobic benefit. With practice, you will learn to develop a rhythm that is both relaxed and aerobic.

GETTING FIT WITH WALKING

Walking has one disadvantage: it doesn't get your heart rate up as quickly or as high as running and other more vigorous aerobic exercises. This means you may have to exercise longer as a walker to achieve the same results that other aerobic exercises offer. Before setting forth, review the exercise principles and warm-up and cool-down routines in Chapter 10, and the FIT aerobic training variables in Chapter 12.

Start each workout by walking at a comfortable pace for about five minutes as a warm-up. Then, increase the tempo of your walk to reach a pace that is within your aerobic target heart rate range. At first, alternate walking brisly with walking slowly until you can walk twenty minutes near your aerobic level. Even if you can only get to within 60 percent of your maximum, that is sufficient for fitness benefit as a beginner. You may notice that your breathing becomes slightly faster and deeper. If you feel tired or out of breath, slow the pace. If your pulse isn't high enough, swing your arms and walk faster.

A typical starting pace is about one mile in twenty minutes. Build gradually until you can walk briskly for at least thirty minutes. Since walking doesn't burn calories as fast as other aerobics, it is helpful to build up to walking for forty-five to sixty minutes at a time. Start out by walking three to five times a week. Later you may walk every day if you enjoy it and have the time. A good goal is fifteen miles a week: three miles at a time, five times a week.

Always walk slowly for five to ten minutes for a cardio-respiratory cooldown. If you cannot walk comfortably the day after your exercise walk, it probably means you are doing too much too soon.

Here is a suggested progression chart for beginner walkers. A beginner walker is someone who has already worked up to walking comfortably for twenty minutes.

Week #	Minutes
1	20 (approximately 1 mile)
2	22
3	25
4	28
5	30
6	30
7	30
8	30–45
9	30–45
10	30–60 (approximately 1.5–3 miles)

WHEN TO WALK

Walking can be enjoyed at any time of day or night. (If you do exercise outdoors at night, be sure to wear a reflector vest.)

Some walkers love the morning workout before going to the office or to school. Stephen Kiesling and E. C. Frederick, authors of *Walk On: A Tool Kit for Building Your Own Walking Fitness Program*, write: "By warming up your body, morning walks also warm up your mind. Without early morning workouts, your body temperature rises gradually from its low point (around 4 A.M.), peaking in the evening and then dropping again. . . .

Exercise helps you fight the early morning 'lows' of temperature and alertness that you'd otherwise have to face." My father walks a fast five miles at 5:30 A.M. every day but Sunday because, he says, "it's the best part of the day."

A moderately paced walk to work for you and to school for your kids will not only improve your fitness levels, but will also help all of you function better mentally at the start of the day.

Walking before meals will also depress your appetite. You are a two-way winner: you burn off calories while cutting back on food intake. Walking after meals boosts your metabolism and increases the amount of calories burned. It also aids digestion. Walking is one of the few exercises your body will tolerate after eating.

Walking is also beneficial for handling emotional stress. A noonday walk at work or school (or afterwards) will help burn off tension. Kiesling and Frederick write that "a brisk walk can produce a sensation of euphoria that results from physiological changes. . . . But in walking—more than in any form of exercise—the good feeling seems to come from taking time to get back in touch with your body, to feel the subtle nuances of training, and to notice the world around you."

Look for ways to make walking part of your daily schedule. Walk instead of drive to do shopping or to run errands. Walk to the movies or theater. Get off the bus or train a few stops ahead of your station and walk the rest of the way. After eating out with your family, go for a walk to sightsee for an hour or so before returning to your car. If you go to some event, park a good distance away, where it is easier to find parking—rather than driving with the traffic; you'll get on the road afterwards more easily too. Always ask, how can I include walking in my activities? Start your kids walking briskly at a young age. I walk so fast that Christopher as a pre-schooler had to skip and run to keep up. Soon, Dad will have to skip and run to keep up, since he really loves to walk briskly now.

Schools should include walking in their physical education programs. Corporations should encourage all employees—not just executives—to stay fit, and walking should be included in their fitness programs. You can, on your own, easily get in a fifteen- to thirty-minute walk around your office area during your lunch break. Bring a healthy, easy-to-eat lunch and go for a walk either before or after eating; use the time saved waiting in a restaurant or cafeteria. You don't need to change your clothes. Just put on your walking shoes, and step out the door.

According to the U.S. Census Bureau, more than 5 percent of America's working adults walk to and from work. I find in New York City that I can cover two miles faster by walking than I can by taking a taxi, subway, or bus. I also walk to important business meetings. This gives me time by myself to collect my thoughts and review my strategies. After the meetings, I usually unwind by walking back to my office or home while going over the meeting in my head. Then I write out my notes highlighting the meeting and the next strategy.

WHERE TO WALK

Cities have one advantage over suburbs and rural areas: sidewalks. In most cities—Los Angeles is certainly one exception—you can walk almost everywhere, slowing down only for traffic lights. There are, of course, areas of cities where it's dangerous to walk and there are places that are congested with traffic, which makes walking unpleasant.

One increasingly popular place to walk is in suburban shopping malls. They are air-conditioned in summer and heated in winter, shaded from the burning sun and the rain or snow, and free of bike and automobile traffic. The walking surface is also smooth.

For these reasons, the number of serious "mall walkers" is growing. They've even started clubs. The Mall Walkers Club in Boynton Beach, Florida, for example, has more than three hundred members who regularly walk around the 1.6-mile circuit of the local mall. The Boynton Mall opens up early every morning to all the mall walkers so they can exercise before the crowds of shoppers come in at ten o'clock.

In Edina, Minnesota, the Southdale Shopping Mall and the Fairview Southdale Hospital co-sponsor a Making Tracks for Health walking program. Walkers are welcome to come into the mall for brisk workouts on a safe, controlled, measured course.

INCREASING THE CHALLENGE

If you have taken up walking and found a good spot to walk—mall, park, street, woods, or track—you may eventually want to increase the challenge of your program. If you are already in good shape—or as you get into good shape—you can make your walks more challenging by walking uphill, up stairs, or over rugged terrain. Besides increasing your heart rate and burning more calories, these activities will also strengthen your leg muscles. You may also want to try walking workouts indoors on treadmills, stair-climbing machines, or even on the stairway of your building.

If you find that you cannot walk as briskly as you want, simply walk longer. Carrying hand weights will increase your workload and strengthen your upper body. Start with one to three pounds. If you swing your arms in a regular pattern while carrying hand weights, you will add to your workout. I recommend hand weights for fitness walking, but not for running. I do *not* recommend ankle weights. They place too much stress on your knees and lower legs.

RACEWALKING

You can also learn to walk faster. To do this, you will need to learn the technique called racewalking.

It is difficult to walk faster than twelve minutes per mile without using racewalking. This is a combination of running and walking. The racewalker drives with the hips and pumps with the arms to propel his or her body forward. But part of one foot is always on the ground. This gives race-walkers their exaggerated motion.

Racewalking is difficult to do properly. You should have someone give you lessons so that you learn the technique correctly. It is an excellent exercise for strengthening muscles in the front and back of the legs, the hips, abdominals, and the upper body.

MARCHING

You may not have thought of this, but marching in a band is also good walking exercise, especially when you consider the amount of conditioning that goes into such marching. This can be a novel way to get in shape and enjoy music at the same time.

William C. Moffit, director of athletic bands at Purdue University, leads marching workouts at a local mall three times a week. He suggests popping some marching music into your tape player and stepping out—pumping the arms, lifting the knees, and keeping step to the music. Look out, Sousa!

HIKING, TOURS, AND VACATIONS

Inn-to-inn hiking is becoming as popular in the United States as it has been in Europe. It can be done in several different ways. Hikers can walk from country inn to country inn, while their suitcases and other equipment are carted ahead by van. The inns are, ideally, about ten to fifteen miles apart. Or, hikers can make reservations at mountain huts—most notably, Shepherd says, across the Presidential Range of the White Mountains of New Hampshire—and hike along the high mountain trails carrying only a lightweight day pack with emergency gear. When you reach the hut, supper is ready at large communal tables. One drawback: Sleeping is in bunk beds, dorm style, women in one room, men in the other.

You can also hike along trails in parks all over the United States. Hikes can be taken by family groups, or as part of a packaged tour. You can enjoy day hikes or backpack into a wilderness area for days or weeks.

Walking clubs around the country will provide you with information about walking trails, tours, and vacations. Every state has its tourist department, and every city its chamber of commerce. They are excellent sources of such information. You can also write: the Walkways Center, Suite 427, 733 15th Street, N.W., Washington, D.C. 20005. If you want to explore marked trails in more than 300 national parks and waterfronts, contact: the National Parks Service, Office of Public Inquiry, P.O. Box 37127, Washington, D.C. 20013 (phone number: 202-343-4747).

WALKING EVENTS

Many areas of the country have walk-a-thons, club walks, fitness walks, and other kinds of fun-walk events that you and your family can join. *City Sports Magazine*, for example, sponsors City Stride in a half-dozen cities around the country. Our family enjoyed one of their events, a seven-mile walk through the streets of Lower Manhattan. Hundreds of families joined in, and Christopher thought that the best thing about it was that he "walked his age"—seven.

Part 6

FITNESS AND SPORTS

20

Pre-schoolers

Maybe we should ban the word *exercise* from this chapter, and substitute *play*. And by play, I mean unstructured activity, family fun, exploring, and learning—all left to when and how a child wishes. According to Dr. David Elkind, a child psychologist who advocates a child's right to be a child, too many American parents in the late 1980s want their young pre-schoolers to be "superbabies." They want them to be in structured exercise classes as toddlers.

I say, let them be babies and children first. After all, before the first grade, children get minimal benefit from planned exercise. They will achieve some degree of motor skill development and muscular fitness, but not much more—if any—than they would get from simply playing regularly.

"Play," as Mark Twain wrote, "is an activity that has great meaning, but no purpose." Part of the meaning of play is as a social activity and as a way of preparing a child to accept enjoyable physical activity (and, later, fitness) as part of his or her life. Thus, what we really need to emphasize here is the value of "pre-fitness for pre-schoolers."

As a parent, you have an important part in your child's play as a role model; the environment you create in your home has tremendous influence. "The average kid sees his parents cemented to the couch growing fatter and fatter," Keith Henschen, a sports psychologist at the University of Utah, told *Health Magazine*, "while the most important thing they could be doing is showing him how to kick a ball or going swimming with him." When your child sees you exercising regularly, this will influence him or her. Ironically, as the opening chapter made clear, if you wait too long you may have to undo bad habits and teach your own kids how to play.

Dr. Paul G. Dyment, chairman of the sports medicine committee of the American Academy of Pediatrics, told *Health Magazine*, "The whole family should be active so that by the time the youngster is of school age, exercising is done together as part of a lifestyle." But to achieve this, you as a parent must set an example and watch your child's play and development closely. This chapter will help. "Parents can play an important positive role in their children's learning," Dr. Elkind told the *New York Times*. "It's healthy to want a child to excel and do well. But you do that by providing a stimulating environment, rather than pushing a small child to master specific skills."

BIRTH TO ONE YEAR: AGE OF SELF-DISCOVERY

A child's first and most important toy is you. Infants like to look at, touch, and smell your face, hands, and body. Physical contact with parents is the child's first step toward developing motor skills.

Infants are fascinated by the newness that surrounds them. They are constantly reaching out to touch and smell. Consider the simple challenge of standing, says Wisty Rorabacher in the *Melpomene Report*:

> New body sensations in muscles which are being stretched and used in new ways.
>
> New sensations from sensory receptors because of the upright position.
>
> A new vantage point for looking out at the world as well as down at one's own body.
>
> New noises from falling, fun noises that can be made at will.
>
> New distances to drop objects.
>
> Changes in body sensations and balance when reaching out to grab something.
>
> For whatever combination of these exciting factors, children are motivated to repeat their wobbly actions hundreds and thousands of times until the new muscles and nerves learn what is required and the child finally masters the new skill.

Rorabacher adds that the task of adults during the child's age of newness and self-discovery is to respond with appreciation, wisdom, and encouragement. Parents "have to learn new appreciations for children's natural physical activities," Rorabacher writes.

> They have to learn how to facilitate children's extended, vigorous involvement in safe, appropriate physical "play." And perhaps the biggest challenge for adults is the same for children—to cope with newness. Children have to cope with a world which changes as bodies and competencies change. Adults have to be "on their toes" to keep up with the changing needs of children.

Birth to Three Months

Here are some specific ways that you can play with your child and at the same time enjoy your child's physical development. You can use a variety of shapes, sounds, and textures. Keep them small enough to grasp and safe enough for your child to put in his or her mouth:

Hold toys far enough away to make the child reach—stretch—and then grasp.

Arouse interest with rattles and other gentle noisemakers.

Put a bar across the crib or playpen and hang objects from it.

When changing diapers, gently push and pull your child's arms and legs to encourage movement.

Three to Six Months

Your child is now probably able to reach and grasp things, shake them, examine them, and bang them. He or she can also probably roll over. More physical play between the two of you is now fun and helpful. You might want to play the old favorite, pat-a-cake, or let baby scramble around on your bed. Playpens also provide a relatively safe and interesting environment, but they should be used only for short periods of time or for naps. Make sure there is nothing along the bars or railing that will scratch or cut and that any hanging toys or objects cannot get caught and snap or choke your child.

At this age, Christopher had a favorite "bounce chair." These are upright and stable, but springy, chairs that allow your child to jump up and down in them. Christopher also loved his Jolly Jumper, which hung safely in a doorway. The child sits in it and jumps up and down with the aid of a spring mechanism and the child's own movement. These look like so much fun you'll wish you were small enough to try it out. Do not let your child play in these for too long or he may get too fatigued.

Six to Nine Months

Here come the tub-splashing years. It's good exercise—try it yourself!—and all you need to do is put down the towels and watch. Shepherd's daughter enjoyed bathing with another little girl, and they would pile in all their rubber toys, splash, and scream with glee. When things got slow, Shepherd played kids' music from the next room, and the little ladies danced in the water.

You will probably also have to "childproof" your house at this time. Your child will start to crawl soon, and join the legions of "rug rats" who scoot from coffee table to sofa to dining table with a speed you would have thought impossible. This is a kid on the move, Mom, and that means putting all family treasures and breakables out of reach. Now you won't have to say, "Don't touch this, don't touch that."

If you don't childproof, then you will soon see that your little baby can hold things very firmly in his hands, pass objects from hand to hand, and even toss them a bit.

Nine to Twelve Months

Now you have a little "erectoid" who is taking steps. He or she will love help "walking" around. Be alert to sharp-edged tables and other obstacles and get them out of the way. Hold baby's hand and help him or her balance and walk.

Walkers on wheels will allow your child to move around and get used to pushing the legs with power. But don't keep the child in the walker too long. Let her cut loose!

AGES ONE TO TWO: WALKING AND RUNNING

During these years, your child may go from crawling to walking to running. He or she may learn to kick a ball, move objects while walking, climb, swing, and jump. You may find your active child tiring you, but remember that this time with your child—as all times—will pass too quickly. Enjoy it and share it.

Allow your child to fall and get back up without help. This is how he or she will get stronger and build confidence. Don't baby your child by making a fuss. One-year-olds are made for falling. When Shepherd's kids fell at this age, he and his wife used to say, "Fall down! Go BOOM!" and the kids would laugh and get up and waddle off, only to fall down again.

You might want to give your child pushing and pulling toys, maybe later even wagons and carts. You also may want to throw soft foam balls to your child, bat around balloons and beach balls, and even engage in a little easy roughhousing by gently swinging your child around, giving him or her piggyback rides, or raising him or her high overhead and down low. By two your toddler can ride a wheeled vehicle without pedals. Christopher was a terror on his plastic motorcycle, which he pushed at full speed with strong little legs.

Hand-eye coordination develops during this period. You might consider playing with your child and a large, fat plastic bat. Throw the ball so it hits the bat and let the child take off running. You can play similar games with a foam kickball—let your child take off running, with you in pursuit.

THE TERRIBLE TWOS

Between the ages of two and three, a child may grow to half his adult height. He or she may become bold and adventurous and learn how to jump with his or her feet together, run efficiently, balance on one foot, walk stairs alone, and zoom up playground slide steps and slide down head first. (I almost died when Christopher first did this, yelling "Supermaaaan!" as he slid down with his arms out front like a diver.) A child will temporarily pass through the so-called terrible twos, which combines his or her increasing physical activity with early efforts to test how far he or she can—or wants to—move away from the early childhood nest.

Your child will need plenty of chances to run, jump, climb, and explore. Look for playgrounds that have more obstacles and adventures than just the standard swings and slides. Let children climb "mountains" wherever they find them. They also love roughhousing. If you can, set aside an area for your child to have as his or her own, where your child can play freely and bounce on an old mattress.

Christopher loved being lifted up and played with at this age. One favorite was "going to the moon," when I would count down from ten to blastoff and then lift him over my head on his "rocket trip" to the moon, and let him drop gently behind me on the bed. "Bye, bye, Chrissy," I'd say. Then I'd hear him giggle behind me and say "It's meeeee! I'm not on the moon." We'd do it over and over again.

Another favorite: I'd lie on my back on the bed, knees flexed, and he would sit on my lower legs as I lifted them up and down fast like a "bucking bronco." Sometimes he'd buck off, and sometimes he would stay on for the whole ride. "Monkey in a tree" was still another favorite: I would lie on my back with my legs straight up and Christopher would climb up my legs until he reached the top and balanced on my feet. Then, "Timberrrrr!" the tree would fall and he would tumble down with a laugh. He'd do these games as long as I could last.

AGES THREE TO FIVE

Here we begin to see the little adult in our child. He or she can pedal a tricycle, skip rope, hop on one foot, and learn to catch and throw a ball overhand. Your child may enjoy learning new activities like cross-country skiing, swimming, or tennis. Around age five is a good time to teach him or her how to ride a two-wheel bike. This is a lifetime skill and a confidence-building activity; don't force it or be tense about it.

Many children at this age enjoy cooperative group games with other kids and will invent games—sometimes elaborately imaginative—to play at the playground or in the local park or woods. If this activity is safe, and perhaps somewhat supervised, this is a good age to free your child to go off and play alone. Many of the imaginative games described in Chapter 14 were favorites of Christopher's at this age.

Physically, your child needs daily outdoor play time. He or she enjoys challenging playgrounds with good, creative design and equipment; or, just an outdoor area that can be safely explored.

PRE-SCHOOL EXERCISE PROGRAMS

Babies and young children spend a lot of their waking hours exercising: stretching, crawling, kicking, and climbing. Most pediatricians agree that this is sufficient exercise for them. One problem is that many parents spend too little time with their children—especially if both parents work—and when home they restrict their young child's exercise opportunities. The child grows up and enters the fitness development years—kindergarten through sixth grade—without a good fitness base or awareness. As I said at the beginning of this book, America's kids spend too much time in cars, strollers, and playpens—not to mention in front of TV sets.

For better or worse, pre-school exercise programs are growing across the country. Are these programs beneficial for pre-schoolers?

The pros and cons of pre-school programs. There are some good things about these programs, and some real cautions.

First the good: Pre-school programs do introduce children to exercise, and for that reason probably help set lifelong exercise habits. The programs also get young children and their parents together sharing a worthwhile experience. Good pre-school programs are fun, emphasizing the joy of play and the interaction between parent and child. Pre-school programs also bring children and mothers—and to a lesser extent, fathers—together. (I was the only father in Christopher's "Mom and Tot" exercise class.)

Nationally franchised programs include Gymboree, Fit-By-Five, Play-orena, and Playful Parenting. In addition, your local YMCA, YWCA, and YMHA all probably offer some form of quality exercise programs for pre-schoolers, sometimes offering spots to kids as young as three months.

Gymboree programs are broken into age groups. Babygym, for example, is for infants from three months to a year and emphasizes massage-like muscle stimulation with scaled-down equipment. Gymboree is for toddlers from one to two-and-a-half years old. It offers lots of climbing, crawling, and exploring. Gymgrad takes in kids up to four years old and gives them elementary gymnastics skills, group activities, and an introduction to sports and games.

Gymboree's founder, Joan Barnes, told *People Magazine:* "We are not little Jane Fonda workouts. Our goal is not physical fitness. It's self-esteem. These children are mastering skills at their own pace with the love and support of their parents. Everyone wants a confident child."

Christopher enjoyed his gymnastics/movement class at New York City's 92d Street YMHA when he was two years old. The class was as beneficial socially as physically: he met other kids in a semi-structured environment. A shy boy, he thrived on the fun and took on challenges—especially the trampoline—because of the fellowship with his playmates. Later, as a five-year-old, he enjoyed a peewee karate class at the Y that combined fitness and the fun of movement.

Not every parent should enroll every child in a formal pre-school exercise or play program. For one thing, most children are already active enough. They do not need structured exercise classes as much as they need parents who will help them turn off their television sets and do the things that kids have always done: actively play.

Pre-school exercise programs where parents and infants or toddlers exercise together can be fun, but they do not necessarily speed the development of your child's motor skills. Parents who think enrolling their child in a pre-school exercise program will accelerate his or her development are in for some sad news. "Most exercise won't hurt a normal child," said Michael Traister, M.D., assistant professor of clinical pediatrics at New York University School of Medicine. "But exercise probably won't make a baby a developmental superstar. In fact, there is no evidence that exercise advances development at all. The only good reason to follow an infant exercise program is that it's fun for you and your baby."

An American Academy of Pediatrics committee two-year study of pre-school exercise programs concluded that they gave children no head start physically. Infants will exercise anyway, if allowed to do so, and parents merely need to supply the space, toys, and attention. Moreover, Dr. Suzanne Haefele, an AAP committee member, does not recommend organized physical activities for children under age six. Instead, she believes spontaneous physical activity that involves the child's parents is an excellent exercise habit. "Adult models in the family," Dr. Haefele told *The Physician and Sportsmedicine,* "are the most influential for children. If the adults are physically active, the children will be active."

Other experts believe pre-school fitness programs can be dangerous both physically and emotionally. Overly competitive or programmed classes discourage a child's natural sense of spontaneity and movement. "These kinds of programs have no proven value," said Dr. Elkind, the author of

Miseducation: Preschoolers at Risk. They are just further "example[s] of children being regarded as a profitable market. Preschool kids normally get all the exercise they need playing around the house."

But that assumes parents have the space, time, and money to encourage their pre-schoolers to play. If they don't, a good program—where children play freely, move to music, and have fun with simple equipment—may be invaluable. This is especially true if the parents actively participate in their child's development.

"The prevailing view seems to be that they [pre-school exercise classes] are of no medical value," says Dr. Paul Dyment, chairman of the sports medicine committee of the American Academy of Pediatrics, "but if they increase the time spent between parent and child, then they can be of great psychological value."

What to look for. Programs for kids under the age of, say, six should be well supervised, fun, and insist on your involvement as a parent. Otherwise, they are baby-sitting operations. The goal is not a super-fit, fast-developing athlete, but fun and activity. I recommend that you take the time to go around with your child and try out several programs. The best program will put you and your child together in a playful situation. You both will like it!

Pre-school programs are also helpful in terms of preparing your child for school programs starting around age five. A good program progresses and helps your child develop a positive attitude toward physical fitness that will carry over during the important fitness years of six through twelve.

I also recommend that you start your child in such a program only once a week. This is not day care. This is a change of pace for your child and a stimulus to you on how to play better and exercise with your child. A good program, therefore, will build an important friendship—a lifelong gift—between parent and child. Also, it will give you the confidence and knowledge to continue physical activity at home and throughout your child's development as he or she approaches school age.

Most important, do not force your child to participate in these programs. He or she may not want to go unless a friend is in the program. If your child cries and does not want to start a class, wait it out. Christopher paid no attention to the instructors and other kids in his first exercise class for the first four weeks. He was happy just watching and then going out and playing on the equipment with me after the class was over. But he was watching closely and felt part of the class. He told his mother about all the things they did that day. By the end, he had joined in with everyone else. He had overcome his shyness and he had taken the first few tentative steps down the road toward fitness.

If you are anxious about such classes, your child will pick this up and be anxious too. You may just need to forget the class and try again when your child is more socially prepared and ready. I assure you, this is not a sign of failure.

So look for several things: your child's willingness to go, a balanced program of semi-structured fun, and parent-child involvement. Add to this your own at-home parent-child playtime, imaginative and unstructured free play, and free time with your child and his or her playmates. The goal is to teach your child that physical activity is a good, fun part of life.

EXERCISE EQUIPMENT, RECORDS, AND VIDEOS

There are a lot of things you can buy for your child beyond the pre-school fitness classes. Fitness toys—miniature weight sets for kids, sit-up boards, aerobic dance costumes—crowd the shelves of many toy stores. They are pushing out such useful items as jump ropes, scooters, sleds, tricycles, and roller skates.

Not all of what is on the shelves is junk. There are some records and videos that, properly used, can help you instill the fun and fitness attitude in your children. The important thing here—as everywhere in the book— is that you have to join in. There is no way you can have a fit child while you continue being an unfit adult!

Christopher enjoyed three pre-school programs with me. I pass them along as examples of what you might consider as you and your child move along this fitness path.

"Mousercise" is a Walt Disney record that stars Christopher's favorite character: Mickey Mouse. In the record, Mickey leads children through a series of fun movements that are designed to develop physical skills in time to music.

Christopher and I enjoyed dancing, jumping, and rolling along with Mickey and the gang. If you are prepared to get down and be a kid again, this record will be lots of fun for you and your child, ages one through six. Don't forget to stretch a little bit before doing something quick and strenuous; you don't want to be a parent with a "Mickey Mouse pull"!

"Fit Kids" is a series of three records (also available in video) of pre-school exercise programs developed by Patty Dow, coordinator of the Discovery Program's Toddler Center in New York City. The programs are set to lively music and aimed toward three age groups: one month to walking; walking to three years; and three years and up.

Each record teaches body parts, warm-ups and cool-downs, and stretching. They contain imaginative games and movements set to music. Christopher's favorites included "Roller Coaster," "Monkey See, Monkey Do,"

"Boogie Woogie," and "The Freeze Game." The records are practical only if you push aside the furniture and get out and boogie with your kid.

"Kids in Motion" is an action-packed video that combines dance, music, poetry, and imaginative play to help young children enjoy exercise. It was developed by Julie Weissman, a dance and movement specialist. The video features a group of enthusiastic kids who do routines like "Tummy Tango," "The Body Rock," and "Animal Action" to groups like The Temptations. You may have seen Christopher demonstrating this program on "The Today Show"—he was the lively frog.

PHYSICAL EDUCATION

A child's activity pattern is learned early in life. Many children have already become overweight and physically inactive before starting kindergarten. There is a growing need to expand the formal physical education program into the pre-school environment. According to a University of Georgia study by L. M. Albertson, six-year-olds scored significantly higher on an educational readiness test after three years of pre-school experience than those who did not attend school at this age. However, the study showed that those who participated in pre-school education would have been better off, in terms of motor skill development, to have stayed at home. Clearly this demonstrates the need for pre-fitness activities in our pre-school educational system.

21

Teenagers

Those of you who have teenage children are certain of at least one fact: that the terrible statistics we all know about teenage drug use, suicide, and physical unfitness tell only half the story. The other half is that most of our teenage kids are really interesting, bright, intelligent, and hopeful individuals. In fact, Dr. Daniel Offer, a psychiatrist at the University of Chicago, declared a "Defense of Adolescents" in an article in the *Journal of the American Medical Association* and in a presentation to the 1987 convention of the American Psychiatric Association. Dr. Offer told the psychiatrists' convention that his research indicates that "the vast majority of adolescents are well adjusted, get along well with their peers and their parents, adjust well to the mores and values of their social environment and cope well with their internal and external worlds."

The struggle between the security of childhood and the independence and responsibilities of adulthood present a difficult time for teenagers. It is a time when parents need to be concerned about both the physical and psychological health of their children.

Statistics and surveys show that since the early 1960s, the general health of today's teenagers—kids ages thirteen to nineteen—has declined. A study of teenage students in Mississippi, conducted between 1965 and 1967 and then repeated in 1982, discovered that blood pressure levels had risen significantly during the seventeen-year interval. "We referred twice as many students to physicians for evaluation of high blood pressure as we had in the 1960s," said Dr. Robert Watson, director of the study.

In 1984, the Office of Disease Prevention and Health Promotion completed a two-year national fitness study for kids ages ten to seventeen. The study found that U.S. teenagers today have a "significantly higher" percentage of body fat than those twenty years earlier, and they cannot perform well on chin-ups, bent-knee sit-ups, or other fitness tests. In 1976, when the AAHPERD conducted a National Youth Fitness Test, 15 percent of high-school students qualified for the Presidential Physical Fitness Award, the highest level. In the same test given in 1983, fewer than 1 percent of those students tested reached this fitness level. Tests in the late 1980s show no improvement. Furthermore, as the fitness standards in Chapter 4 indicate, fitness scores for the average teenager—especially girls—decrease after age fifteen. Teens enter adulthood with a declining fitness profile.

In 1988, four prominent groups involved in health education announced the results of the first National Adolescent Student Health Survey.* While some of their findings are very encouraging, some are disturbing. For example, the survey revealed that suicide is a serious problem among teenagers in the late 1980s: one out of every seven teenagers has attempted suicide. The survey also showed that more than half of all eighth-graders and two-thirds of all tenth-graders in the United States have smoked cigarettes, and that 80 percent of all teenagers have tried alcoholic beverages. The survey also reported that one out of six eighth-grade kids and one out of every three tenth-graders has smoked marijuana. One out of every twenty eighth-graders and one out of every ten tenth-graders has used cocaine.

These kids also face difficult decisions about their personal health and safety. Most of them understand about AIDS (Acquired Immune Deficiency Syndrome), sex, refusing sex, and preventing pregnancy. But one out of three said they did not know where to go for medical care, and 44 percent said they would be embarrassed to ask their doctors questions about personal health and/or sex.

More than half of the girls and about one-third of the boys reported difficulty dealing with stress, and said that stress at home and school was particularly troubling. They also reported stress of another kind: almost half of the boys and one girl in every four reported having been in a physical fight during the past year. One out of every three students said that someone had threatened to hurt them; 14 percent had been robbed and 13 percent attacked at school or on the school bus in the past year.

What does all this have to do with fitness and this book? For one thing, the National Adolescent Student Health Survey showed that half of all U.S. teenage girls and one-third of all boys do not eat breakfast regularly. Another study reports that half of high-schoolers skip the school lunch. Nutrition and personal health are not being taught to these kids!

I also argue that our teenagers are not getting enough exercise of the

---

*The American School Health Association, the Association for the Advancement of Health Education, the Society for Public Health Education, and the American Alliance for Health, Physical Education, Recreation, and Dance.

right kind—and that good exercise and nutrition go together. The enforced discipline of structured fitness programs—running, swimming, biking, walking—might help them physically and mentally. But in too many of our middle and high schools, teenage kids think exercise is for athletically gifted students. By high school, 90 percent of our kids have assumed the role of spectator; their only exercise is cheering on their physically gifted classmates. The result is the dismal statistics above.

WHAT CAN WE DO?

It is helpful to understand some things about teenagers, particularly their growth and exercise. By age twelve, your child should understand the benefits of physical exercise and be active aerobically on a regular basis. If not, your problems are compounded, but not hopeless (I'll get to them in a minute).

I believe that regular exercise, coupled with instruction about good nutrition and health, could benefit almost everyone of our adolescents. They also need about nine hours of sleep per night. I also believe we should push—and push hard—to get a national fitness program started among our teenage kids. How much more warning do we need than the statistics and studies cited above? The four keys to improved health for our teenagers are: diet, exercise, sleep, stress.

I'd like to see every kid who is physically able running about two miles every other day at age fourteen. Other quality aerobic activity is also acceptable.

I would like schools and parents to start activity programs at a young age when children love to play and run around. If you can help your children stay active and motivated, then the teenage years will be somewhat easier. Over the long run, your child will be healthier and happier. Continue to urge your children to learn and use lifelong exercise skills. Rowing, biking, running, squash, cross-country skiing, and other such activities are going to benefit your child every day of his or her life.

I would like to see middle and high schools institute no-cut policies on their teams. That means that any kid who wants to play a sport could play on a school team. The uncoordinated kid who gets cut from the soccer or basketball team may in fact turn out to be the better player. That's why no-cut policies are so valuable; they give the kids filling out from rapid growth a chance to work on their development. They take into consideration the feelings and physical development of teenagers. For example, the Hanover, New Hampshire, High School (where Jack Shepherd's children graduated) has such a policy. Soccer is an enormously popular autumn sport for both the boys and girls. In the middle school, ages twelve to thirteen or so, there are boys' and girls' teams lettered A through C. Any student who wants to play soccer in the fall plays. In high school, there are varsity, junior varsity, and freshman teams; there are junior varsity B teams and freshman B teams when needed. In the autumn of 1988, three out of every four students were playing inter-scholastic sports—soccer, cross-country, football, and field hockey—at some level of competition. More important, three out of every four students were exercising after school every day all autumn long!

Hanover, and its sister town, Norwich, Vermont, across the river have extensive community exercise programs that start kids out playing on the town greens at age five or six. What is the result of such a program? Five members of the 1988 U.S. Winter Olympics team came from these two tiny New England towns! More important, the school is graduating more teenagers who will be fit for life.

Watch Our Kids

Such programs can be put in place almost anywhere. But to be successful, they must stress two things: everyone plays and the kids are not pushed into winning. There is a third point to remember: teenage kids are also rapidly growing and their musculo-skeletal systems can be hurt (sprains, stress fractures) by too much exercise. We should be alert to growth spurts, generally in girls between ages eleven and thirteen, and in boys ages about thirteen to sixteen. These will cause postural changes, tighter muscles, temporary loss of coordination, and other physical and sometimes mental stress. During these years, encourage your child to stretch regularly to maintain flexibility (it will also feel very good) and do some easy muscular development work such as sit-ups and push-ups.

Watch and listen to your child. If he or she is on a team and suddenly drops out it could be an alert signal. It may mean there is too much coaching or peer pressure in his or her life, or it may mean that your child is being distracted by (or attracted to) something else. That may not always be good—drugs, kids who put down exercise, etc. It could be that your child suddenly believes that he or she cannot compete or is somehow incompetent. Or perhaps your child has been pushed too hard and now hates exercise. Or the cause may be something as simple as locker room blues: lack of time to change clothes and get ready for classes, not having the required gym clothes, boring activities, locker room harassment by peers— all these turn off kids to physical education. High schools must be urged to allow kids more time to dress after exercising and get ready for their next class. Some high schools have schedules like colleges, where students have classes and open hours scattered throughout the day.

Adolescents who have chosen a self-paced lifelong sport are by far the best off. They will stick with the activity and make it their own.

Pay Attention to Them

Talk to your kids and any other teenagers you meet. You'll discover a human being, not a statistic. You'll also discover someone with raw, untried ideas, serious thoughts, and a great capacity to love (offered openly and without conditions).

Expect explosions, arguments, rebellion, stubbornness. Just remember the old saying, If all the world's a stage, home is backstage. Let the kids storm and rage, but be there when they want to talk. Dr. Joseph Zanga, chairman of the American Academy of Pediatrics' Committee on School Health, indicated that most parents spend little time with their teenage children. The average is—are you ready for this—ten to twenty minutes a day. "Furthermore," said Dr. Zanga, "most of this is one-way communication, with the parent criticizing or giving orders." As a result, adolescents frequently go through the emotional turmoil of their lives without adult guidance, listening, or help. A good time to chat with your teenager is while enjoying exercise together. The exercise relieves tension between parents and teen and serves as a common point of interest.

Eat with Them

Our teenagers grow at different rates. Chronological age may be the same among all of them but their biological ages are vastly different. Just think of the various sizes that thirteen- and fourteen-year-olds come in. Kids who are large for their age at thirteen or fourteen may simply be average size at sixteen or seventeen. This is to say that growth during puberty is best promoted by increases in the quantity and quality of food. The adolescent's whole hormonal system is rapidly developing and needs adequate nutrition.

Providing teenage kids with a good meal or two should not be difficult for American adults. Our stores have the food our kids need. Yet, for various reasons, too few parents bother to feed their kids. They send them off to school without breakfast, the kids don't have a lunch from home and skip the school lunch, and they return home to snacks and TV. Donald Ian Macdonald, administrator of the Alcohol, Drug Abuse and Mental Health Administration, told *Reader's Digest* that "increasing numbers of families do not eat dinner together. The children eat as they watch TV, and their dinner is too often snack-oriented."

You want to do something for your kids? Feed 'em good food, and eat it with them.

Exercise with Them

In 1960, most states required that their high-school students take four years of daily physical education classes. Now only Illinois and New Jersey have such a requirement. Most high schools offer no physical education—no exercise—to their students after the tenth grade. This is often a double whammy, since many high-school P.E. classes also included health and nutrition education. So our kids are getting less and less exercise or health and nutritional information.

This puts the burden back on you. If you have pre-teenage children you may be better off—in this chapter anyway—than if you have teenage children who have no exercise background and no P.E. classes in high school. If your kids are not yet teenagers, you may still get them involved in family and community fitness workouts. But by the time a kid is thirteen or fourteen, he or she may be indifferent to the benefits of regular exercise unless it is associated with a team or with friends (or friends' opinions). "You can't tell a sixteen-year-old anything," says Dr. Paul Dyment of the American Academy of Pediatrics, "let alone to run three miles, three times a week to prevent a heart attack when he's forty."

What to do? First, analyze what your kid is at this moment. A couch potato? Neo-sloth? Or perhaps someone who still rides a bike occasionally, hikes in the park or countryside when there's a chance, or plays a ferocious game of tennis, handball, or squash. Shepherd, at age thirteen, was told (by a coach) that he was the worst baseball player in the eighth grade. He went on to become a starting varsity shortstop in college. He was also cut from his high-school soccer team every year he tried out; he went on to play four years of varsity soccer in college, including one year when his team upset the number one nationally ranked Navy team and won its division.

Second, encourage your kids to do anything physical: ride bikes, play intramurals, join community groups for any exercise (hiking, swimming, whatever they like). Encourage, make things available, but don't push. Shepherd played junior varsity baseball throughout high school, and intramural soccer. He grew eight inches in one year, and he took four years to fill out. His parents simply made a soccer ball and a baseball backstop available around the yard. His own interests did the rest. There are two lessons here: Watch what your kids like to do and encourage them to do it. Maybe there's a third lesson: Join them.

22

Girls and Women

Why a chapter on girls and not boys? For the same reason that I coach an all-women's elite running team. Girls and women are not equal participants in sports and fitness—despite making up more than half of our population. This is wrong. As the data and studies in this chapter make clear, girls and women can hold their own in fitness and sports—and should have the opportunity to do so. The women's team I founded in 1980 is named Atalanta, after the Greek mythical figure who was intelligent, beautiful, and athletic. To win her hand in marriage, a man had to beat her in a foot race; to lose meant death. I can think of some male athletic directors who should race against the goddess Atalanta.

"Sport has always been the prerogative of the male," said Dr. Dorothy Harris, vice president of the Women's Sports Foundation. "A double standard exists in society. Males are socialized to use their bodies to please themselves, while females are socialized to use their bodies to please others. Physical prowess, team sports, that's male turf."

That turf is starting to be shared with girls and women. But there is still a long way to go.

HISTORY

In many communities and schools, girls and boys playing sports together is frowned on; even girls and women exercising vigorously remains, in some regions of the country, unusual. The old cliché still holds: Men perspire, women only glow.

Yet, a paradox exists. Since Title IX of the Education Amendments Act*

---

*Title IX guaranteed equal opportunity for girls and women in programs in federally funded schools and colleges. In 1984, the U.S. Supreme Court held that Title IX applied only to a specific program and not the institution or school as a whole. In 1988, Congress restored Title IX's equal opportunity in all school programs, including athletics, under the Civil Rights Restoration Act.

was passed in 1972, there has been a revolution in women's sports. In 1974, just 2 percent of college and university athletic budgets was designated for women and only sixty colleges offered athletic scholarships to women. Today, college women get one-third of all athletic scholarships and 16 percent of the total athletic budget.

More girls and women than ever before are playing sports or exercising regularly. A study by American Sports Data, Inc. shows that "women now make up a majority of all new participants in physical conditioning, weight training, running and fitness bicycling, not to mention the already female-dominated activities of aerobic dancing and exercise to music." Between 1971 and 1985, the number of girls playing high-school sports jumped fivefold. In 1985, more than 1.7 million girls took part in thirty-three sports—more than two out of every nine girls participating, according to Carl Ojala at Eastern Michigan University.

There is still a long way to go, however. Boys still outnumber girls by two to one on our high-school playing fields. A 1984 National Children and Youth Fitness Study showed that boys still spend about 10 percent more time in physical activity than girls.

Girls and women are generally not as physically fit as boys and men. The 1988 Wilson Sporting Goods–Women's Sports Foundation survey showed that while 82 percent of the girls polled said they did some sports or fitness activity, the number fell sharply with age: 87 percent of girls seven to ten and 84 percent of girls eleven to fourteen said they were involved in sports. But only 75 percent of girls fifteen to eighteen said they played sports or exercised.

Although fitness scores for boys improve through their teens, those for girls decline—except for flexibility. "They get to age fourteen and they quit," said Guy Reiff, director of the President's Council on Physical Fitness and Sports' 1985 study. They lose interest and become more sedentary. According to national fitness test scores, the fitness level of boys continues to increase from age fifteen to eighteen, but girls' scores decline from age fifteen on.

Why Do Girls Quit Exercising?

The 1987 Wilson Sporting Goods–Women's Sports Foundation survey, "Moms, Dads, Daughters and Sports," listed several reasons: competing interests distract them; 51 percent of the dropouts felt they were not good enough at the sport; 58 percent said they did not have the time for sports or exercise; 25 percent of the girls responding in ages fifteen to eighteen said that sports are more important for boys, but only 10 percent ages seven to fourteen gave the same reason.

A 1987 conference of three national girls and women's sports groups* examined the reasons why girls and women stop playing sports or exercising. They identified several psychological factors as barriers to participation:

- conflicts with sex-role identity;
- perceived incompetence in sports;
- early or late physical maturation;
- social pressure in coed competition;
- embarrassment because of body changes;
- peer pressure to be more "feminine";
- found fitness or sports activities too challenging or not challenging enough;
- lacked motor skills to enjoy sports.

Three major themes emerge here. Somewhere after puberty girls get the notion that they are not good at sports, and they quit. They reach what frustrated physical educators call "the puberty barrier." There is, secondly, a lot of strong peer pressure to take on more traditional feminine roles, such as cheerleader rather than player. Third, several of the studies mentioned above cite lack of support from parents and school as strong reasons for girls or young women dropping out of sports or exercise programs.

The Parents' Role

Here is an area where parents—and especially fathers—can play a major role in their daughters' health and fitness. According to the Wilson study, 87 percent of today's parents accept the idea that sports are equally important for boys and girls, and 97 percent believe that sports and fitness activities provide benefits to girls who participate.

The Wilson study showed that parents who play sports or engage in fitness activities as adults tend to have daughters who play or who exercise regularly. Almost half the daughters polled said the fact that their parents participated in fitness activities or sports influenced them to do so too. But while mothers encourage daughters of all ages, only 27 percent of the young girls said their fathers encouraged them.

According to the National Children and Youth Fitness Study II, mothers of children ages six to nine exercise with sons and daughters with equal frquency. But while fathers spend at least fifty days a year exercising with sons, they spend only thirty-five days exercising with their daughters.

*The Girls Clubs of America, National Association for Girls and Women in Sport, and the Women's Sports Foundation.

Fathers tend to encourage sons to play sports and keep fit, but not daughters—at least not until they are high-school age. Then, according to the Wilson study, about 44 percent of girls fifteen to eighteen in this study said their fathers encouraged them to play sports or participate in fitness activities.

This may be, I believe, because fathers perceive their daughters at age fifteen or older as athletes; they get the same vicarious thrill and enjoyment from their daughters' successes on the playing fields as from their sons'. Either that, or they have overcome their own bias in favor of boys as athletes, and girls as spectators and cheerleaders. "If dads stepped in earlier," said Kathy Button of the Women's Sports Foundation advisory board, "daughters might be better skilled and less likely to give up sports."

SHOULD PHYSICAL ACTIVITY BE COED?

Before Puberty

By the time they reach elementary school age, children have often learned that active sports are "masculine" and not "feminine," and that masculine games have more prestige among adults. Increasing girls' participation in all sports and at an earlier age can help overcome these sex-sterotyped ideas. Physicians from the American Academy of Pediatrics (AAP) agree that there is no reason to separate children by gender in sports, physical education, or recreational activities before they reach puberty. The AAP doctors say that girls can compete against boys in any sport if they are matched by size, weight, degree of physical maturation, and skill.

This really means that most boys and girls can play on teams or take gym together—if they are matched by skill level—until they reach puberty, since they are almost the same size and weight. Before puberty only slight differences in body structure and motor skills exist between girls and boys. The opportunities for improving performance, or sustaining injury, are almost identical. In fact, girls at this age have similar aerobic capacities but a slight edge over boys in speed and strength.

The differences in skills between girls and boys at this age, however, are largely reflective of difference in opportunity to learn those skills. According to a study at the University of Virginia, girls improved in sit-ups, long-jumping, and other exercises when placed in a coed setting, whereas the abilities of the boys remained about the same. The reason: Girls were exposed to activities that allowed them to catch up with the boys. "There are no biological differences that affect girls' capability to participate in sports," according to the Girls Clubs of America's booklet Sporting Chance. "The socialization process is the only limiting force, and can be changed."

There are, however, some psychological issues to consider when placing girls and boys together in fitness or sports activities. Most parents worry about how the girls will hold up, but in fact it is the boys who are under the most stress. According to Rainer Martens, author of *Joy and Sadness in Children's Sports*, defeat by girls may damage a boy's feelings of self-worth. He is expected—by adults—to beat a girl in competition. Yet, as such competition becomes more commonplace, and girls are playing on previously all-boy teams (even in high school), "the psychological threat (especially to boys) of competing with the opposite sex will dissipate."

As things now stand, however, most play in elementary school is sex segregated. Boys who dare play with girls are taunted by their male peers, as Christopher has learned.

After Puberty

Girls enter puberty around ten or eleven years of age and experience a growth spurt that peaks around thirteen or fourteen. Boys enter puberty about two years later than girls and their growth spurt peaks around fifteen or sixteen. It is not uncommon for girls in the ten to thirteen age range to have a size advantage on boys the same age and to excel in sports compared to the boys. When the boys' growth spurt occurs, however, they catch up with the girls and gain in strength, speed, and power. At this point, girls often fall behind in comparative athletic ability. This race between growing adolescents should be carefully explained to them by their parents. At one point, boys may feel inferior to girls who are larger and quicker than they; at another, girls may actually stop playing sports because they can no longer compete with boys who at thirteen or older are faster and stronger.

I believe this is the time to separate the girls and the boys into separate fitness classes and teams. According to the physicians at AAP, because puberty gives boys an advantage both in strength and size, safety and fairness dictate that boys and girls should no longer compete against each other at that point. The AAP warns that girls should not play against boys in collision sports because of the risk of injury due to their lesser muscle mass and body weight. Whether or not they should compete as members of the same team remains in debate. The AAP doctors agree that girls can be allowed on previously all-boys teams—for example, soccer. It makes no sense, however, to allow a girl who is good enough to play on a boys' team to do so if her school has a girls' team in that same sport.

Boys and girls can therefore compete together to about age eleven to twelve, as long as coaches and parents are aware of gender-related sensitivities. In the best of all possible worlds, girls age twelve and under should be able to play on teams with all girls, or a mixture of girls and boys. After puberty, boys and girls should probably compete separately, but on teams with equal equipment and coaching. Teenagers can play together on a low-key basis in gym classes, recreational camps, and on teams playing soccer, volleyball, or softball. They can—and should—enjoy non-competitive fitness activities such as running, biking, walking, and swimming together. A natural coed activity: dancing.

Adult Coed Sports

Sharing fitness classes and sports with men has become in the 1980s a pleasant and new reality for women in the United States. According to a study by Miller Lite and the Women's Sports Foundation, coed sports have become commonplace. There are three reasons: the efforts of women to find sports partners of equal skill, regardless of gender; the belief "that women have something to teach men about humane competition"; and "abundant evidence of strong self-confidence among athletic women, a clear conviction that sports participation does *not* diminish femininity."

One of the early ways men and women came together for fitness and sports competition was running. In the early 1970s, most road races contained 90 percent or more men. Women were not allowed to run with men in most events. My friend Kathrine Switzer was almost wrestled out of the 1967 Boston Marathon when she tried to run in a previously all-male event, causing quite a lot of nationwide publicity. Another friend, Nina Kuscsik, became the first official female division winner of this event in 1972, when women were finally accepted.

Now, several major running events around the country have as many or more women participants as men. The key here is that they compete at the same distance and time, but are scored separately for awards. Thus, there are two separate races at the front of the pack, and plenty of fun for the coed masses in the back—not to mention the post-race partying. Still, the women-only L'eggs Mini Marathon in New York City's Central Park attracts more than eight thousand women, including, I'm sure, hundreds of women who are uncomfortable running and competing among men.

More and more women and men exercise together—and get fit together—in popular activities like running, walking, and biking. They exercise and talk with one another (remember my rule about the talk test) and fitness workouts become ways of meeting new friends.

The Results

The Miller Lite–Women's Sports Foundation report makes very clear that girls and boys playing together before puberty is good for the girls. Those athletic women who played with boys or mixed girl-boy teams in childhood, the study found, were far more likely to have positive body images, take leadership positions in sports, and participate more actively in sports and fitness as adults.

Sex segregation of play harms boys. Researchers now are exploring whether or not boys' "masculine" free-time activities—building, competitive sports—may explain why they are six times more likely than girls to have difficulty learning to read. One study under way in Maryland indicated that boys' severe reading problems could stem in part from sex stereotyping. Boys who engaged in the most sex-segregated play performed least well in communications subjects. Moreover, when girls don't participate in games with boys, it appears to harm the development of their spatial skills (the ability to visualize three-dimensional objects in space). Unfortunately, we continue to separate girls and boys and to give them sex-stereotyped fitness roles.

According to the AAP, moreover, girls also benefit physically from sports. Their conditioning, agility, strength, endurance, and sense of well-being improve. The AAP also points out that such activity has no adverse effect on a woman's menstruation, future pregnancy, or childbirth.

In fact, the Women's Sports Foundation survey found that those women who as girls played with boys had better body images and were more competitive than those who had not. According to the Girls Club of America's booklet *Sporting Chance*:

> Participation in athletics can teach assertiveness, which in turn can have a favorable impact on females: studies have shown that women will act assertively only if they believe the situation permits them to behave that way, or if they can act anonymously. Studies of female entrepreneurs suggest a positive link between early play patterns, including sports participation, and late achievements in life.

There are some certain benefits to girls and women for participating in sports at an early age. As mentioned, assertiveness is one. Also, researchers say that women who played sports as girls develop a lifestyle that reduces their risk of breast and uterine cancer. They are more likely to have a lean body, eat a low-fat diet, and remain active through menopause. Studies at Rockefeller University in New York City and Harvard University's School of Public Health indicate that by their mid-fifties, sedentary women have a two and a half times greater risk for cancer, of the reproductive system, twice the risk for breast cancer and 3.4 times the risk for diabetes. Some of these risks are reduced by exercise.

OBSTACLES

There are some obvious hurdles to having more girls and women participate in fitness and sports. Most schools have limited budgets to spend on sports and fitness. Girls' sports are considered less important, partly because boys' sports programs attract more crowds and therefore more money and prestige to the school. The girls, as a result, tend to get less money, poor equipment and facilities, and off-hour practice and game times.

The majority of coaches in coed and girls' teams are men. This appears to be true even on the high-school and college level. In fact, over the last few years the number of women coaching girls' and women's teams has decreased. Women should get more involved as coaches, officials, and administrators to establish role models for girls. But even here we need to work on attitudes. *Sporting Chance* reports: "Equity research shows that male and female teacher/coaches give more instruction and correction to boys and more praise for effort to girls." It is as though they expect boys to go on to be athletic and that girls are somehow doing something they shouldn't.

The Women's Sports Foundation, in its *Parents' Guide to Girls' Sports*, states:

> The chance for females to participate in athletics is often diminished because there is not equal societal support. However, girls and women will participate if given the opportunity. In some instances women have developed their own teams and leagues in order to compete. The family needs to investigate the opportunities in their schools, the local private clubs, Y's and local teams such as Little Leagues. If equal opportunities are not available, find out how to make them available. Equal opportunity is the law.

MALE VS. FEMALE: THE DIFFERENCES

Right from the beginning, there are exhibited differences between boy and girl babies. According to Crystal Branta, a speaker at the 1987 New Agenda II women's sports seminar, female-male differences in play occur as early as thirteen months of age and develop in a particular way. Boys seem to take risks more than girls during games. Girls tend to be more sedentary and their play "more nurturant and self-grooming." Here, again, parents seem to play a role: mothers tend to allow males to cry longer in their cribs before comforting them and to cuddle females more than male children.

Studies of sex differences show that after about age eight, boys generally run faster and jump farther than girls; but girls hop better than boys. These same studies, reviewed in *Sporting Chance*, indicated that boys spent more time outdoors in movement and took more space in play than girls, which gave them a distinct advantage in learning most sports activities.

These studies reached a very interesting conclusion: since girls mature earlier than boys, they should begin physical activity programs earlier than boys, to increase the influence that exercise has on them. Traditionally, however, girls are organized in sports much later than boys.

I agree that girls and boys should exercise and play together up to a certain age, about twelve or so. I also agree that girls should be given the chance to start organized exercise activities as soon as they are ready, perhaps around age six. But I also say the same thing about boys. I agree with many researchers who are now concluding that most differences in performance between boys and girls are learned, not the result of physiological differences. Before puberty, there are no physical reasons for boys to be better than girls in fitness or motor skills. I believe that up until age twelve or so, children should be treated as exercising individuals, not as girls or boys. Learning to run, bat, kick, and throw should be the right of each child and should be taught equally.

The difference, of course, comes at puberty. Up to about age twelve or thirteen, boys and girls on average differ little in either height or weight. In the eight-to-twelve age group, girls are about two years ahead of boys in physical, bone, and hormonal development. Not until about thirteen or fourteen do boys begin to surpass girls in height, weight, and muscular development. Then the differences are more pronounced, and separate competitive sports activities are needed.

There are other differences. On average, men are about 40 percent stronger than women. Between ages seven and seventeen, however, the difference is far less. We also know that girls and women have the potential to develop much higher levels of strength than those found in sedentary females.

In terms of cardio-respiratory endurance, girls and boys are again similar if not identical. Recent studies indicate that endurance among girls and women does not drop much compared to men, nor is it markedly below men of similar age levels.

Motor skills and athletic ability among boys and girls—with the exception of throwing—are much alike up to age twelve. In tests of running and speed, boys and girls are about equal up to twelve or thirteen. Boys do outperform girls in motor skills, but as I said above this may be due to practice rather than physiology.

While some researchers argue that physiological differences separate girls and boys athletically after about age twelve, others disagree. They attribute the differences as much to what society expects of teenage girls as to physical differences. As Lawrence Galton wrote in *Your Child in Sports:*

It should be noted that although the differences exist, there are girls and women who can hit a ball farther than many boys and men, and boys and men who cannot swim as fast as most girls and women can.

One thing is certain: Girls and women have just begun to approach their athletic potential. They have some catching up to do since they started later than males, and they are catching up.

In swimming and running, recent tests on women are showing remarkable results. In fact, women now hold some long-distance running records for both sexes. They have improved their running marathon times consistently since the mid-1970s, when they began competing in races with (but not against) men. During ultra-marathons of fifty miles or longer, women have run men into the ground. "The evidence suggests that women are tougher than men," says Dr. Joan Ullyot, a physiologist at San Francisco's Institute of Health Research and a world-class master's marathon runner.

Injuries

There are many reasons, usually given by male teachers, coaches, and athletic directors, why older girls and women should not participate in sports or vigorous fitness activities. One has to do with injury to their bodies and the other with the impact on their reproductive abilities. This is serious, nineteenth-century thinking.

Some male coaches and athletic directors argue that women are somehow more fragile than men. I would like to remind those men—and any others out there—that a man's scrotum and testicles are far more vulnerable to injury than a woman's ovaries. Nor are a woman's breasts easily damaged. Dr. John Marshall, director of sports medicine at New York City's Hospital for Special Surgery, once told *Time* magazine that "There is no evidence that trauma of the breasts is a precurser of cancer." Most important, scrotum or breasts can be easily protected.

Another canard concerns a woman's menstrual cycle. Some coaches argue that the cycle prevents peak performance—yet world and Olympic records have been set by women during their periods. Some researchers do contend that physical performance is somewhat better during the time immediately following menstruation up to about the fifteenth day of the cycle. But this varies so greatly from woman to woman as to be inconsequential.

Some women who run long distances or take on hard training over long periods of time find that their menstruation stops. This is called amenorrhea and it occurs in about 45 percent of women who run more than sixty-five miles a week. It is also found among dancers, cyclists, ice skaters, gymnasts, and rowers, and medical studies indicate that it may be due to the loss of body fat during exercise. A cutback in training, with the concomitant gain in weight, usually restores the normal cycle.

Another concern is pregnancy. Most physicians now approve exercise for women after they have become pregnant at least through the first six months—unless they were not exercising at all when they became pregnant. That is, an exercise program should not be started after a woman has become pregnant.

Equipment

Girls and women playing sports do need some special equipment. Some progress in design has taken place—the "jogbra," for example. But for the most part girls and women can wear whatever boys and men wear—socks, shorts, shoes, pants, sweatshirts, jerseys—simply cut to their somewhat different body shape.

Some sports need special equipment—field and ice hockey, softball, lacrosse—and may require strength training on equipment designed for men. Girls and women should use special caution and discretion here, and work out under the close supervision of a qualified coach. Seats on bicycles are also designed differently for men and women, and women should select a bike seat contoured to the dimensions of their pelvic bones.

Coaching

According to the Women's Sports Foundation, "Worries about coaching girls because they are 'different' are unnecessary. It should be remembered, though, that in many cases girls have not had the opportunity to learn fundamental sport skills at an early age. Coaches (and parents) need to be sensitive to this fact and be prepared to drill the basics, if necessary." Donna DeVarona, the Olympic swimming gold medalist, agrees: "If my father had not treated me just like my brother—always telling me I was capable of the best in whatever I did—I would never have made it to the Olympic victory stand."

My experience coaching the Atalanta women's running team is similar. Many of the women don't start running until they are in their twenties, thirties, and even fifties. They are emotionally ready to train hard, but lack the long-term development that provides a base of muscle fitness. I tend to be more conservative with them than with men until they have trained with me for several years. Then, when they are ready, I intensify their training to at least the level of men of similar ability. An example is Angella Hearn, who started running in her thirties, and at age forty-one—training one hundred miles per week—ran a world-class 2:39:55 marathon.

I'm often asked the difference between coaching men and women. To me, there are two differences: Women need to be held back more when first starting due to their lack of experience in sports; and women appreciate coaching and improve much faster than men—perhaps because they listen well and train better.

Where does all this leave us?

There appear to be few physical differences between young boys and girls, and certainly none that would mean they cannot and should not play and exercise together. After age thirteen or fourteen the gap widens somewhat in terms of motor skills, speed, and strength. But I still believe that girls should play on some boys' sports teams—those without body impact—if they want to and no similar girls' team is offered. Certainly, without exception, girls and boys, and men and women, should exercise together for fitness and fun. And, as summarized by Dr. Dorothy Harris after reviewing the encouraging 1988 Wilson Report on attitudes surrounding girls and sports: "The word tomboy is going to become obsolete. No longer will girls who play sports be considered unladylike."

23

The Health Impaired and Physically Disabled

Many parents who have a health-impaired, or mentally or physically handicapped child, are too protective of him or her. I believe that most chronic medical problems should not prohibit a child or adult from exercise and sports. Generally, the benefits of exercise for most handicapped individuals far outweigh the disadvantages.

My experience working with handicapped children and adults indicates that an exercise program specifically designed for them improves the quality of their lives. Often it also improves the handicapped person's ability to deal with his or her medical problems. Some handicapped people—asthmatics, diabetics, epileptics, for example—have been world champion athletes. Many physically and mentally handicapped boys and girls and men and women can compete against each other in a variety of sports.

The problem is that we, as parents, and society at large tend to protect and coddle our handicapped children. Under the care of a knowledgeable and concerned physician, most handicapped people can enjoy physical activity. Any limitations they might have, in my opinion, should be viewed more as limits on their skill at a specific activity rather than limitations on their ability to enjoy exercise.

I also believe that our handicapped children should be placed in regular physical education classes in school whenever possible. An exercise program for the handicapped should be based on what is medically acceptable for each person's particular condition. The condition, limitations, and medical guidelines for each handicapped person should be thoroughly communicated to all coaches, teachers, and family members who might be involved in the individual's physical activity program. The handicapped person should be told of the risks in each activity. This includes any physical health risk as well as risk to the person's self-image.

While the physical risks are small, given careful medical attention, there are serious psychological and emotional risks. Positive support and reinforcement are very important to the child learning to overcome his or her physical limitations. The child needs help in learning to deal with his or her handicap, and especially in learning to deal with being treated differently. Self-image and social acceptance, especially important to children, can be enhanced by letting them participate in sports and physical activity. Whenever possible, they should also be "mainstreamed" into school physical education programs, sports teams, and so on.

Overprotective but well-meaning parents and teachers can have a negative effect on a child's acceptance of his or her handicap. By not letting the child do whatever he or she can, the parent or teacher actually increases the problem: the child feels "different"; his or her motor skills and physical fitness decrease; the child feels socially detached from her or his peers. Sometimes, a child will use the excuse of the handicap to get out of physical activity. The result may be poor fitness levels, lack of motor skills, and low self-esteem.

MAINSTREAMING

I believe that almost every handicapped person should have some form of daily physical activity. In fact, rigorous physical activity has been shown to increase physical fitness among the handicapped, enhance the person's ability to deal with the handicap, and create greater social and psychological independence. In my own work, I have seen dramatic changes in the ability of handicapped men, women, and children to function better in society by improving their physical fitness level.

According to the law, handicapped kids should be placed in regular physical education classes whenever possible. This is called mainstreaming. They should first be placed in a regular school setting. Teachers might make adjustments to help the child, without singling the child out. Or, if that is inappropriate, the child should be in a program similar to the regular school setting. Extremely handicapped kids may be placed in special education classrooms with trained teachers. They should have the chance to be with the other students, however.

The idea is to allow handicapped kids to join activities in an unrestricted environment. The purpose is to give these children the opportunity to reach their potential as students—and to have fun and get fit along with their non-handicapped peers. The handicapped child is a participant in an individualized goal system. This measures their progress only against themselves. They set the goals and work to attain them.

Not all kids can do this. Chronic illness can damage the child's ego:

"Why can't I do things like other kids?" The dependence on medicines, special diets, or the attention of anxious parents are seen as signs of weakness. Overprotection here is almost as bad as no protection at all. This is a common reaction to feelings of guilt and insecurity as parents try to shelter their child from his illness.

Well-meaning teachers, peers, and family often try to restrict handicapped kids from tasks they are capable of performing. Dependence may become a habit and a source of frustration. Handicapped kids need to participate in as much of normal life as their illness allows—and with as little special attention as possible. The goals of physical education and fitness are no different for the handicapped child: develop and maintain a good level of physical fitness and motor skills. Each child needs to test competence and develop independence, and physical fitness and motor skill development help. Self-confidence, leadership, and social interaction are of equal importance to handicapped kids.

THE ACHILLES TRACK CLUB

When Dick Traum walked into my office in 1975, I was shocked. He wanted a fitness test so he could take my beginner runner's course. Dick, then thirty-four, had been gaining weight, and was under increasing stress as his business grew, and he had decided to register for my YMCA fitness program. He was typical of any other businessman entering my program—except he had only one leg. How should I help this man run? I asked myself.

I decided to treat him just like everyone else, with one adjustment. Instead of riding the stationary bike for the cardio-respiratory fitness test, I had him hop up and down on a bench. Dick scored about the same as other men his age: he was in fair to poor shape on every test. His biggest handicap wasn't the lack of one leg, but his twenty pounds of excess weight and his sedentary lifestyle.

"Can you run?" I asked him.

"Sure," Dick replied. In fact he hadn't run a step since losing his leg in an automobile accident ten years earlier, in 1965. But he wanted to get started and he did not want to get turned down for the fitness program just because he was an above-the-knee amputee. That evening, Dick later told me, he practiced running and hopping with his prosthetic leg along the hallway of his apartment building. He waited until it was late at night so that his neighbors wouldn't see him.

In my class, Dick Traum quickly progressed from beginner to intermediate to advanced levels of the Y fitness program. I challenged him to start running outdoors and to enter a five-mile race in Central Park. He did, finishing last in seventy-two minutes. But when he crossed the finish line, the other runners loudly cheered him. He was hooked. Dick next trained for longer races, and got more cheers as he crossed more finish lines. Then he took on the ultimate challenge: a marathon. Within the next fifteen years or so, Dick ran several New York City Marathons, with a personal best of six hours, forty-four minutes.

I wrote a story about Dick Traum for the January 1977 issue of *Runner's World*. A twenty-two-year-old Canadian, who was about to have his leg amputated above the knee in an effort to halt the spread of cancer, read that story just before his surgery. Encouraged, Terry Fox vowed to run across Canada to raise money to fight cancer. In 1980, he began his trans-Canada run and logged 3,339 miles in a personal "Marathon of Hope." In June 1981, however, two-thirds of the way to his goal, Terry Fox died from the disease. He had raised millions of dollars for cancer research, and the books and television movie about his life inspired many men, women, and children—both able-bodied and disabled—to start a fitness program themselves.

After attending a Terry Fox benefit run in Canada in 1982, Dick Traum came to me with a radical idea. Inspired by the interest over Terry Fox's fitness challenge, Dick wanted to start a fitness program for the physically disabled. "We just need to get the word out that through exercise many of the obstacles to leading a normal life can be removed for the handicapped," he said.

I selected the name for the program: Achilles, after the Greek god who had a powerful body but one weakness, his heel. This is the way I see handicapped men, women, and children. Certain parts of their bodies are impaired, but they can still benefit from exercise. And exercise can be used to help them build confidence in the rest of their lives. Dick got the New York Road Runners Club to sponsor the program. We were off and running.

With their physicians' approval, hundreds of men and women of all ages and with a wide range of disabilities started exercising with the Achilles Track Club in New York City. They established other chapters in countries around the world—including Poland and Russia.

We found that aerobic exercise is an excellent way to improve the physical and mental health, energy, and self-esteem of people who have physical handicaps. In many cases, their disabilities actually lessened from the regular exercise. For example, Sandy Davidson, a Scotsman working at the United Nations, was partially paralyzed by a stroke and forced to walk with a cane. After a few years of running, however, he no longer needed the cane, and now gets around without it.

While the emphasis of the program is running for fitness, not for competition, every year about one hundred members of the Achilles Track Club compete in the New York City Marathon. One of my favorite stories concerns Linda Down, who has cerebral palsy. In 1982, Linda ran the New York City Marathon using "Canadian Cane" crutches, and finished in the dark after eleven hours. President Ronald Reagan watched Linda on television and invited her to the White House. "I discovered," she said, "that I can stress my worst aspects—my legs and my body—and still be successful. And if I can take the worst aspects and be a success, then imagine what I can do with my best aspects. The focus is on what I'm able to do rather than what I can't do."

Dick Traum, president of the Achilles Track Club, has this to say about the physically disabled: "Their real disability is not being blind or whatever, but being out of shape. They get reinforcement and a sense of self-esteem from physical accomplishments." Patty Lee Parmalee is the Achilles coach and an irrepressible optimist. "I gradually have learned that any kind of disaster can be overcome," she says, "or, with the right attitude, turned to advantage."

Physical exercise can be of immense emotional and even spiritual therapeutic value to the physically handicapped. I believe that the really disadvantaged people in life are those who could exercise if they wished, but prefer to live a sedentary lifestyle.

THE ACHILLES TRACK CLUB YOUTH PROGRAM

In 1987, Dick Traum got another brilliant idea. Working with the New York City Board of Education's Division of Special Education, he started a running program for handicapped boys and girls. By 1988, Dick had reached more than three hundred young people, ages five to twenty, with a wide range of disabilities; the kids came from more than twelve schools in all parts of the city.

These young Achilles members have special running classes during school hours, supplemented by workouts with the adult Achilles Track Club. At first, they set modest goals. Instructed by physical education teachers specially trained to work with handicapped people, the youngsters build up to running twenty minutes for fitness. When they reach that target, they receive an Achilles Track Club T-shirt and start participating in low-key races and fun runs.

The kids are bused to races. In 1988, Christopher participated in the New York Road Runners Club first one-mile youth fitness run, which I directed. As about fifty kids lined up, ages six to twelve, two busloads of Achilles Track Club youngsters—wearing their team T-shirt—unloaded and lined up with the able-bodied kids. I announced to the children that these "special guests" were physically disabled, but that was no reason for them not to have the same goal as everyone else: to earn a ribbon by finishing the one-mile course.

The children applauded loudly and made their new running friends feel very welcome. Running on crutches, with artificial legs, in wheelchairs—some partially dragged by volunteers—all the disabled children completed the first one-mile run of their lives, to loud cheers from the other children and parents. Christopher was very touched by his involvement in this event. "It made me feel so good when I saw their faces when they got their ribbons," he said. "I never knew handicapped people before. I mean—wow, they were so great!" Over one hundred Achilles youths and their families were bused in to enjoy our 1989 Post Raisin Bran Family Fitness Festival.

The Achilles Track Club South, a chapter in Miami, Florida, also started a youth program. One of their first members in 1987 was little five-year-old Jeffrey Leon, who spends most of his life in a wheelchair suffering from spina bifida. In his first race, Jeffrey started a mile from the finish line of a ten-kilometer run and wheeled himself across in a large clumsy wheelchair. Runners who passed him went on to finish and then turned around and ran back, cheering wildly, to escort Jeffrey across the finish line.

The emotional scene inspired the race sponsor, Sunset Commercial Bank, to start a fund to raise money to help Jeffrey train. Because of the fund, Jeffrey Leon woke up on Christmas morning in 1987 to find an apple-red racing wheelchair in the family living room. His father, Miguel Leon, told the *Miami Herald:*

> When you have a boy, you think "We'll play baseball together." When he was born I closed up. I wondered, "Why does it have to happen to me?" Now we know better. The disabled play baseball and basketball, too.

Jeffrey has developed more independence as a result of his wheelchair racing. For a boy who was not supposed to live much beyond birth, his progress has been miraculous. The doctors had told his mother, Maria, when she was eight months pregnant, that Jeffrey would probably be born dead. The Leons prepared for his death, and when Maria gave birth the nurse came to Miguel: " 'He died, but would you like to see him?' He was actually born not breathing, and they decided not to do anything," said Miguel. "But he started crying by himself. The nurse came back and said, 'He has a very strong heart.' " Now Jeffrey is committed to a lifetime of physical activity and making others cheer.

Dick Traum believes that encouraging disabled youngsters to enjoy the benefits of exercise gives them a new lease on life. They enhance their chances not only to prolong their lives, but also to improve their quality. "If they work hard at it and achieve success," says Dick, "they can carry it over into other areas of their lives."

> They'll develop what you could call a success history. They'll be mainstreaming, rubbing shoulders with people who are not disabled. They will be treated as adults. They will have a sense of growth. They will share the high of running and finishing races.
>
> But most of all, these youngsters will have a positive outlook on life and be ready to accept and overcome challenges they encounter in all areas of daily living.
>
> So much of their lives they hear about what they cannot do. Now they start seeing what they *can* do. It's a wonderful vehicle for mainstreaming. A disabled kid who is trained to run can go a longer distance than an able-bodied youngster who is not trained. It's like a metaphor for life.

FITNESS FOR THE HANDICAPPED

Generally, a handicapped person should compare himself or herself to other men and women of comparable age and fitness level. A person is either in shape or out of shape. A handicapped person may have spent years being inactive. So have most men and women. There is, however, one basic difference: the handicapped person thinks that he or she is out of shape because he cannot exercise. But he can!

If you are handicapped or the parent of a handicapped child, check with your doctor to find out what limitations, if any, might be placed on an exercise program. If your doctor doesn't exercise and is against you or your handicapped child undertaking an exercise program, get a second opinion. Find a doctor who believes in exercise, understands the psychological value of it to you, and listen to his or her advice.

A handicapped person may have to adjust his or her training program by starting more slowly and progressing at a more conservative rate than programs offered to others throughout this book. You can find specific help for exercise and sports for your specific handicap from organizations like those listed in the appendix. Here is some general information about specific handicaps and exercise.

THE ORTHOPEDICALLY IMPAIRED

These conditions of musculo-skeletal impairment include muscular dystrophy; spina bifida; neurological impairments like cerebral palsy; and impairments associated with trauma, including amputations and injury.

(One of the leading causes of traumas among children is abuse by adults.)

No one should be barred from physical education classes or fitness work-outs or even sports teams because of any impairment. The orthopedically impaired can use artificial legs, as Dick Traum did, or crutches and wheel-chairs to participate in most activities. Wheelchair basketball leagues, for example, exist across the United States. Special programs for men, women, and children with particular disabilities are increasingly available, but as much as possible any impaired person should be put into regular fitness and sports programs.

An excellent example of a handicapped person who benefitted from such programs is Jim Abbott, the star pitcher for the 1988 U.S. Olympic baseball team and Sullivan Award winner as the best U.S. amateur athlete. Jim was born without his right hand. But as a child he was allowed to participate in sports with his friends. He learned how to throw a baseball with his left hand after tucking his glove under his right armpit. After releasing the ball, Jim quickly slips the glove onto his left hand, fields the ball, slips off the glove, and throws the ball again.

We are going to see more of Jim Abbott, and other kids like him, in the future. In 1988, Jim was selected by the California Angels baseball team in the Major League baseball player draft. He started playing professional baseball in the minor leagues; if he makes it, or if he doesn't, will depend not on any handicap, but only on his ability.

Another person who did not let his handicap keep him from enjoying sports or a successful career is amputee Robert Kerry, Democratic senator from Nebraska. Joseph Kennedy, Jr., son of Senator Ted Kennedy (D-Mass.), is a skier and fitness enthusiast despite having had a leg amputated because of bone cancer.

It is almost impossible to have a physical disability so severe that you cannot exercise. Robert Wiegand "runs" marathons despite having no legs. He picks up his body with his arms and moves it forward; although it sometimes takes days, Wiegand still finishes any marathon he starts. Bill Reilly and Dan Winchester have no use of their arms and little use of their legs. Yet they sit in wheelchairs and kick at the ground with their feet to propel themselves backward to the finish line of marathons. Most disabled people can at least push a wheelchair to build fitness. After all, little five-year-old Jeffrey Leon has already proved that even the smallest person can have a big heart through exercise.

THE HEARING IMPAIRED

People who have hearing loss or impairment may be in poor physical condition for two reasons, says Toshika d'Elia, a world-class masters runner whom I coach, and a teacher at the New York School for the Deaf in White Plains, New York. First, they often don't breathe well, perhaps because they have never learned to breathe and vocalize. Second, they may have been held back from physical activity all their lives.

A hearing-impaired person's disability often affects their sense of balance. They lack the confidence to run or even to move quickly. To restore that confidence, I suggest a walking program that gradually moves to fast walking and then to running. Or, the hearing impaired may want to try stationary bicycling or rowing, or swimming—where they are safe and supported in water.

The physical education program at the New York School for the Deaf in White Plains serves as an excellent model for the handicapped. State law requires daily physical education for deaf schools—a mandate not currently in place for regular public schools—and the White Plains school administration firmly supports that concept. According to Jody Cole, physical education instructor for elementary school children, language skills for the deaf children can be improved through physical activity, since they learn best through doing. Thus, there is a very valuable carryover value from physical activity to academics. The school's physical education program starts with three-year-olds, who are taught to enjoy walking, running, skipping, hopping, and other basic movements which come naturally to most pre-schoolers. Deaf children, however, most often do not have much physical activity experience because parents tend to overprotect them due to their disability. Cole exposes the elementary school children to many types of activity so they can find ones that they can enjoy for their lifetimes. Included in their curriculum are daily aerobic fitness runs and weekly swimming classes (which are particularly helpful to teach breath control, since deaf children don't learn to breathe naturally through speech). The focus of the fitness program is the school's participation in the American Heart Association—AAHPERD's Jump Rope for Heart program.

THE VISUALLY IMPAIRED

Many blind runners have participated in my fitness classes. One, Mort Schlein, says: "Most people think it's incredible that a blind man can run. I don't know why. Blindness doesn't affect my feet, only my eyes. I move my feet like everyone else."

Partially sighted people can participate, with some limitations, in many physical activities. Those who are totally or nearly sightless can exercise by walking or running while holding a rope attached to a sighted running mate. Or they may walk or run close enough to touch or be touched by a sighted runner.

Like the hearing impaired, blind people might work out on stationary rowing or bicycle machines. They can also swim in pools where a light current can be set up to serve as a "trail" or guide for them to follow. All it takes is determination, a little imagination, and maybe a friend or two to get started. Says the feisty and independent Mort Schlein: "I don't want anyone to feel that running with me is their good deed for the day."

ARTHRITIS

There has been increasing concern among runners that this fitness activity will somehow cause osteoporosis or arthritis, particularly in the knees, later in life. Research studies indicate that exercise actually minimizes the risk of developing arthritis. In addition, regular and non-strenuous movement has also been shown to relieve the pain of arthritis.

Probably the best exercise for people suffering from arthritis is swimming. The movement and the flow of the water seem to combine to ease the pain associated with this disease, plus, of course, giving fitness benefit.

ASTHMA

Few handicaps cause such debate among fitness experts and physicians as asthma. Can an asthmatic person exercise aerobically? Should he or she? What are the benefits and risks?

Asthma is one of the most common respiratory diseases. It afflicts about eight million Americans. As three researchers wrote in *The Physician and Sportsmedicine:*

> Although exercise provokes bronchiospasm in most asthmatics, the severity of exercise-induced asthma can be reduced by several factors: control of exercise duration; less intense, intermittent exercise; warm-up, warmer, humid inspired [inhaled] air; aerobic fitness; and drugs.

> Regular vigorous exercise increases fitness, enhances tolerance to attacks, and provides more social and psychological independence. The development of protective medication has made such activity possible for many asthmatics.

Physicians from the American Academy of Pediatrics have stated that the asthmatic child may participate in school and recreational activities and sports programs with minimal restrictions. It is important that asthmatics engaging in exercise use their medication consistently and according to the direction of their physicians. When Shepherd coached his high-school freshman boys' soccer team, there were two asthmatics on the squad. The boys brought their inhalant spray to the games, but Shepherd had them in such excellent physical condition that they never needed the medication. In fact, neither had any problem with his asthma—until several months after the season had ended and they had stopped their conditioning. Can asthmatics excel in sports? Jackie Joyner-Kersee showed the world they can by winning two gold medals in track and field at the 1988 Olympic games.

CANCER

No single word—with the possible exception of AIDS—strikes such fear into us as *cancer*. We have come to associate cancer with death, despite the fact that many forms of cancer are now being defeated with early detection and treatment.

Exercise will not prevent or cure cancer. Exercise will help cancer patients feel and look better, and will give them both the strength and the optimism to battle their disease. Moreover, if you are a regular exerciser who then discovers that you have cancer, you will bring a healthy body and spirit to the crisis.

Previously sedentary men and women who have developed cancer have started exercise programs. I recommend doing so, with the permission and cooperation of your physician. We have several cancer amputees running with the Achilles Track Club. The exercise gives them the strength and confidence they need in this big battle.

CARDIAC REHABILITATION

Until the early 1960s, heart-attack patients were confined to bed and rest for months. The advice was to take it easy. Now we know that bed rest over long periods of time actually does more harm than good.

Today, patients with uncomplicated heart attacks are out of bed in a few days and home within five to ten days. They are often put into a gradual exercise program like the one I directed under the supervision of cardiologists at New York City's West Side YMCA. Most patients in coronary rehabilitation programs start with a walking or biking regimen. They are carefully supervised. The goal is to get the patient in good shape—in many cases much better shape than before the heart attack—and to live a more normal, active life. This not only gets the exercising cardiac rehab patient fit, it also gives him or her confidence to lead an active life. This creates a positive outlook.

DIABETES

Exercise cannot cure diabetes or make insulin injections unnecessary. The diabetic exerciser must still take insulin at regular intervals to stay well.

Regular exercise may help lower blood sugar and lessen the amount of insulin needed, however. Complications from diabetes are best controlled by taking the right amount of insulin, eating the appropriate kinds and amounts of food, and getting regular exercise. Diabetic exercisers should coordinate their diet, medicine, and exercise under careful medical supervision.

EPILEPSY

Epileptics, like asthmatics, have been overly and unnecessarily sheltered and protected. They are often prevented from participating in sports or exercising in a normal, regular way.

In 1977, a young woman named Patty Wilson decided to do something about this attitude. Patty had suffered her first epileptic seizure in the third grade. Afterwards, her friends had teased her and were afraid to play with her. Even her own father was frightened of Patty's affliction.

On her own, Patty Wilson decided to become a runner. Her doctor encouraged her and she always ran with someone—a good idea for women in general. In high school, Patty won several cross-country races. She then ran some ultra-long distances with her father, including a five-hundred-mile run from her home to San Francisco.

At that point, Patty and her dad decided to publicize the fact that epileptics can be physically active. They decided to run from Los Angeles to Portland, Oregon—a distance of about thirteen hundred miles. For most of the run, Patty and her father averaged thirty-one miles a day. When they reached the Oregon border, high-school track teams and members of local running clubs joined them. People with epilepsy stopped and talked with her. "She was a light for them," said Patty's father.

Patty's dramatic run demonstrated that epileptics—or other handicapped people—can and should be on the road to fitness with everyone else.

OBESITY

Being overweight is largely a function of heredity, one's attitude toward exercise, and simply eating too much. Calories consumed must be burned off by exercise or they become fat. If you and your kids think an exciting afternoon consists of potato chips and TV, chances are you are overweight.

Bored, undirected, non-exercising people are often bored, undirected, non-exercising fat people.

Obese individuals should start an exercise program in conjunction with a diet. Here, you need special help under medical supervision. Swimming, stationary biking or rowing, and slow walking are probably the best first exercises for you to do. Start slowly and build gradually. As you begin to lose weight, you may want to add a gradual weight-training program, to tighten up loose skin. This is especially true if you have been grossly overweight.

With regular exercise, obese individuals can see their bodies gradually slim down and fat turn to muscle. There are no miracles here. Your program must be gradual. And you must recognize another important fact: obese people are notorious back-sliders. If you start losing weight through a diet-exercise program, stick with it. You cannot win if you do the program, lose the weight, and then stop. The fat will pile back on faster than it went off.

THE EMOTIONALLY DISTURBED AND MENTALLY HANDICAPPED

Exercise programs have been widely used among institutions—schools, residence facilities, and hospitals—sheltering emotionally disturbed children and adults. Most of the research shows that regular exercise can cut down the anger and aggressive behavior of disturbed individuals and give their lives a focus and support previously missing.

Let me cite one example here. The San Diego Center for Children is a residential treatment facility for children ages six to thirteen who have severe emotional and behavioral problems. Research there shows that an exercise program can cause a sharp decrease in aggressiveness of disturbed children. Many of the children who exercised regularly could be taken off their medication as long as they continued the exercise program.

There is also some evidence that regular exercise programs help children and adults who have more severe mental handicaps. I have worked with the Special Olympics, for example, and have witnessed the joy and confidence that comes from the regular training and exercise required to participate in those games for the mentally handicapped.

All of this is to say that regular aerobic exercise should not be considered beyond the reach of even the most severely handicapped person. I think of people like Jeffrey Leon, Jim Abbott, Jackie Joyner-Kersee, and even Robert Wiegand moving along without legs—and I ask you: Have you any excuses left?

Youth and Sports

Team sports for our kids have come under tremendous criticism during the last few years. In junior-high and high-school football, for example, some parents and coaches have created dishonest, harmful, and win-at-all-costs systems in which the players—the kids—come last.

Although I have criticized team sports in this book, I am still a sports advocate. Properly managed, little else can match team sports as an exciting and rewarding experience for your children. As detailed in Chapter 2, goals are set, training is directed toward those goals, and a group of peers is gathered together to try as hard as they can to train well and achieve something. There may not be a more noble or worthwhile human endeavor. In addition, team sports can also serve as a "fitness lure"—getting kids into the habit of exercising regularly for some clearly stated goal.

Why, then, do team sports come under so much criticism? I believe there are two fundamental answers here: team sports too often only benefit school athletes; and coaches and the players' parents emphasize winning over playing. There are other important issues:

- Most school physical education programs emphasize sports skills rather than fitness. Our kids don't learn important lifetime fitness skills. (The answer to this problem is detailed in Chapters 5 through 9.)
- School sports programs often benefit only the athletically gifted. Other kids don't try out for teams, or they get cut or ride the bench. The few play, the many sit. Community programs also often follow the star system. The solution, I believe, is a no-cut policy: any kid who wants to play on a school sports team can do so; just add more teams to the program. Younger children especially need as much playing time as possible, and programs for them should be open to all kids interested in playing, not just the select few.

- Parents and coaches confuse being athletic with being fit. They think that if a child is active on a football or baseball team he is getting sufficient exercise. He is not. The solution is to include fitness training in every sport. Teams should emphasize stretching, push-ups and sit-ups, and aerobic exercises—and then practice the techniques of the sport. Fitness should come first, sports play second.
- Adults interfere too much with sports programs. We pressure kids too much about winning. We give them poor role models with our bad behavior at games. We over-organize school sports programs for our benefit and glory, and too often neglect our kids' real need: to have fun.
- Too many coaches model themselves after professional coaches. They are insensitive to the psychological and emotional needs of children. Do you want a Billy Martin clone coaching your kid?

Joe Paterno, the football coach at Penn State University, once remarked that when he returned home from a game as a youngster, his father never asked him whether he had won or lost, but whether he had had fun. That is the key in team sports—or any exercise: enjoyment; having fun while learning how to improve, having fun while striving to win, having fun while participating in a common physical activity with friends and family.

The Youth Sports Institute at Michigan State University surveyed approximately eight thousand students ages ten to eighteen on why they participated in nonschool and school sports, why they dropped out, and how the programs would have to change to lure them back in. Vern Seefeldt and Martha Ewing, the study's researchers, made four recommendations for improvements in youth sports programs based on the students' responses:

- Adult leaders of sports activities should gauge the amount of time spent in practices and games to the overall scope of activities that children want to explore.
- Program goals should be matched with children's expectations, including enjoyment, physical fitness, and the positive aspects of competition.
- Skilled coaches should also be available to younger children.
- Competent and "sensitive" coaches should be the top priority for successful youth sports programs.

We don't need to eliminate team sports for kids because of problems by adults. We need to give sports back to the kids. We don't need to replace sports with fitness. Instead, we need to achieve a balance between fitness, sports, and fun that will most benefit our children.

PARTICIPATION

More than 30 million boys and girls play in some form of community or school sports programs. But only about 5 million play in organized school sports; the rest are in other programs. This means that one-sixth of our active boys and girls get the greatest attention; somehow we should be rewarding the other five-sixths too.

On the plus side, the number of boys and girls playing sports has been increasing each year since 1983. But it has not returned to the all-time high of 1977–78, when some 6.5 million boys and girls played on high-school sports teams.

Despite the adult trend toward lifetime individual fitness sports, our boys and girls still prefer team sports, according to a 1988 Wilson Sporting Goods survey. Boys' high-school sports on the rise include basketball, baseball, football, and soccer, while for girls, soccer is expected to be the major growth sport.

The following charts show the ten most popular sports for high-school boys and girls for 1987–88, according to a survey by the National Federation of State High School Associations.*

WHEN SHOULD KIDS START PLAYING TEAM SPORTS?

Some children understand competition as early as age three or four. They seem to know what it means to do better than another child, according to the Parenting Advisor's booklet *Competitive Sports and Your Child*. That doesn't mean they are ready for adult-style competition and sports teams.

The American Academy of Pediatrics feels that children do not begin to acquire the concept of teamwork until about four or five years of age and that they should not begin team sports until at least six years of age. Of course, as I have said earlier, not all children grow physically and emotionally at the same rate. Some will be ready sooner than others. I've found Christopher and his friends ready for "watered down" competition by ages five or six, but most were certainly not ready for serious games based on winning and losing.

Young kids need to ease into win/lose games. I play baseball and basketball with Christopher and let him win until he is ready to handle the

*Reprinted with permission of the National Federation of State High School Associations, P.O. Box 20626, Kansas City, Missouri 64195.

Ten Most Popular Girls' Sports		**Ten Most Popular Boys' Sports**	
Schools		Schools	
1. Basketball	16,196	1. Basketball	16,769
2. Track & Field		2. Track & Field	
(Outdoor)	13,804	(Outdoor)	14,246
3. Volleyball	11,834	3. Football	14,068
4. Cross-Country	8,747	4. Baseball	13,589
5. Tennis	8,426	5. Cross-Country	9,823
6. Softball (Fast Pitch)	8,314	6. Golf	9,360
7. Swimming & Diving	3,897	7. Tennis	8,844
8. Golf	3,719	8. Wrestling	8,358
9. Soccer	3,697	9. Soccer	6,159
10. Track & Field (Indoor)	1,165	10. Swimming & Diving	3,919
Participants		Participants	
1. Basketball	392,047	1. Football	949,279
2. Track & Field		2. Basketball	524,606
(Outdoor)	326,694	3. Track & Field	
3. Volleyball	292,883	(Outdoor)	431,009
4. Softball (Fast Pitch)	208,344	4. Baseball	407,630
5. Tennis	126,566	5. Wrestling	246,771
6. Cross-Country	104,975	6. Soccer	208,935
7. Soccer	103,173	7. Cross-Country	157,306
8. Swimming & Diving	83,964	8. Tennis	136,083
9. Field Hockey	47,701	9. Golf	124,486
10. Softball (Slow Pitch)	40,539	10. Swimming & Diving	94,199

possibility of losing. When he first played against friends, I made sure the games either weren't scored or ended in a tie. By about age seven the kids started demanding more accurate scoring. They were ready to accept winning and losing. Even at this age and beyond, however, kids need plenty of praise and support, win or lose.

"Children should not be involved in intense athletic competition before they are 10," Thomas D. Fahey, professor of physical education at California State University at Chico, states in *Competitive Sports and Your Child*. "Childhood and adolescence are periods of development and learning. Early competition may, in fact, result in cutting off the learning process prematurely. Five-to-ten-year-olds should belong to organized teams only if those teams provide an atmosphere for learning a variety of movement fundamentals and for developing a love of the sport." (For example, see "Sports Club," Chapter 25.)

Kids should start with individual sports like swimming, biking, and running and then move along as they wish to team sports. A good introduction to team sports for kids are low-key games like tee-ball baseball and soccer. Both can and should be made up of coed teams, with no scoring and everyone playing for equal lengths of time.

To get everyone interested in the game and playing a lot, alternate players by innings (with unlimited substitution). To keep the kids interested, I suggest substituting in soccer by minutes played: Johnny plays the first five minutes of the second quarter, Mary Beth the last five minutes; then reverse for the next quarter.

Dr. J. J. Gugenheim, M.D., told the American Running & Fitness Association:

> We must establish sports programs that are appropriate for the physical and psychological benefits of [our children's] development. From age six to 10, we should foster an emphasis on awakening interest in sports, having fun, learning basic skills, and socialization. There should be reinforcement of positive results with compliments and rewards, not comparing performance between children.
>
> From 11 to 14 years, the emphasis should be on developing versatility, proper techniques, and tolerance for increased training. Highly organized sports before age 12 retard spontaneity and probably lead to early burnout.
>
> During age 15 to 18, we should emphasize increased training, such as strength and endurance or individual sports, and begin extensive competiton.

CHOOSING A SPORT

How should your child choose a sport that is best for him or her? For one thing, your child will choose the sport, not you. You can only be supportive of your child's decision, which may include not choosing a sport at all! You should be a good listener and discuss the various options. Help your child to measure his or her own interests, physical strength, and skills. Never discourage your child's participation; if she wants to play tackle football, let her try. Advise her of both the advantages and disadvantages of the sport.

As your child's interest in a sport develops, talk to the coaches and to other parents whose kids play on that team. Often your child will want to play a team sport because his or her friends play. That's fine if your child likes the sport and you like the coaching. (More on this further on.) Keep in mind that individual sports—track, cross-country running, tennis, squash, handball, swimming, gymnastics, or wrestling—may benefit your child more than team sports. They allow for more individual goal-setting and achievement. Ideally, your child will choose a blend of team and individual sports to gain the benefits from both activities.

I believe that kids benefit most by playing as many sports as possible—both team and individual—for as long as they can. Let them have fun learning lots of sports and skills before applying their talents to a more specific activity. By high school, most kids will have selected one or two sports they like best. They may only play them on the intramural level, or as recreational activity, but at least they are exercising, having fun, and perhaps starting a lifelong fitness pattern.

You might encourage your child to play different sports during each season. Here are some suggestions:

Autumn: cross-country running, soccer, football, field hockey.

My favorite is cross-country, which is a great aerobic conditioner and offers individual achievement within a team sport. Kids usually don't start this sport until junior high school. Some youth teams compete at earlier ages.

Soccer, the fastest-growing sport in the United States, is also a good aerobic conditioner that encourages overall skills and team play. Youth leagues are a lot of fun if your child is ready from about age nine. Football is dangerous, but attracts the crowds and headlines. Although youth football programs exist for young kids, I don't think a child should play until at least age thirteen. If your child insists on playing at a younger age, make sure that the league divides players into programs based on weight classification.

If the choice were mine, I would encourage a child into soccer and/or cross-country running.

Winter: swimming, gymnastics, wrestling, basketball, volleyball, ice hockey, cross-country skiing, squash, and indoor tennis.

The best sport for fitness on this list is swimming, which can be done by almost everyone, including the physically handicapped. I also like gymnastics, because it promotes muscular fitness and young kids can do it as exercise before using it as a competitive sport.

Wrestling is a great conditioner—physically and mentally—and is open to boys of all sizes, since competition is by weight class. (You should not allow your son to make his weight class with drastic dieting.) I suggest this sport only for teenage boys and older.

Basketball, another one of my favorite sports, can provide boys and girls with aerobic training, motor skills, teamwork, and fun. Youngsters can start early with small basketballs and lowered rims. Most programs begin around age eight to ten.

Volleyball is a great team sport and, like basketball, an excellent conditioner if played vigorously that can be played well into adult life.

Ice hockey is popular where frozen ponds, lakes, or indoor rinks are available. Played informally as a pick-up game, it is a good exercise. Played on a team, it can be a vicious and ugly sport, with little conditioning benefit because of the rapid substitutions. Shepherd's son Caleb played ice hockey in high school to get into condition for spring lacrosse. The sport's fans disgusted him; he particularly remembers an away game at a New Hampshire high school where the parents of the opposition players spat on him and his teammates as they entered the rink.

Cross-country skiing, squash, and indoor tennis offer good workouts where available. Cross-country skiing is a lifelong sport and if it is offered in your high school you might encourage your kids to try it. Even one season of playing on a freshman or junior varsity team will give your child enough experience to retain the skill for the rest of his or her life. The same is true for indoor tennis or squash, although neither offers the conditioning level of cross-country skiing.

Spring: track and field, baseball/softball, lacrosse, field hockey, spring soccer, tennis.

Long-distance running in track is the best aerobic conditioner. Short-distance runners and field event specialists (long jump, shot put, pole vault) need to balance their training with aerobic workouts.

Baseball is another favorite of mine and, of course, it is the national pastime. It has been marred recently by greedy players and childish coaches. But the game itself, played quietly during the summer without benefit of electronic scoreboards or rock music between innings, has a wonderfully seductive, challenging rhythm and intensity that those who play it come to love. It's now Christopher's favorite sport too. Kids can start to play around age six in pick-up games or loosely structured leagues that have no pitching; the ball is placed on a tee, where the young player whacks it with a bat. From then on it's just like the regular game. Unless you use the games I discuss earlier, baseball offers little in the way of fitness, but does provide strategy and hand-eye coordination.

Lacrosse for boys and girls offers excellent fitness benefits and team play. More and more high-school boys' and girls' lacrosse teams are employing weight training along with aerobic running as conditioning. The game requires good stick handling, hand-eye coordination, and motor skills, and the play is quick and aerobic, although there is extensive substitution for midfielders.

As mentioned, tennis is a good lifetime, individual sport that can be learned from a young age. Golf falls into this category too. But it is not aerobic and should not be considered as physically challenging.

I would add to these traditional team sports another choice that I feel offers good value: martial arts. Christopher took a peewee karate course at age five and learned a lot about fitness and discipline. The teaching, however, must be low key, friendly, and focused on defense—not on what you can do to a block of wood or an enemy. Keep your kids away from the tough-guy karate schools that echo the "Karate Kid" movies. In addition, I would encourage judo, aikido, and t'ai chi ch'uan training, both for the movement and the relaxation benefits. None of these, of course, is aerobic, but they are good lifelong activities.

Are any sports more preferable than others for school-age children? Pediatricians and sports psychologists give high marks to soccer and swimming because they offer good movement skills, all-around fitness, have low injury rates, and can be enjoyed by a wide range of people. Gymnastics, although it has a somewhat higher injury risk, can help a child learn a wide range of movement, control, and balance skills.

Keep in mind that the selection of a sport or sports is your child's, not yours. You are a guide only. If your child is not ready for team sports, do not push it. If your child does not feel very athletic, at least get him or her to participate in an after-school program for exercise.

DROPOUTS FROM SPORTS

Children quit playing team sports for many reasons. If your child decides to drop out of a team sport, you should listen carefully and, in most cases, go along with the idea. The Youth Sports Institute study showed that 45 percent of all U.S. ten-year-olds participated in organized sports. That's the good news. But by age seventeen, only 26 percent were still playing. The decline is much sharper in team sports than in individual sports like swimming, gymnastics, cross-country skiing, tennis.

Why do kids drop out of team sports? They may develop other interests—music, scouting, community service—that are equally worthwhile and leave little time for sports. They may decide to pursue individual lifetime fitness activities like biking or skating instead of team sports. Or they may feel abused by the coaching, confused by the adulation of adult fans, even distracted by teenage love.

According to the National Youth Sports Research and Development Survey, released in 1988, the leading reasons for team sport dropouts included excessive pressure on the kids, inadequate coaching, and lack of fun. Another study, published in *The Physician and Sports Medicine*, showed that kids nine through fourteen quit team sports for two primary reasons: too much time spent sitting on the bench, and the feeling that they were not successful at their particular sport.

Bench-sitting is a serious accusation and addresses one of my favorite topics: no-cut teams that let everyone play. The Youth Sports Institute study also showed that about 90 percent of children playing team sports said they would rather play on a losing team than sit on the bench of a winning team. I believe that the best sports program would allow all kids to play on any team they wish and get into every game played. This is much better than emphasizing winning above all else. That may be why I like cross-country and track so much: all the kids run in various levels of competition.

What to do?

If your child decides to drop a team sport, encourage him or her to substitute some other form of exercise. Parents must allow their children to make their own choices of how they want to spend their time. Part of your discussion, however, should include your child's commitment to his or her team and teammates and the effect of quitting on them and their team.

Talk with your child. Ask why he or she wants to quit. Listen carefully. Watch: there may be some serious signs of stress, like vomiting, loss of appetite, headaches, loss of sleep, or withdrawal. These symptoms indicate that the stress is such that withdrawing from a team sport is warranted.

Remember that this is basically your child's choice. And your child needs to learn—along with winning and losing—what quitting means. Sticking it out is not always in your child's best interests. But quitting something simply because it is difficult is not a good lesson either. You should discuss ways to resolve the problems and issues raised by your child's decision. You may want to take steps, short of your child's dropping off a team, to remedy the problems. Can the problems be worked out? Search for alternatives, discuss them with your child, listen to your child's response, and then reach a decision together about what would be best for your child, the team, and his or her teammates.

GETTING CUT

As I mentioned in Chapter 20, Shepherd was cut from his high-school soccer team every year for three consecutive years. (He finally got the message his senior year and became editor of the school newspaper!) He played intramurals and went on to start on his college varsity soccer team for four consecutive years. He was also cut from the varsity baseball team after batting .391 as a junior varsity third baseman. He went on to start at shortstop for two years on his college varsity. Even though the cuts had rather happy sequels, those did not come until Shepherd was in college. Having been cut off his high-school soccer and baseball teams, Shepherd went through his high-school years hurt, humiliated, and angry. He never forgot the painful experience.

There are lessons here about coaches, teams, and cutting. I prefer no-cut sports for all schools. The Allen-Stevenson School model in Chapter 8, for example, allows for A and B teams so that all kids have the chance to play. The sad fact about cuts is that, as Shepherd's case illustrates, those kids cut sometimes turn out to be good athletes. They could and should be playing. These are the kids who need a chance to grow in team sports.

What should you do if your child is cut from a team? The first thing is to understand that your child has suffered a painful rejection, whether or not he or she shows it. Your child needs your love and support, and you need to sit and listen to the whole sad and humiliating story; this may take several nights of sitting on the edge of the bed, gently asking questions, waiting for tears to subside, listening, being there.

Everyone faces disappointments, and I believe that disappointments make us stronger. You make this disappointment easier for your child by making certain that he or she knows your love and esteem is not diminished in any way by this setback.

Here's a good chance to put sports into perspective: maybe team sports are not that important after all. You might ask your child who else was cut, and would they want to join your child in individual sports such as running, biking, or rowing? Or, you and your child might search for options in other sports programs. The important point here is sympathy and love for your child at a painful time, and using the moment to teach a lifelong lesson in bouncing back, searching for more interesting alternatives, setting new goals.

I still think a no-cut policy would save all this pain.

SPORTS-RELATED STRESS

The pressure to win creates stress. I think this is the wrong way to measure your child's team sports performance. The better yardstick should be effort. Leave winning and its stresses to professional adult athletes.

Parents can control team sports stress for their children. They can be sure that kids are put in groups of the same age and skill levels; for contact sports, I would add height, weight, ability, and maturity. Sports rules can be changed to make the game fairer for all to play; nets can be lowered or races shortened.

Parents can also teach their kids that success does not mean winning, but achieving personal goals. (More on this further on.) These are not the goals of coaches, adults, or even their parents; they are goals your child and you have set together. If you stress goal setting, effort, trying your hardest, you will relieve much of the stress on your child that comes from team sports where winning is emphasized.

Can sports hurt a child? I'm not talking about physical injury. I'm talking about other hurts.

Jon C. Hellstedt, Ph.D., associate professor of psychology at the University of Lowell (Massachusetts), wrote in *The Physician and Sports Medicine* about the negative experiences some children have in team sports. He cited three general causes: low self-esteem, aggressive behavior, and excessive anxiety.

"Children worry about how their parents, coaches, peers, and teammates will evaluate their performance," says Dr. Hellstedt. "Children who receive negative verbal and nonverbal messages can develop low self-esteem." This may cause some children to drop out of sports. When coaches use positive encouragement, he said, players have higher self-esteem.

Aggressive behavior also turns off kids, who hear coaches and parents yelling at officials, players, and each other. In sports like football and hockey, kids are told to hit hard and be aggressive and violent to win. Some have trouble doing this and feel badly both because they are told to be more aggressive and because they cannot respond.

Some anxiety is present in all sports and in parts of life. A certain amount of anxiety, in fact, can motivate players on teams, but this is usually at the level of arousal to play rather than a fear of playing or of being hurt. When arousal becomes fear or anxiety, performance falls. The fun goes out of the game, and the child quits.

The result is a kid who is overwhelmed by the demands of competition and training, and wants to escape. Dr. Hellstedt lists symptoms a child may manifest when he or she has suffered from what he calls sports burnout: signs of agitation and depression, sleep disturbance, skin rashes, nausea, headaches, muscle rigidity, lack of energy, sadness, frequent unexplained illness, and loss of interest in training and competing.

"In this emotional state," he warns, "an athlete is very susceptible to injury. Injury can be seen as a socially acceptable way to exit from the pressure.

"I believe that competitive stress and burnout result from excessive adult pressure to win or excel." Children who are under such stress, he says, usually have parents or coaches who behave in specific ways:

- The parents or coaches evaluate the child's sports performances negatively.
- The parents or coaches give "inconsistent feedback" and the child is confused by the mixed messages—for example, saying that "winning isn't everything" and getting angry when the child loses.
- The parents or coaches over-protect the child.

Removing this stress can be easy. First, parents should let their children select their own exercise methods, and either individual sports or team sports. Second, parents should always put fun and fitness first; winning is always secondary. Third, parents must listen to their children; if your child doesn't want to play on a team, don't force him or her to do so. Fourth, parents should always praise their child's *effort;* they should never comment on *performance* unless the child specifically asks to be evaluated.

WINNING AND LOSING

If stress and bench-sitting are two major reasons kids quit sports teams, what is the message they are giving us, their parents and coaches? I believe it has to do with winning and losing. Stress and bench-sitting are both characteristic of a team sports program that emphasizes winning.

Winning at all cost is for professional athletes, who are paid handsomely to play under stress or to ride a bench in an effort to win. Wanting to win, striving to win, are healthy goals. Being obsessed with winning is not. John Wooden coached the UCLA basketball team to ten college national basketball championships in a twelve-year period from 1963 to 1975. He was a winning coach, but did he win at all cost? He once told a group of parents and coaches:

> You cannot find a player who ever played for me at UCLA that can tell you that he ever heard me mention "winning" a basketball game. He might say I inferred a little here and there, but I never mentioned winning. Yet the last thing that I told my players just prior to tip-off, before we would go on the floor, was "When the game is over, I want your head up, and I know of only one way for your head to be up. That's for you to know that you did your best." No one can do more. . . . You made that effort.

When Christopher was a pre-schooler, I let him and his friends beat me in everything we played. It made it more fun for them—and, frankly, for me, since playing to lose was new. Losing—and winning—are things we all need to learn to handle, but not at the pre-school level. As Christopher entered the first grade, he gradually began learning about winning and losing. He came home and at first said that he didn't enjoy "winning games." By playing in a low-key program, he gradually adjusted. He has come to understand better the school motto: "Everyone is a winner if he tries."

I gradually introduce winning and losing to our Sports Club programs. But I keep the teams balanced so the games are close and all the teams win about the same number of times. At the end of the season we play an "all-star game" against the parents with each kid being selected to the team. Guess who wins?

I've coached several youth sports teams and every one of them had a winning record; many won league titles. A Babe Ruth League baseball team of thirteen- to fifteen-year-olds coached by my brother and me while we were college students completed a perfect 14-0 season. But I never, on any of my teams, made winning more important than teaching. By stressing the fundamentals, teaching the game, motivating players to hustle, I was able to develop teams that won regularly because we were well-prepared for making a *team* effort.

Children, and their parents and coaches, must understand that to be successful you don't always win and that losing does not mean you are a failure. Sure, the goal is to win and you should *always* try your best. As John Wooden says, you walk off the floor with your head high: you know you tried your best. That's what counts most.

Fred C. Engh, president of the National Youth Sports Coaches Association, told *USA Today*:

> Sports gives the opportunity at an early age to learn discipline, training, desire to succeed and the ability to work with others. But sometimes the lesson plan goes wrong. Children are naturally competitive, but they're not cheaters or win-at-all-costs. Parents too often teach them that, because we've created scoreboards, championships and all-stars for the young ages.

How do you handle wins and losses with your child?

I believe that all of us should be humble in victory and generous in defeat. By that I mean we should accept congratulations for victory with humility, and we should offer congratulations to the winners when we lose.

Winning is sometimes as difficult to accept well as losing. We need to teach our kids to reach out to those they have defeated in sports, and not to rub in the victory or gloat. When our kids lose, we hope their opponents will do the same.

Each loss is different, and each child reacts differently to each losing experience. As a seven-year-old, Christopher was often sad and on the verge of tears. But within five minutes he would be laughing and playing with members of both the winning and losing teams.

It is natural to be upset after losing. After all, if we didn't care about the outcome we wouldn't try hard. Parents and coaches need to respect those feelings, especially if a child takes a loss hard. A hug or other gesture, a kind word later about effort, will let your child know that you support and love him or her. Be alert to the fact that parents often take losing harder than their kids, the players. But listen carefully and be patient.

I remember when the Little League team my brother played on went to the New York State finals. They lost a tough game they could have won. The kids cried almost all the way home. They were embarrassed to return to their little town of Dansville, which had treated them like heroes after a string of victories over much larger towns and cities across the state. But when they arrived at the edge of Dansville after losing, the players were loaded into an old locomotive vehicle and escorted into town with police car and fire engines blaring. A long procession of cars, horns honking, followed them for a tour of the streets, where the townspeople cheered them. The players didn't come home as losers, but as winners. They had done their best, and little Dansville was proud of them!

The American Coaching Effectiveness Program trains school and community coaches in the United States. In its course textbook, *Coaching Young Athletes,* a sound philosophy of coaching ("Athletes first, winning second") is explained:

> Every decision you make and every behavior you display is based first on what you think is best for your athletes, and second, on what may improve the athlete's or team's chances of winning. . . .

> When winning is kept in perspective, sports programs produce children who enjoy movement, who strive for excellence, who dare to risk error to learn, and who grow with both praise and constructive criticism.

> When winning is kept in perspective, there is room for fun in the pursuit of victory, or more accurately, the pursuit of victory is fun. With proper leadership, sports programs produce children who accept responsibilities, who accept others and, most of all, who accept themselves.

SPORTSMANSHIP

Sports is also a way of teaching sportsmanship. This may transfer into a moral code of life. Competitive team sports often create situations in which moral decisions occur, and these provide opportunities for children to learn moral behavior and for adults to teach it. For example, we sometimes read about professional golfers who admit that they placed the wrong ball into play; we see examples of soccer and basketball players who signal their own fouls.

There are rules to the games we teach our children. Following rules, playing within them, striving to do our best without stretching or breaking those rules is sportsmanship, and also the first lessons of moral behavior. I once asked Christopher what sportsmanship meant to him. He replied: "Trying your best, not cheating, not making fun of anyone if they don't do good, loving everyone after the game. It is stupid to hate people after a game. After all, it's just a game!"

Parents and coaches carry responsibilities here, too. Criticizing players, arguing with officials, swearing, and other inappropriate behavior all make an impression on kids (and parents). What makes your behavior as a parent and a parent-coach all the more important is what these same kids see taking place during college and professional sports play: players fighting, coaches yelling at referees or throwing chairs and equipment, fans booing and shouting or chanting obscenities. Parents and coaches need to ask: "How will my behavior be interpreted by young athletes?"

Here, too, I think inappropriate behavior comes from the stress and pressure of win-at-all-cost athletic programs, whether those programs are in high schools or in colleges. I would even argue for severe penalties on professional coaches and players who fight, scream, spit on, or kick dirt at an opponent or umpire, or perform other kinds of abusive behavior. They, too, are role models, and they are giving us and our kids awful moral and sportsmanship lessons.

Little League baseball is an organization that has been stereotyped as representing all that has gone wrong with kids' sports in the United States. Parents and coaches scream and yell at opponents and umpires; kids play at increasingly professional levels on fancy diamonds in televised games. What's being taught here?

As a former Little League player and coach, and now a Little League father, I believe that Little League is no better and certainly no worse than any other U.S. sports program. Its value lies with the morality and sports-manship of the adult coaches and the parents. Adults need to put the kids first, not their own egos. I strongly support Little League baseball as it once was played and as it should be played again. Perhaps the adults involved with Little League should stand before every game—maybe before every inning!—and recite the Little League pledge:

I trust in God.

I love my country and will respect its laws.

I will play fair and strive to win.

But win or lose, I will always do my best.

THE PARENTS' ROLE IN YOUTH SPORTS

I have discussed in several different ways here your role as a parent of a child playing on a sports team. There are some other specific points to be made.

I believe that it is your role, as a parent, to guide your child into fitness activities and sports that are safe, fun, and challenging. The National Youth Sports Research and Development survey indicated in 1988 that most parents (89 percent) think they play a key role in their child's success in sports, but most (75 percent) also think adults get too involved in kids' sports programs. The Miller Lite–Women's Sports Foundation survey found that 87 percent of parents thought winning is important for them and their kids. It is natural to look at your child's participation in sports as an extension of yourself, your childhood. When Christopher hits a home run or strikes out—so do I. Don't let this natural ego problem interfere with your child's enjoyment of sports. Learn to control the monster within you. I agree, it isn't always easy.

Maybe one rule should be to step back from your kids' sports play— and remember that it is only play.

Also, as I have said before, you need to be an effective role model by being physically active yourself. To this I have added in this chapter: you also need to live in a sportsmanlike, moral way.

That means using team sports to teach lessons about life—right and wrong, cheating, winning and losing—to help your kids mold their own moral character.

- Play with your kids more. Learn the games they enjoy. Volunteer your time for sports your kids enjoy. Watch other sports contests together. Attend as many of your child's games as possible. But also attend the school plays, concerts, and parents' nights.
- Don't force them to play if they don't want to. So what if baseball is your favorite sport and your child plays tennis instead? Maybe the child is sending you a message: "I'll choose my own sports, so don't pressure me."
- Praise your child's efforts, not performance. Watch for improvement, and if your child asks your opinion, give it. Otherwise, keep quiet.
- Make game day a special family experience. Give the kids plenty of family support and go out afterward for a meal or treat.
- Introduce yourself to the child's coach. Try to get to know him or her on a personal, non-interfering level.
- Then, leave the coaching to the coach. Be careful of what you say and

do along the sidelines. This is, after all, only a school sports game. It is not the Super Bowl, World Series, Final Four, or Armageddon.

- Avoid, if possible, coaching any team that your child plays on. Both Shepherd and I have done this, and it is difficult to remain objective. You also lose the chance to discuss the game afterwards, since you both were so intimately involved in it. If there is no alternative, be sure to treat your child exactly—no better, no worse—as you treat the other players.

The lessons of this chapter really focus on how you and other adults treat your child. The answer is easy: with respect, honesty, care, and concern for him or her as an individual. The issues of bench-sitting, winning and losing, and fairness and morality would all be easier if we simply encouraged our kids to play hard and honestly and told our schools to play every kid who wants to play in every game.

I am not the only parent/coach concerned about sports and kids. There are many, and some of them have come up with excellent guidelines in the area of team sports, parenting, and coaching. Here are their codes for athletes, parents, and coaches.

CODES OF ETHICS FOR ATHLETES, PARENTS, AND COACHES

I believe that children have fundamental rights in sports. They certainly have the right to enjoy themselves free from adult interference. The "Bill of Rights for Young Athletes" was drafted in 1977 by the Youth Sports Task Force of the AAHPERD. It offers some basic guidelines for parents and coaches as they work with our children.

The Women's Sports Foundation adapted the AAHPERD Bill of Rights for their booklet "Parent's Guide to Girls' Sports." Their newer version is somewhat more focused and detailed:

1. The right to determine when to participate and in what sports, and to what degree of intensity and involvement.
2. The right to play in every game, no matter what her degree of physical ability or the relative importance of the game in terms of league competition.
3. The right to be taught the fundamentals of the sport by a qualified teacher/coach and to play on fields, courts, and rinks that have been adjusted proportionally to children.
4. The right to be coached by those who have been trained in or who have been made aware of the various stages of emotional and psychological development in children, and to be treated on a level equivalent to her emotional and physical maturity—not by standards of collegiate or professional sports.

Bill of Rights
for Young Athletes

1. Right to participate in sports
2. Right to participate at a level commensurate with each child's maturity and ability
3. Right to have qualified adult leadership
4. Right to play as a child and not as an adult
5. Right to share in the leadership and decision-making of sport participation
6. Right to participate in safe and healthy environments
7. Right to proper preparation for participation in sports
8. Right to an equal opportunity to strive for success
9. Right to be treated with dignity
10. Right to have fun in sports

5. The right to have a coach who places the child first, the team second, himself/herself third, and winning fourth; to feel free to laugh after a defeat and to have fun participating even while playing on a losing team; to be able to use play as an opportunity to test life; and not to be subjected to adult-imposed pressures to win.

6. The right to have a coach who is patient and supportive, as opposed to one who believes in a harsh, negative, "professional" approach; a coach who takes time to work with each athlete, regardless of ability or potential, and who offers periodic evaluation of the child's physical improvement and emotional growth as the season progresses.

7. The right to be treated as a member of a democracy, not a dictatorship, including the freedom to voice opinions openly to the coach without fear of repercussion.

8. The right to proper medical treatment and the right to play in a safe and supportive atmosphere.

9. The right to report to coach or parent any physical pain or emotional concerns such as fear or rejection without fear of ridicule or loss of esteem.

10. The right to freedom from physical and emotional punishment by her parents or the coach. Punishment leads only to fear and inhibition. The purpose of sports should be to help a child grow, feel expansive, and realize his or her potential.*

*Reprinted by permission of the Women's Sports Foundation, December 5, 1988. Address: 342 Madison Ave., New York, NY 10173.

As parents become increasingly interested in their child's participation in team sports, guidelines are needed. Since we parents must be role models both of fitness activity and moral behavior, the following Code of Ethics for Parents, from *Parenting Your Superstar* by Robert J. Rotella and Linda K. Bunker, may be helpful:

Code of Ethics for Parents

1. I will help my child learn to enjoy sport and develop the skills that he or she is capable of performing.
2. I will learn the strengths and weaknesses of my child so that I might place the young athlete into situations where he or she has a maximum opportunity for success.
3. I will become thoroughly familiar with the techniques and rules of the sport my child chooses.
4. I will do my best to learn the fundamental teaching skills and strategies related to my child's sport.
5. I will practice and help my child so that he or she will have an opportunity for skill improvement through active participation.
6. I will communicate with my child the rights and responsibilities of others who are involved in sport.
7. I will protect the health and safety of my child by insisting that all of the activities under my control are conducted for his or her psychological and physiological welfare.
8. I will treat each player, opposing coach, official, parent, and administrator with respect and dignity.
9. I will uphold the authority of officials and coaches who are working with my child. I will assist them when possible and use good judgment if I disagree with them.
10. I will become familiar with the objectives of the sport programs with which my child is affiliated.
11. I will strive to help select activities that uphold our family values.
12. I will help my child develop good sportsmanship and a desire to strive for success.

Next, I believe coaches need guidelines too. The National Youth Sports Coaches Association has issued its own Code of Ethics Pledge:

Code of Ethics for Coaches

I will place the emotional and physical well-being of my players ahead of any personal desire to win.

I will remember to treat each player as an individual, remembering the large spread of emotional and physical development for the same age group.

I will do my very best to provide a safe situation for my players.

I promise to review and practice the necessary first-aid principles needed to treat injuries of my players.

I will do my best to organize practices that are fun and challenging for all my players.

I will lead, by example, in demonstrating fair play and sportsmanship to all my players.

I will ensure that I am knowledgeable in the rules of each sport that I coach and that I will teach these rules to my players.

I will use those coaching techniques appropriate for each of the skills that I teach.

I will remember that I am a youth coach, and that the game is for children and not adults.*

Take a few minutes to think about these rights and codes. Something is happening in sports in the United States that means our kids are missing the basic lessons of play. These codes are designed to draw us back to that goal, where winning wasn't everything and how you played the game counted most.

*Reprinted by permission of the National Youth Sports Coaches Association.

25

A Model Youth Sports Program

As Christopher started in first grade, I faced a dilemma. He wanted to play on a baseball team. Not just a scrub pick-up team in the park, but a team with bats, helmets, and uniforms. I had played and coached Little League baseball. I knew how exciting sports could be for a child and how it could create positive lifelong lessons and friendships. But the sports programs I knew in New York City seemed to lack a sense of community. Kids from all over the city and various schools got mixed together on teams that sometimes seemed stages for showing off individual performances rather than team effort.

Christopher was also very nervous about starting in a new all-boys school with kids he had never met before. I decided this was a good time to organize a sports program for him and his new classmates. They could play and they could get to know each other better. He needed an anchor, and since he loved sports I figured that perhaps I could use that medium to help him adjust. Thus, he and I together founded Sports Club. We had no idea at the time that it would serve as a model sports program for this book. But like all good ideas, it grew and took on a life of its own. Christopher once told me that Sports Club was more important to him than his birthday and Christmas together.

STARTING A SPORTS CLUB

Christopher and I started a baseball program after school on Fridays. Several of his new buddies joined us. The parents were thrilled about the program and how it helped the boys adjust to school and each other. It was also great for Christopher's confidence.

I was encouraged by the way the boys accepted my watered-down imaginative version of baseball. Their skills developed quickly, and so did an infectious love for the game and for exercise. We decided to expand Sports Club to a school-year–long program, playing baseball in the autumn and spring, and basketball in winter.

Not everyone has the chance to take off on Fridays and play baseball and basketball with first-grade boys. (I believe that everyone *should* have the chance—but that's another topic.) I think this Sports Club program has a lot to offer as a model for programs that your child may participate in or which you may choose to develop. It can also serve as an example of how to introduce your child (particularly if he or she is five to ten years old) to team sports and competition in a gentle, educational, fun way.

Success-oriented Philosophy

The key to the Sports Club was its *success-oriented* philosophy. By this I mean that every player, boy or girl, succeeds. No one sits on the bench or strikes out. The rules of the game are modified—for first-graders often beyond recognition—in order to create many successful experiences for kids of all skill levels and to keep the kids moving, rather than sitting or waiting for a brief moment of activity.

Enthusiasm and team spirit dominate rules and serious competition. Rules and equipment are modified to meet the needs of smaller people. Why play with adult-sized equipment if you have small hands? Why shoot at a ten-foot-high basket if you are only four feet tall? Why play by adult rules when you are just learning a game and care more about having fun?

We make each game a special event and include a lot of pizazz in our playing. The goal is simple: to make the kids feel special while learning to have fun playing a game and exercising.

SPORTS CLUB BASEBALL

When Christopher and I set up the Sports Club baseball program, we wanted to include some fitness work and plenty of fundamentals. But we also wanted to make it fun. So, we put together the following program.

First, we walk the half-mile from school to Central Park and then run at least a half-mile to work some fitness exercise into our baseball program. Then we take a juice break and discuss any problems that occurred in the previous game. This makes the kids an integral part of the sports program; we encourage, listen to, and incorporate their ideas. I let them air their worries, and they understand my role as a friend and coach.

Because we limit the size of the program to six kids per coach, twelve kids per game, the boys actually learn the fundamentals of the sport more thoroughly than in a larger, more structured program using adult equipment and rules. They can now lay down a bunt or slide into base with more skill and confidence than most kids in more competitive programs. The bottom line is that each kid gets treated equally as a developing athlete. He receives plenty of individual instruction and encouragement. Fun comes first, then learning, then competition and learning to win and lose.

Next, we work on skills before playing the game. The kids learn how to run bases, slide (a very exciting event!), throw, catch, bunt, bat, and pitch. We keep this part of the program brief. They want to start playing. Then we divide the boys into two teams of comparable ability. As pitcher and umpire, I juggle things around to keep the games close. We try to play an eight-game season, and I try to make sure every kid is on a winning team about half that time. We play in all kinds of weather, and use rubber baseballs in the rain.

We use small bats (twenty-six inches) and tennis balls to make the game fun and manageable for the kids. Hardballs sting and are more difficult to throw. As the kids grow, we move to larger bats. Tennis balls don't sting and they fly through the air when hit; right away, the kids love batting. For fielding and throwing practice, we use soft baseballs that have the feel of the real thing. We also move the bases out to sixty feet from home. This allows plenty of room for running. To add excitement, we put up some plastic cones in the outfield to create a home run fence. With the tennis balls flying, almost every kid hits one "out of the park" for a home run— and gets met at home plate by his classmates for "high fives."

I pitch and another coach or parent catches. This speeds up the game. The game moves faster and there are no walks or strike-outs. I quickly throw pitch after pitch underhanded; I aim for the bat. Kids want to hit the ball and run the bases. If a batter is in a slump and having trouble getting a hit, we have him bunt.

Any ball hit back to me is a foul ball. Fielders are positioned so that almost every batter can get to first base each time up. More skilled players are shifted around, rather than positioned where they can get most of the other players out.

As the kids get better and older, I pitch overhand. We also let the kids do some catching with youth-sized catchers' equipment. I don't use a real baseball until at least the third grade. What's the rush?

Although we stretch and change some of the rules, the kids do learn the basics. They know right away to throw to the correct bases. Runners advance and when a throw is made I call "time out" and hold the runners to the base. They are not allowed to advance too far. Teaching time outs are also called whenever a lesson needs to be discussed—such as throwing to the right base, or fielding the ball the correct way.

Each kid gets to bat twice each inning. There are no recorded outs. The boys are praised every time they hit the ball and every time they field the ball. An inning ends after every player on a team has been up twice; we adjust if the number of players on a team is not even. The batting order is also changed each inning. Every kid plays a different position in the field each inning. All players are treated equal. We try to play for at least an hour. We try to end on an exciting play so the kids aren't bored.

We use liberal rules and as the kids get older and more skilled, we will gradually enforce some of the regulation baseball rules more strictly. Having fun and boosting confidence are far more important than the rules. When in doubt, I say, the runner is always safe. Outs are called if a ball is clearly caught on a fly—coaches cannot catch fly balls—or if the runner is tagged out after a throw is made. Chasing after a runner and tagging him out is not allowed.

We end each game by walking a half-mile to a playground. The kids run around and have fun in free play—a good release after such structured activity. When their parents arrive to take them home, each child is praised in front of his mom or dad.

We do several things to create team spirit and fun. Kids love uniforms, and so we bought simple bright yellow T-shirts with "Sports Club" written on them. The boys wear them everywhere and they boost team spirit, identity, and self-esteem.

The highlight of the baseball season is the all-star game. Everybody makes the all-star team, and we practice for the big game against the parents. At the game, each kid is dramatically introduced to the applause of the fans—moms, dads, sisters, and brothers. We sing the national anthem and "Take Me Out to the Ball Game." At first we asked the parents to let the kids win. Now we don't have to; second-graders can really hit the ball! After the game, the winning team members run to hug their parents—and the parents know they won, too, since they take home a very happy boy.

We also build spirit by putting together a newsletter and mailing it to each boy's parents after every game. In it are dramatic highlights (I have a vivid imagination), funny experiences, and lessons learned. Each boy gets his name mentioned several times. The boys take the newsletters and put them into a scrapbook—just the way Christopher's proud grandfather does. We also made up a bubble gum baseball card with the team picture and name. It is a real baseball card and includes all their names. The boys love to pass them out to friends and family. Who knows, maybe a Christopher Glover Sports Club team card will be worth something in the next century.

Fitness is the essence of this program. The game is treated as a special event to make the boys and their parents feel good about sports, exercise, and each other.

SPORTS CLUB BASKETBALL

This program follows the same fun/fitness philosophy as baseball. Here are some highlights of this type of program:

Before playing basketball, we stretch and perform strengthening exercises like push-ups and sit-ups. Then we run a half-mile. This is followed by relay races. After fitness, we play basketball.

Using equipment that fits the size of the players lets the boys focus on developing proper technique instead of trying to control a large ball and throwing it at a high and distant basket. We use mini-balls and six-foot-high mini-baskets. This lets the boys learn how to pass, catch, and shoot. By third grade, they can be eased into a junior-sized basketball and eight-foot baskets. Between the fourth and sixth grades, they can be eased into regulation-size basketballs and ten-foot baskets.

Practices include learning to pass, dribble, shoot, and play defense—as well as team cheers. Up to six boys are assigned to a coach and one coach is assigned to each basket. Contests are held before the games to generate interest in learning to shoot. First, we have a lay-up contest and award one point for hitting the rim, two for making a basket, and three for a well-executed layup. Then, we have a foul-shooting contest. The boys stand six to ten feet from the basket for foul shots, and they get a point for hitting the rim, two points for a basket, and three points for a swish shot.

At first, the games are played full court with the boys (in two shifts of five to six players) against the coaches. That's usually six against two. The boys take turns in being the shooter in the order of a numbering system. The ball must be passed at least twice before shooting. Double dribbling is not called, but we encourage them to attempt to dribble correctly.

Later, we gradually introduce them to playing against each other. We limit three to a team on the court at any one time, to coach them better. They cannot block shots or play too aggressively yet. At first, defensive players have to stand next to a cone and not move from it in order to let the offensive team have a chance at moving the ball around. During games, we award one point for hitting the rim and two for making a basket. This makes the scoring higher and the game more fun. We also give three points for an outside swish shot—one that doesn't touch the rim before going through the net—and for well-executed layups.

If a boy hasn't scored in a while, he is awarded a foul shot. We believe that all players need to get on the scoreboard and feel successful.

At first, we apply basketball rules rather loosely. Then, as the boys improve, we apply the rules more closely. The emphasis is on fun, and any rule that gets in the way is put aside until the boys understand it and their level of play warrants its use.

As in the baseball program, we try to balance the number of "victories" among the players. We also use teaching time outs frequently to explain the game or work on fundamentals. Fouls are not called at first. Instead, we call a time out and explain why what happened was a foul. Later we ease into fouls and foul shots, but no one is allowed to foul out of a game.

After the game, we give each player a basketball for free shooting. This is the free-time equivalent of the playground after the baseball program. The boys use their imagination to imitate Magic Johnson, Larry Bird, or Michael Jordan. They practice layups and foul shots, as well as fancy hook shots. They yell "Downtown!" and yelp with delight when they toss in a shot from way outside. As their parents arrive to pick them up, the boys keep them in the gym with "Watch this shot!" and "Did you see that, Mommy?"

Here, as in baseball, the highlight of the basketball season is the all-star game. Again, everyone makes the team and practices for the big game against the parents. At the game, each child is introduced to the applause of parents and the cheers of little brothers and sisters. After the national anthem, team photos, and team cheers, the kids beat the socks off the parents and later celebrate their victory.

Adam Cohen's father, Martin, summed up the feeling of the parents who participated in our first basketball program when he wrote to me: "Last Friday afternoon I experienced something that will last in my memory for a long time. The sense of sportsmanship, teamwork, spirit, and accomplishment displayed by our first-graders was overwhelming."

FAMILY SPORTS DAY

During each baseball season we go to a New York Mets game as a team and family—players and parents. For the basketball season, our extended family enjoys a New York Knicks game and a Harlem Globetrotters performance. After these events, the kids return to the diamond and court ready to try new moves—and new fun.

26

Injury Prevention
and Treatment

Most sports programs for children are safe. Kids are not more likely to be injured in a sports activity than they are in normal daily play. But injuries do happen—to both parents and children.

All people who exercise overcome two physical obstacles: the diseases of inactivity, discovered when one starts to get into shape; and then the diseases of excellence that sometimes come from exercising too much or from sports competition. Some injuries are just bad luck. Others come from trying to do too much too soon, or from trying to excel in sports competition before you are ready for that effort. However it comes, injury is part of an active life, but it can also be avoided or minimized.

As adults, we are prone to injuries of inactivity. Our children, however, are more prone to injury from excess or excellence. Some sports that our children play carry greater risks than others. Football leads the injury list for boys, while softball, gymnastics, and running head the girls' list. But, as Dr. James G. Garrick of Phoenix found in a study of high school sports injuries, kids get hurt at the rate of one injury for every 650 hours of participation. This is minor. "It is difficult to imagine any activity," said Dr. Garrick, "that would not result in one injury for every six hundred fifty hours."

Nor are boys more injury prone than girls. Dr. Garrick and Ralph K. Requa of the University of Washington Sports Medicine Division found that about 24 percent of all boys playing sports got injured each season compared to about 22 percent of all girls. Two-thirds of the injuries were sprains and the girls and boys returned to action within a week. No injuries involved breasts or genitalia—a concern that we parents should finally put to rest.

A study by Dr. Christine E. Haycock of the New Jersey Medical School and Joan V. Gillette of the Office of Intercollegiate Athletics of the University of Nevada, Las Vegas, reached similar conclusions for college-age women. "It would appear that, in general, women athletes sustained the same injuries in relatively the same numbers as their male counterparts," said the Haycock-Gillette survey, "with only injuries related to the patella (kneecap) and joints occurring more often in women—only a few of the injuries were unique to women."

SPORTS AND YOUTH INJURIES

Most sports injuries involve the soft tissues of the body, not the bony skeleton. Only about 5 percent of sports injuries are fractures. Most are sprains and strains. Physicians at the American Academy of Pediatrics (AAP) describe sprains as injuries to ligaments, the tapelike connectors between the bones, and strains as injuries to the muscles. Here are some surprising statistics:

- About one million U.S. school children are injured each year while playing in team sports, according to the AAP.
- About 700,000 kids ages five to fourteen are treated in emergency rooms for injuries from playing baseball each year.
- Over 300,000 children are treated in emergency rooms for injuries from bike riding and about 600 of them die.
- About 200,000 injuries involving playground equipment are serious enough to require emergency room treatment each year.
- About 40 percent of all drownings happen to children under age eleven.
- The *Journal of Orthopaedic and Sports Physical Therapy* reports that speed sports like skateboarding and ice-skating make up one-third of all adolescent injuries. Non-contact sports like tennis, swimming, and running have a much lower incidence of injury.

Football is responsible for one out of every five injuries in organized sports—twice as many as basketball or gymnastics. It is by far the leading cause of head, neck, and spinal injury in organized sports. These injuries are also most likely to result in long-term disability.

Many pediatricians advise against tackle football until after puberty. The AAP also recommends that no young person engage in boxing because of the high risk of brain damage.

YOUTH INJURY CAUSES

All activities carry with them some risk. You can even get hurt waving your arms to hail a taxi.

Overuse is a major cause of injury to the musculo-skeletal system in children, according to Dr. Lyle Micheli, an orthopedist and director of the Division of Sports Medicine at Children's Hospital in Boston. Overuse occurs when joints and bones with soft growing surfaces are repeatedly subjected to small bumps and stress. This may be painless, but after prolonged periods of use and exercise, sufficient damage is done unless the child gets proper training, conditioning, and rest.

Overuse rarely occurs when kids play freely or during school physical education. It is far more common in organized sports where repetitious training is required. Children who are experiencing adolescent growth spurts—especially boys between the ages of twelve and fourteen—are less flexible and more likely to suffer overuse injury, says Dr. Micheli.

Because a child's bones are still growing, they are more susceptible than adults' to certain other types of injury. They may also suffer injuries that can complicate the growing process. Ligaments in children, which join bone or cartilage and strengthen joints, are two to five times stronger than the ends of the bones to which they are attached. They can rupture or become injured more easily than those in adults.

Overuse and complications from children's growing process are causing special medical problems. "We're beginning to see a lot of injuries in kids that we've typically seen in adults," said Dr. James C. Puffer, head doctor of the 1988 U.S. Summer Olympics team, at the 1987 American Academy of Family Physicians annual convention. The cause, he believes, is an upsurge in children doing repetitive exercises and strenuous athletic events such as marathon running and triathlons.

So, now that we know kids get injured, how can we prevent and treat those injuries?

PREVENTING INJURY

Many exercise and sports-related injuries to children and adults can be prevented. Here are some guidelines to make participation in sports and fitness activities safer for you and your child.

Pre-exercise Health Evaluation

The American Academy of Pediatrics recommends that every child who wants to play in a sports program get a check-up and evaluation from a physician. I suggest the same for every adult who is starting an exercise program. For the sports program, your child should be evaluated by a physician who understands sports and is familiar with the potential hazards (as well as benefits) of this special activity.

The physician should screen for congenital problems, previous injuries, biomechanical weaknesses (especially in the feet and knees), unequal leg length, muscular imbalance, and of course general fitness and health. Youngsters who are growing rapidly—those boys and girls ages about ten to fifteen—should be carefully checked to be sure that their levels of bone, muscle, and joint development are adequate to meet the rigors of the sport they wish to play.

Physical Conditioning

Many injuries that occur in sports and fitness exercising could be prevented with a proper conditioning program.

You and your child should do several things to avoid injury. First, always warm up and cool down correctly before participating in any sport or exercise. You can follow the examples set forth here in Chapters 10 through 12. Second, always ease into strenuous activity. Give your body time to adjust to increased levels of physical stress. Third, get into a proper training program before undertaking any strenuous exercise. Sports should not be played until after you are in good shape. This includes team sports and individual sports like tennis or squash. You risk injury just stepping into play without conditioning yourself first. A good training program—which emphasizes improving muscular strength and endurance, flexibility and cardo-respiratory endurance—allows time for your ligaments, muscles, and bones to adapt to the stress of sports activities.

Be alert to the fact that just because you are in good shape for one sport, you are not necessarily in shape for another. A fit runner, for example, will need to do special exercises to prevent injury before playing basketball or going skiing.

Pre-season conditioning should not differ from any other pre-activity workouts. Conditioning drills should be progressive, not punishing, workouts. Improper exercise routines cause more injuries than they prevent. For example, running stadium steps is a traditional form of exercise (and sometimes punishment) for soccer, football, and lacrosse players. The exercise is supposed to develop your leg muscles, especially your quadriceps (those muscles at the top of your thighs). But you can do this more safely with a weight program and hill running, and avoid the risk of tripping going up or down stadium steps. Second, exercise such as running laps or doing push-ups should never be used as punishment. Coaches send the wrong message doing that. These exercises are important to your conditioning and not mechanisms for punishment. I do not believe that athletes, especially young ones, need punishment: they need good teaching.

Nutrition, Drugs, and Sleep

Nutrition is important to performance. Never do a "crash" diet to lose weight or to make weight for a sport like wrestling. This will set you up for injury. If you are undernourished and underweight you may have muscle weakness that could also cause injury. Being overweight does increase the likelihood of being injured. You can lose weight and get in shape faster by a combination of moderate and progressive exercise linked with a careful diet, rather than any crash program.

Use of alcohol and tobacco is detrimental to fitness and sports performance. A lot of baseball players put a pinch of tobacco (or more) between cheek and gum. But evidence increasingly shows that nicotine in any form—cigarettes, cigars, *and* chewing tobacco—is cancer causing. There is no evidence that tobacco improves athletic performance. Neither is there any evidence that drugs improve performance on the playing fields, tracks, or roads. Here, too, the evidence swings in the other direction: that drugs actually diminish your ability to perform well, not to mention their effects on your overall health.

Studies do show that good, careful nutrition and plenty of sleep improve performance. An adequate amount of sleep—for adolescents that may be as much as ten to twelve hours a night—helps prevent injury by making you rested and able to perform better. If stress is preventing sleep, or if you find yourself under a lot of stress, back down on your training for a while.

Protective Equipment and Facilities

Almost 20 percent of sports injuries to children involve equipment. Always use proper equipment in good repair for every sport or activity— for example, wearing a protective helmet while biking. Protective equipment includes: head gear, padding (for contact sports), gloves, eye guards, proper shoes, and fitted mouthpiece. Equipment like tennis racquets and baseball bats should also be modified to the size of the kids. All equipment and gear should be checked out and properly fitted to each athlete. Used equipment should be used only when it is in excellent repair. Check to see if the equipment passes safety standards and is endorsed by a recognized governing sports body.

Clothes and even uniforms must fit. I suggest loose-fitting clothes, since tight clothes restrict movement and can thereby cause injury. Don't wear jewelry while playing sports—it can get caught in something and injure you. Eyeglasses should be made of plastic safety material.

Always wear proper shoes for your exercise activity. Tennis shoes are not running shoes. Soccer shoes differ from football shoes, although either may be worn for lacrosse. But in that case, match shoes to surface: there are special shoes for artificial surfaces and for dirt fields. I like biking shoes for serious bikers putting in long distances and high-topped basketball shoes for that sport, since the shoes give good ankle support.

Finally, make sure the facilities you use for sports and exercise are safe. This includes proper lighting for playing and running safely; avoid dark parks and paths when out running. Coaches should check and repair or remove any dangerous obstacles on the playing surface, such as broken glass, discarded bottles, weakened goal posts, or basketball supports. Some playing fields, especially those available for freshman and junior varsity sports, have dips and gullies that players should be aware of. Also, make sure that posts are padded on courts and all movable obstacles like bikes and benches are well away from the out-of-bounds lines.

Supervision

Many injuries occur during practices. Any coach supervising team practices must be alert to things that might cause injury—obstacles mentioned above, the weather, fatigue of players, and so forth. Proper warm-up and cool-down will help prevent injury in practices and games. Good skills also minimize the chances of injury and should be taught and repeated. "Horseplay" can cause injury, especially around equipment, and should not be allowed.

At games, coaches and officials need to act with authority to keep the contest fun and rewarding. Shepherd took his freshman soccer team off the field twice during one away game when the referees could not control parents along the side lines and the opposing team became too physical. Pulling players who would rather fight than play is sometimes also necessary, and a good lesson to all. But basically, officials need to enforce the game's rules to keep the game safe.

Coaches and officials should also modify or even discard rules in the interest of safety. Rules are there to protect players from injury, and should be enforced and changed to meet that need. One example: not allowing young kids to pitch in baseball and limiting the frequency that older kids can pitch.

Participants in youth sports should be matched by size, weight, strength, maturation, and not just age. This is particularly important in contact sports, but is also applicable to soccer and baseball. A youngster who is big for his or her age may injure smaller, less-skilled participants. Kids should compete on an equal basis. This makes the games more fun and safer for them.

As mentioned in Chapter 24, before puberty kids can and should play on coed teams. After puberty, however, the size, strength, and speed of boys increase quickly, and boys and girls should be divided into separate teams.

The Overuse Syndrome

More is not always better in exercise and sports. If runners, for example, keep increasing their mileage, applying more and more stress, they get fatigued, burned out, or injured. They seldom get better. Baseball players, swimmers, tennis players, and other athletes who specialize in a sport can practice the same skills over and over, using the body in the same way and overstressing it. Overuse injuries in sports have developed special medical terms: "runner's knee," "jumper's knee," "swimmer's shoulder," "Little League elbow," "tennis elbow."

Balance your exercise program. Don't do too much too soon. Seek variety in your activity. For several reasons, kids should play various sports in season to use a wide range of muscles and movements.

Caring for Your Own Body

Children, and particularly teenagers, need to be educated by parents and coaches about their responsibilities to their own bodies. Professional athletes may "play through pain," but children and adults should not. Youngsters need to stand up and protect their own bodies; they need to admit it when injured, tired, or burned out. They need to feel comfortable about telling coaches they are injured without the fear of losing playing time or being benched.

When your child gets injured, you can respond in one of four ways. You can ignore the injury and have him or her continue exercising, often making the injury worse. You can have your child quit exercising and hope that the injury will go away; this is sometimes effective. You can try to treat the injury yourself. You can seek medical help. Most parents deal with injuries to their children (and to themselves, for that matter) in this order: ignore it, quit for a few days, self-treat it, and finally see a physician.

For most minor injuries, this order is fine. For more serious injuries, medical help should be sought quickly. How can you tell the difference? Usually by going through the four-point sequence, either quickly (within an hour or two) or over time (within a day or so). In the absence of an obvious serious injury, time often dictates how you treat yourself or your child when injured.

Teach your kids that all injuries should be immediately reported to both parents and coaches. Adults and coaches need to be alert to signs that kids are injured, and educate them. Keep injury in perspective: it is much better to take time out and be able to return than to ignore an injury and risk a longer layoff.

Anyone who exercises or plays sports and gets injured needs time to rehabilitate the injury. This is often done under medical supervision. You or your child should gradually ease back into training. You should follow the routine similar to the conditioning program used when you started (see Chapters 10–12), and practice your sport skills gradually before returning to full practice and competition. If you do not return gradually you risk re-injury, which may be worse than the original injury. Favoring an injury often results in a second or third injury to another part of the body. For example, an ignored foot injury in a runner may cause him or her to continue running in an exaggerated or crooked manner, which might injure his or her back.

Injury prevention in kids is really pretty simple. Do not let them overdo their sports programs and exercise. Make sure their equipment is good, working well, and protective. Treat any injuries seriously and quickly. And keep listening to how your kids describe their exercise programs and sports teams and how they are doing.

EMERGENCIES

A physician or other medical emergency person should be present or available during games, particularly of contact sports or in very hot weather. Clear policies should be made and followed regarding procedures for first aid and treatment of injuries. Coaches and parents should know how to administer emergency first aid (CPR training is a must) and how to reach the nearest emergency medical help. Basic first-aid equipment should be present and easily available to all practices and games. Coaches should also have emergency phone numbers for family members of each player on the team.

Most injuries are minor strains, sprains, and pains that can be treated with *R.I.C.E.*

R is *rest*. Stop any exercise immediately after injury. Continuing to play or complete your exercise will probably make the injury worse. You may need to stop exercising for several days to allow the injury to heal.

I is *ice*. Apply cold, either in the form of ice or cold compresses, to the injured area as soon as possible. This shrinks the damaged blood vessels and helps stop internal bleeding, thus decreasing swelling and bruising and minimizing the injury. Apply the cold treatment immediately for about thirty minutes. Then repeat several times a day until healed.

If you have active kids around your house, or expect kids home during vacations and holidays, keep a couple of the gelatin ice packs in the freezer compartment of your refrigerator, just in case. When you use these packs, or ice, be sure to wrap them first in a soft, dry towel to keep the cold off the skin area.

Note: heat applied to the injury will have the opposite effect. It will encourage blood flow to the injured area and stimulate circulation around it. Heat may indeed be desirable for some injuries, such as pulled muscles.

C is *compression*. Wrap the injury firmly, but not too tightly, with an elastic bandage or cloth to minimize swelling.

E is *elevation*. If possible, the injured area should be raised above the heart so that gravity will help drain excess fluid. This should also minimize the swelling and pain.

You should start the *R.I.C.E.* routine immediately after an injury. This can be done without waiting for an ambulance or a doctor, although be cautious about wrapping the injury at this time. The ice pack alone is good emergency procedure for most injuries. Later, with your physician's approval, a non-prescription analgesic, such as aspirin or ibuprofen, will help minimize the pain and swelling and promote healing.

Injuries that are worse than minor sprains, strains, and bruises should be treated by a physician. If what seems like a minor injury doesn't improve within a few days, see your doctor.

Any severe twists or falls in young children—especially injuries to the head, joints, or bones—should be examined by a doctor. Since children are still growing, especially during early puberty, an injury to a bone, for example, could slow that bone's growth or produce incorrect growth.

LISTEN TO THE WARNING SIGNALS

Sports injuries to a child tend to increase when that child is not enjoying playing sports. There are some well-known physical and emotional warning signs. These include:

- Stomachaches, headaches, vomiting, depression, fatigue, withdrawal.
- Reluctance to participate.
- Obsession with "winning."
- Alcohol or drug abuse.
- An increased number of "minor" injuries such as mild sprains, twists, muscle spasms.
- Physical symptoms suggesting more serious injury, such as dizziness, blurred eyesight, difficult breathing.

There are other warning signs of injury that exercising parents should watch for in themselves and their children. These include:

- Mild tenderness or stiffness that doesn't go away after a few days of rest. Poor performance in workouts or an uncharacteristic lack of interest in training and games.
- Fatigue after a full night's sleep or a sluggish feeling that lasts several days.
- A continued thirst despite replenishment of fluids. Check your urine. Normal urine is almost clear and odorless. Dehydration will darken your urine.
- A significant loss of body weight.
- A feeling of sore throat, fever, or a runny nose—any sign that your body is fighting infection.
- Muscle cramping (due to mineral depletion).
- Increased irritability, feeling of tension, depression, apathy.

All of these symptoms should be warning signs of doing too much. Take a few days off, or encourage your child to take some time off from his or her sports activity and do something else.

HEAT INJURIES

Children may not tolerate extremes of temperature well. A young body is not fully developed, and its thermoregulatory system, which maintains body temperature, may adjust slowly to extremes of heat and cold. If you or your children are exercising in hot weather, take several precautions.

First, try to exercise in the shade and in the early morning or late evening. Avoid the hot, midday sun.

Drink plenty of fluids before, during, and after exercise. Make sure that the coaches of your children's teams understand this. Water breaks should be frequent for kids (and adults) during workouts in hot weather. Water should *never* be denied as punishment to a child or team. Water should also be poured over the head and body to help keep you cool. A hat and a kerchief soaked in water will also keep the body cool for a while. But the best thing is to hydrate yourself with fluids.

Clothing should be lightweight, loose fitting, and white to reflect the sun. If possible, keep yourself lightly covered to avoid sunburn.

The length and intensity of workouts should be cut back on hot days. If games are played in hot weather, substitutions should be made more frequently. Practices and games for young kids should be cancelled in exceptionally hot, humid weather. Take the day off and hit the water somewhere.

When exercising in hot weather, increase your intake of fruits along with fluids. Make sure your diet is well balanced and contains natural sources to replace lost fluids, sodium, potassium, magnesium, and other minerals. Water, natural fruit juices, and a balanced diet will replace what you have lost.

Heat and humidity are killers. Exercising in hot weather can be dangerous. You may suffer from muscle cramps, fatigue, heat cramps, or heat exhaustion. You should learn the symptoms of these afflictions.

Heat exhaustion occurs when hot, humid weather combines with exercise to overwork the cardio-respiratory system. Its symptoms include profuse sweating, dizziness, weakness, and dehydration.

Heat stroke, a far more serious problem, occurs when the heat regulatory system suppresses sweating. The skin feels hot and dry, you have dizziness and nausea; convulsions, collapse, or coma—and death—may follow.

Understand the warning signals of heat: headache, dizziness, disorientation, decrease in sweat rate, and a pale, cold skin. Stop exercising immediately. Find shade and pour water over yourself or the victim. Lie down, raise the legs, get medical help.

Heat is a killer. It has killed young athletes playing football and other sports on hot, humid days. It killed two men, ages twenty-three and twenty-four, in races I was associated with in New York City. Both men were not properly trained and yet they ran hard in hot weather. They rolled the dice—and lost.

When exercising in hot weather, you should consider air temperature and humidity together. The key to body heat removal is sweat evaporation, and when the humidity is high little sweat can vaporize. Your body has difficulty losing heat. An air temperature of sixty degrees Fahrenheit with 95 percent humidity could be more dangerous to you than 90 degrees in a dry climate.

COLD INJURIES

Exercising in cold weather requires some precautions too. But as long as you keep moving and do not get wet, you should be all right. Windburn and frostbite are dangers. To prevent injury from either of these, keep covered, dry, moving, and avoid strong headwinds, especially if you get wet.

Dress in layers to help your body trap heat. Then, you can unzip or take off layers as you get heated up and replace them as you cool down.

Frostbitten skin is cold, pale, and firm to hard to the touch. The first step in treatment is to warm rapidly without excessive heat. Water about body temperature is good. Do not massage or, in the case of toes, walk on the injured area. Seek first aid immediately.

Another cold-weather danger is hypothermia: the lowering below normal of your central, or core, temperature. As the body temperature falls, you respond with shivering, which is your muscles' way of trying to produce heat. If you do not reverse this body temperature decline, you may become incoherent and then lapse into a coma, or die. Hypothermia usually occurs when you are wearing wet clothing. You should get inside quickly, take off wet clothing immediately, and get warm, perhaps with a hot bath.

Generally, exercising in cold weather can be fun. But if you do have any of the above signals, or if you become soaking wet, be sure to stop exercising and get dry and warm. Also, never exercise in cold weather and then stand around outside. Get indoors, take off the sweaty clothing, and get warm.

COLDS AND FLU

Exercise that raises a good sweat may help get rid of colds, but it can also weaken you to infection. When you overstress yourself, you become susceptible to a cold. I'm most vulnerable during the two weeks after a marathon or the pre-race build-up before one.

Exercise tends to break up the congestion of a cold. But colds are warning signals. Says Dr. George Sheehan, the running cardiologist: "I treat colds with respect. It is my feeling that they represent a breakdown of the defense system. The cold is an early warning symptom of exhaustion."

Viral infections, such as the flu, are something else. There are documented cases of people who persisted in exercising heavily despite having a viral infection, and died. If you get one, or have a persistent cold, cut back on your exercise. Never exceed the limits of your energy.

Fever, especially with flu, is also dangerous. The body is weakened and it doesn't need the additional stress of your exercise or sports regimen. Rest completely and then return slowly to a normal schedule. I once spent an entire summer bothered by flu. I never gave in, and suffered three relapses while trying to return to my exercise training. Listen to your body, or your stubborn mind can lead you astray.

Part 7

WELLNESS

27

The Holistic Approach to Health and Fitness

You and your children can be fit and still not be healthy. Despite following all the exercise guidelines in this book and passing all the fitness tests in Chapter 4, you may not be leading a healthy life.

Exercise is essential to good health, but it is only one facet of a wellness program. Dr. Kenneth Cooper, the aerobics expert, warns of the "myth of invulnerability"—the belief that the more we exercise, the healthier we become. We believe we are impervious to coronary illness and other diseases that plague our stressful and sedentary society. In fact, we need to do more than simply exercise.

We need a holistic approach to life to enjoy the benefits of both a family fitness and family wellness program. Fitness is not health. A total wellness program is a marriage of fitness and good health practices.

What do I mean by wellness? Wellness emphasizes the positive aspects of health and fitness, and it incorporates them into a lifestyle that contributes to an increased longevity and the improved quality of our lives. Poor health practices and a lack of exercise result in the opposite of wellness: illness. As the shocking statistics of Chapter 1 illustrate, heart disease and other illnesses often start before the first grade. To bring wellness into your life, therefore, you will need to start it in your very young children.

According to *Preventive Medicine* magazine, a long-term study of seven thousand people identified seven basic health practices that will contribute to living a longer, healthier life:

1. Adequate sleep;
2. Maintaining your recommended weight;
3. Not smoking;

4. Not drinking or drinking moderately;
5. Regular, vigorous physical activity;
6. Eating a regular breakfast;
7. Eating regular meals, avoiding frequent snacking.

The study found that individuals who followed six or seven of these good health practices lived on the average eleven and a half years longer than those who followed none or up to only three of them. As the study is a demographic and statistical analysis of a large group of Americans, it does indeed make good health sense to take the seven steps to a healthier life.

The fitness aspect of a wellness program also includes some health-giving exercises to promote relaxation, improve flexibility, strengthen key muscle groups, and increase your cardio-respiratory endurance. A program to achieve fitness in all of these components has been the central theme of this book. Now I want to add wellness to that theme.

To do that, we must examine the health aspects of your family's total wellness program: stress management, nutrition, weight control, drug and alcohol consumption, smoking, sleeping habits, blood pressure, medical care, the concept of your Self, and heredity. I consider you and your family wellness oriented if you can do most of the following:

- Meet the minimal fitness goals of this book. That is, each of you exercises vigorously at least three times a week, emphasizing relaxation, flexibility, muscular strength and endurance, and aerobic conditioning.
- Properly balance the stresses and joys of family, work, and exercise.
- Deal well with the stress in your daily lives by taking minor upsets in stride and seeking family support or professional help to deal with the more serious stresses. Take frequent time outs—vacations, exercise breaks, regular family activities—from those stresses.
- Eat a balanced diet low in calories, fat, sugar, salt, and cholesterol, and high in fiber and complex carbohydrates (see nutrition guidelines in Chapter 29).
- Start each day with a healthy family breakfast.
- Eat regular meals and avoid unhealthy snacking.
- Maintain a healthful weight.
- Do not abuse alcohol or drugs or use tobacco.
- Sleep seven to eight hours a night (more for growing adolescents).
- Have an optimistic attitude and high energy level.
- Watch over your health and that of your family.

- Have frequent medical exams, including tests for cholesterol or triglyceride levels, blood pressure, and body weight.
- Have a thorough medical exam before starting an exercise program or a new sport season.
- Monitor all heart disease risk factors if you have a family history of heart disease.

Some of the above are simply good common sense. Certainly you should have your blood pressure monitored every time you see your doctor. Following safety precautions at home, work, and during exercise should be second nature to you. Protecting your family's health is an integral part of your daily living. The point I am making here, however, is that you should strive for the level of wellness awareness where all of the points are commonplace to your life. You do them as part of daily living.

Neither exercise nor good eating habits alone will guarantee disease prevention, longevity, happiness, and productivity. Wellness—the combination of fitness and positive health practices—is the key. If you combine exercise with good lifestyle habits, you and your family will take a major step toward total well-being. This is not to say you will live longer—although the studies previously cited show that, statistically at least, you probably will. But the quality of the life you are given will increase.

Let's look at some specific guidelines, much as I suggested fitness guidelines in Part III. The following Wellness Quiz is published by the American Running & Fitness Association, a public service organization for which I serve on the board of advisors. The quiz is designed to be used to evaluate the wellness lifestyle of you and your family. You should take the quiz semi-annually and use it to motivate you to lead a more wellness-oriented family life.

Please understand that wellness, like fitness, does not happen overnight. You can reduce your health risks one factor at a time with gradual, partial changes. To be effective, the entire family will need to be supportive of each family member who wants to make such basic behavioral changes.

WELLNESS QUIZ

Exercise:
1. How much time do you spend walking briskly, running, cycling, swimming, aerobic dancing, rowing, cross-country skiing, or doing other aerobic activities (nonstop, vigorous exercise) per week? To be considered, the activity must be done for a minimum of 20 minutes at a time, and must roughly double your resting heart rate (to around 120 beats or more per minute).
   (a) 150 minutes or more per week . . . . 18 points
   (b) 90 to 149 minutes per week . . . . 17 points

    (c) 60 to 89 minutes per week .... 16 points
    (d) 30 to 59 minutes per week .... 8 points
    (e) 15 to 29 minutes per week .... 4 points
    (f) 0 to 14 minutes per week .... 0 points
2. If you exercise regularly:
    (a) Do you stretch after you exercise?
        Always .... 2 points
        Sometimes... 1 point
        Never .... 0 points
    (b) Do you exercise in spite of pain? .... −5 points
    (c) Do you alternate hard and easy (or rest) days?
        Always .... 2 points
        Sometimes... 1 point
        Never .... 0 points

Nutrition, Diet:

3. Do you eat a wide variety of foods—something from each of the four basic food groups: meat, fish, poultry, dried legumes or beans, eggs, nuts; milk products; whole grain breads or cereals; fruits and vegetables?
    (a) Every day.. 4 points
    (b) At least three times a week .... 2 points
    (c) Once a week .... 0 points
    (d) Once in a while .... −2 points
4. Do you limit the amount of animal fat (butter, fatty meats, fried foods) in your diet?
    (a) Avoid animal fat................................... 2 points
    (b) Try to avoid, but occasionally have some .... 1 point
    (c) Never really pay much attention to this; don't try to avoid... 0 points
    (d) Love fatty foods; eat frequently...................... −1 point
5. Do you limit the amount of refined sugar products in your diet?
    (a) Avoid refined sugar products........................ 2 points
    (b) Try to avoid, but occasionally have some .... 1 point
    (c) Never really pay much attention to this; don't try to avoid... 0 points
    (d) Love refined sugar products; eat frequently .... −1 point
6. Do you limit the amount of salt or salty foods in your diet?
    (a) Avoid salt or salty foods .... 2 points
    (b) Try to avoid, but occasionally have some .... 1 point
    (c) Never really pay much attention to this; don't try to avoid... 0 points
    (d) Love salt or salty foods; eat frequently .... −1 point
7. Do you eat a good breakfast (juice, cereal, and milk, for example)? Pick one that's closest to what you do.
    (a) Daily, with a light lunch and moderate dinner .... 2 points
    (b) Four days a week, with a light lunch and moderate dinner.. 1 point

(c) Skip breakfast in favor of light lunch and heavy dinner.. 0 points
(d) Eat snacks during the day and a heavy dinner .... −1 point
(e) Eat snacks plus heavy meals .... −2 points

Weight:
8. Are you overweight? (To calculate your "ideal" weight: Men should take their height in inches, multiply it by 4, and subtract 128. Women should take their height in inches, multiply it by 3.5, and subtract 108.)

(a) Under "ideal" weight by 11 or more pounds........... −3 points
(b) Under "ideal" weight by 6 to 10 pounds .... 0 points
(c) Within "ideal" weight +5 to −5 pounds .... 8 points
(d) 6 to 15 pounds overweight .... 0 points
(e) 16 to 25 pounds overweight .... −1 point
(f) 26 to 35 pounds overweight .... −2 points
(g) 36 to 50 pounds overweight .... −3 points
(h) 51 or more pounds overweight...................... −6 points

Smoking:
9. Do you smoke?

(a) Never .... 4 points
(b) Quit two or more years ago........................ 3 points
(c) Quit within the last two years .... 2 points
(d) 1 to 10 cigarettes or cigars per day, or pipe .... −1 point
(e) 11 to 20 cigarettes or cigars per day................... −3 points
(f) 21 to 40 cigarettes or cigars per day................... −6 points
(g) More than 40 cigarettes or cigars per day .... −9 points

Alcohol:
10. Do you drink?

(a) Never .... 0 points
(b) Social drinker only .... 0 points
(c) 1 to 2 drinks per day.............................. 1 point
(d) 2 to 4 drinks per day.............................. −1 point
(e) 5 to 6 drinks per day.............................. −3 points
(f) 7 or more drinks per day .... −5 points

11. Do you get drunk?

(a) Never .... 2 points
(b) 1 to 3 times a year................................ 0 points
(c) 4 to 6 times a year................................ −1 point
(d) 7 to 12 times a year .... −3 points
(e) More than 12 times a year......................... −5 points

Drugs:
12. Do you use illicit drugs?

(a) Never .... 2 points
(b) Infrequently...................................... 0 points
(c) Occasionally .... −1 point

    (d) Frequently . . . .   −3 points
    (e) Regularly . . . .   −5 points
13. Do you use prescription drugs?
    (a) Rarely needed . . . .   2 points
    (b) Used occasionally, as needed and prescribed by a
        physician . . . .   0 points
    (c) Don't follow prescribed dosage or schedule . . . .   −1 point
    (d) Regularly use mood-altering drugs . . . .   −3 points
    (e) Use mood-altering drugs combined with alcohol or other
        drugs . . . .   −5 points

Stress and Relaxation:
14. How much stress do you experience in your life?
    (a) Very little . . . .   2 points
    (b) Occasional mild tension . . . .   0 points
    (c) Frequent mild tension . . . .   −1 point
    (d) Frequent moderate tension . . . .   −2 points
    (e) Frequent high tension . . . .   −3 points
    (f) Constant high tension . . . .   −4 points
15. How secure and relaxed are you?
    (a) I'm always secure and relaxed . . . .   2 points
    (b) I'm usually secure and relaxed . . . .   0 points
    (c) I'm occasionally anxious or tense . . . .   −1 point
    (d) I'm anxious or tense most of the time and have difficulty
        relaxing . . . .   −2 points
    (e) I'm anxious, tense, and unable to relax most or all of the
        time . . . .   −4 points
16. How much sleep do you get?
    (a) 7 to 8 hours a night . . . .   2 points
    (b) 8 to 9 hours a night . . . .   1 point
    (c) 6 to 7 hours a night . . . .   1 point
    (d) 9 hours or more a night . . . .   −1 point
    (e) 6 hours or less a night . . . .   −2 points

Self-Concept:
17. How do you feel about yourself?
    (a) I feel good about myself and generally am confident
        about my future and my abilities . . . .   2 points
    (b) I'm comfortable with myself and will probably do well
        in the future . . . .   1 point
    (c) I'm usually comfortable with myself, but have my ups
        and downs . . . .   0 points
    (d) I'm not too happy with myself and seem to make too
        many mistakes . . . .   −2 points
    (e) I don't like myself and can't seem to do anything right . .   −4 points
18. How do you feel about your job (housewives are professionals
too!)?
    (a) It's challenging and I enjoy it . . . .   2 points

    (b) It's sometimes challenging and I'm usually content with
        it .... 1 point
    (c) It's a living.. 0 points
    (d) I don't like my job.................................. −2 points
    (e) I hate my job .... −4 points

Medical Care:
19. How often do you visit a doctor for a checkup?
    (a) Once or twice a year .... 2 points
    (b) About once every four years or so .... −1 point
    (c) Rarely or never .... −4 points
20. Do you do breast self-exams/testicular self-exams?
    (a) Monthly... 2 points
    (b) Occasionally .... 0 points
    (c) Never .... −2 points

To tabulate your wellness score, add or subtract the points to the right of each of your answers. If your total score is:

    50 to 64   You take excellent care of yourself and are in excellent shape.
    25 to 49   You take good care of yourself and are in good shape.
    0 to 24   You take reasonable care of yourself and could be in better shape.
 −31 to −1   You do not take good enough care of yourself and you are in risky shape.
 −32 or less Your lifestyle is hazardous to your health.

Reprinted by permission of the American Running & Fitness Association.

Wellness principles should be taught to children from an early age at both home and school. I suggest starting at home and then later seeing how your school's principal and teachers respond to these new ideas. Some may find them too unusual and threatening. Take the task one step at a time: exercise and fitness first; wellness and health care next.

In 1979, a Louis Harris poll showed that 93 percent of those questioned agreed that: "If we Americans lived healthier lives, ate more nutritious food, smoked less, maintained proper weight, and exercised regularly, it would do more to improve our health than anything doctors and medicine can do for us." A 1988 Harris poll, conducted for *Prevention Magazine*, showed that we did not take our own advice. Although the respondents to the poll knew more than ever about good health practices, few did anything to change. *Prevention*'s Thomas Dybdahl summarized: "It really raises the question 'Are Americans living more healthfully?' "

The answer is probably no. That means that the challenge to you and your family is not simply to read and understand the information in this book. Yes, aerobic exercise is very good for you; and yes, a more healthful lifestyle would prolong your life. But now you have to make the commitment. Start with exercise first and incorporate that into your life. Then move on to wellness and incorporate this into your increasingly healthful family lifestyle—one that your children will pass on to their children and future family generations.

There are other things you can do immediately to improve the way you live and get you started on the road to fitness and wellness.

SMOKING

Cigarette smoking can injure and kill you and your loved ones. Shepherd and I can attest to this first-hand. As a young boy, I can remember my father lying on a couch in the living room struggling to talk to me after having surgery to remove a cancerous growth from his throat caused by years of cigarette smoking. I was scared. I was afraid he would die. *His* father had smoked so much that when he died from cancer his fingers and dentures were stained yellow. My father was luckier. His cancer has never returned. But his message was clear: he asked me never to smoke and I never even tried.

Shepherd watched his sister die slowly from cancer. She had smoked two packs of cigarettes a day for about twenty years. She tried to stop, but couldn't, and the cancer slowly consumed not only her lungs, but also her kidneys, heart, and finally—mercifully—her brain. Over the course of seventeen months, she shriveled up until she was sustained by medication and machine before dying in her sleep one morning.

We cite these family histories as warnings. You can tell us of friends you know who have smoked for decades and are healthy as oxen. But, my friends, the odds are against you. Any form of tobacco—the "smoke-less" cigarettes that came out in 1988, cigars, or chewing tobacco—contains nicotine, tars, and carbon monoxide. They are killers.

According to the U.S. Surgeon General, cancer is the second leading cause of death in the United States; tobacco use, generally through cigarette smoking, accounts for almost one-third of all cancer deaths. Cigarette smoking is the single most avoidable cause of death in our society and the most important health issue of our time.

Tobacco use, particularly cigarette smoking, causes birth defects, heart disease, lung disease (emphysema and chronic bronchitis), and increases your heart rate and blood pressure. Smokers have more sore throats, colds, coughs, headaches, sinus problems, and irritated eyes and nasal passages than non-smokers.

Smokers live seven years less than non-smokers and have a 20 percent greater chance of getting lung cancer.

Smokers miss more work days due to illness; those who smoke twenty cigarettes or more a day take twice as many days off from work each year as non-smokers.

In 1988, Dr. C. Everett Koop, the U.S. Surgeon General, concluded that nicotine was as addictive as heroin and cocaine. He argued that the use of tobacco in any form should be viewed as a serious addiction rather than simply a dangerous habit. He added that the habit was responsible for about 320,000 deaths a year in the United States alone.

Dr. Koop's study reversed the 1964 Surgeon General's report that found that smoking was a habit but not addictive. "Shouldn't we treat tobacco sales at least as seriously as the sale of alcoholic beverages," he asked, "for which a specific license is required and revoked for repeated sales to minors?" Senator Bill Bradley (D-N.J.) introduced legislation in 1988 calling for labels on all tobacco products that would read: "Warning: Smoking is addictive. Once you start you may not be able to stop."

Kids and Smoking

The American Health Foundation found, in a survey, that about half of all U.S. elementary school kids have smoked cigarettes at one time or another. A National Adolescent Student Health Survey indicated that 51 percent of all U.S. eighth-graders and 63 percent of all U.S. tenth-graders reported also having smoked cigarettes. Although teenagers are cutting back on smoking, 18 percent of high-school boys and 21 percent of high-school girls were smoking one or more cigarettes a day in 1987.

Why do our kids smoke? For one thing, they take after their parents or other adults: there are about 50 million adult smokers in the United States; that's about 30 percent of all adults, or about one in three. Kids see them puffing away and think cigarette smoking is a sign of maturity. Children of smokers are far more likely to smoke than children of non-smokers. Studies also show that the younger a smoker starts, the harder it is to quit and the greater the number of cigarettes smoked each day.

Kids also smoke to be rebellious, to show their independence, to join their friends who smoke. And, as Dr. Koop suggested, kids and adults smoke because cigarettes are easy to buy.

Smokeless tobacco. A growing number of our young people are trying chewing tobacco, which the industry sells as "smokeless tobacco." Between 1977 and 1988, the use of chewing tobacco among young men in the United States doubled to reach about four million users under age twenty-one. Most of these users are boys and young men.

Many young boys chew tobacco to copy major league baseball players, who appear in national advertisements for the product. Dental researchers from Farleigh Dickinson University in New Jersey and the University of

Alabama estimate that half the baseball pros and 6 percent of U.S. teenagers are long-term users of chewing tobacco.

"Many teens—even parents and school personnel—think smokeless tobacco is more acceptable than using drugs or smoking cigarettes," said Dr. Curtis Creath, a pediatric dentist, in the *Journal of the American Dental Association*. Chewing tobacco is not a safe alternative to cigarette smoking, however. Users have an increased risk of oral cancer and gum disease. And there have been tragic examples of high-school baseball players who chewed tobacco to copy major leaguers, and ended up with cancer of the cheek and jaw bones.

Passive smoking. This is the involuntary inhalation of cigarette, cigar, or pipe smoke by someone other than the smoker. It is particularly dangerous to non-smokers, whose lungs will absorb the smoke and its harmful ingredients faster than a smoker's already-damaged lungs. The Surgeon General has determined that "environmental tobacco smoke" inhaled by non-smokers can cause heart disease, cancer, and other serious diseases in them.

For example, studies show that infants in their first year who live in homes where parents smoke suffer twice as many respiratory illnesses as infants in non-smokers' homes. The *American Journal of Epidemiology* reported that a person married to a smoker has a 1.6 times greater chance of getting cancer than a person who is not married to a smoker. A study published in the *Journal of Pediatrics* showed that non-smoking teenage athletes exposed to cigarette smoke for at least two hours a week coughed more and had greater lung dysfunction than athletes not exposed to smoke.

Harvard researchers tested the lung function and growth rate of 7,834 non-smoking children. Those children living with parents who did not smoke had both the highest level of lung function and growth rate. Not surprisingly, those children who lived in homes where one or both parents smoked at least one pack of cigarettes a day had weaker lung function and reduced growth rate.

Two things are clear. Parents should stop smoking, for both their own health and that of the children. And we should also continue banning tobacco smoking in public places such as airplanes, restaurants, and offices. At the same time, we should educate our kids about the dangers and addiction of smoking and we should help them and their parents stop smoking immediately.

How to stop smoking. All of us must realize that quitting isn't easy. It's far easier never to start smoking.

"For many smokers," said Dr. Koop, "a genuine desire to quit and, if necessary, persistent and repeated attempts to quit may be all that is necessary. For others, self-help material, formal treatment programs and nicotine replacement therapy may be needed and should be readily available."

We non-smokers can help by giving smokers who want to quit lots of support and love. That may mean a child's love and encouragement of his or her parent's efforts to quit smoking. It may mean the love and support of parents for each other, or for a child's efforts to break the addiction. Sometimes, as Dr. Koop suggests, stop-smoking clinics are helpful.

In the end, however, one of the best methods to stop smoking is to change the way you live. Stop making cigarettes, cigars, or your pipe the focus of your daily life. Break the stimulus-response reaction—that is, eating and then smoking, reading and smoking, and so forth. My recommendation is to substitute love for smoking (love by you for your smoking teenager; love of your child for you, the smoking parent) and substitute exercise for smoking.

How can you substitute exercise for smoking? You could follow the fitness programs detailed earlier in this book, in Parts Four and Five. As you slowly increase your fitness time or distance, you would correspondingly decrease your consumption of tobacco. Your health—wellness, if you will—increases as your unfitness (disease, smoking, alcohol, obesity, and so forth) decreases. I suggest, therefore, substituting love and exercise for unfitness and smoking.

The benefits. Stopping smoking reduces all the dangers (cancer, respiratory problems, heart disease) and the ugliness (yellow teeth, stained fingers, clothing and homes that smell of tobacco, bad breath, and body odor).

The benefits accrue quickly. Your high risk of heart attack drops rapidly when you stop. The heightened risk almost disappears when you stop for two years or more. According to a study directed by Dr. Lynn Rosenberg of the Boston University Drug Epidemiology Unit, the risk of a non-fatal heart attack is three times higher among current smokers than among those who have never smoked. Men who have stopped smoking for more than one year, but less than two, have double the risk. But when former smokers quit for at least two years, their risk appears to be about the same as that of people who never smoked.

Now you know what smokers have to lose.

ALCOHOL AND DRUG ABUSE

There is a thin line between legal use of alcohol and drugs and illegal abuse. I enjoy a cold beer. Shepherd prefers a glass of wine at times. Some of you may like one or two mixed drinks on occasion. But a lot of beer, a couple of bottles of wine, or anything beyond two mixed drinks may indicate alcohol abuse, perhaps even alcoholism.

The same is true of legal drugs. There are times when over-the-counter drugs are needed and helpful. There are times when prescription drugs are essential to make us well or even save our lives. But the over-use and abuse of these drugs is harmful and illegal. Of course, there are other drugs that are clearly illegal no matter what the use: marijuana, cocaine, heroin, hallucinogens, and any legal drugs obtained and used illegally.

Unfortunately, people who strongly believe in sports and fitness may also abuse drugs. We read a lot about athletes taking steroids, such as Ben Johnson at the 1988 Olympics, to gain strength for sports. That, too, is drug abuse. I know of runners who drink a lot of coffee or cola before races for the caffeine's effect. Is that a form of drug abuse? What about using over-the-counter pills to stay awake when driving or studying?

Both alcohol and drugs can damage our bodies. When we become dependent on them—to blur out parts of our lives, numb us to stress, or aid our performances—we are using them illegally. We are abusers. We have lost sight of the reason for living: to take on and feel all that life offers and to care for ourselves and our loved ones.

Unfortunately, both drugs and alcohol are widely abused in the United States. This is increasingly true among our young people: the average beginning age for alcohol abuse is between twelve and thirteen years of age; 30 percent of all thirteen-year-old boys and 22 percent of all thirteen-year-old girls admit that they drink alcohol "regularly." The statistics go on and on:

- Motor vehicle accidents involving alcohol are the leading cause of death for our teenagers and account for 45 percent of all teenage deaths. Every five seconds, a U.S. teenager has a drug or alcohol-caused traffic accident.
- Perhaps one in every ten U.S. adolescents is dependent on drugs or alcohol.
- The National Adolescent Student Health Survey reported that 80 percent of all U.S. teenagers have tried alcoholic beverages; about 33 percent reported having five or more drinks during a single occasion in the previous two weeks.
- About 58 percent of all U.S. high-school seniors have used drugs; 16 percent have tried cocaine. Fifteen percent of all U.S. eighth-graders and 35 percent of all tenth-graders reported having tried marijuana. About one out of every fifteen U.S. adolescents has tried cocaine and one out of every five has tried sniffing glue. Most of these drugs are purchased at school.

We as parents can help our kids say no to drugs and alcohol by helping them understand fully what drugs and alcohol can do to them. We also need to help them understand that they will be accepted by the friends who count even if they refuse to drink or use drugs.

Woman's Day published some helpful warning signs to alert you to whether or not your child is abusing drugs or alcohol:

- Your child is not going to school regularly, cuts classes, suddenly starts getting poor grades, or becomes a discipline problem.
- Your child seems uninterested in you, the family, and his or her old friends or activities.
- Your child suddenly becomes accident prone, isn't sleeping well, or shows severe mood swings.
- Your child makes new friends who seem the type who would drink or use drugs. Use your own intuition here—being careful to avoid stereotypes (boys with long hair or earrings).
- Your child changes his usual behavior and starts to lie to you, steal from your home, or leave home without telling you where he or she is going.

What can you do? Turn off the TV and take the phone off the hook. Talk to your child and listen hard. Look your child in the eyes. Sit close together. Try some scenarios out on him or her, starting with "What would you do if . . . ?" That is, what would you do if you went to a party and all your friends started drinking a lot of beer? What would you do if you were too drunk to drive or a friend was too drunk to drive you home? The "what if" removes the risk from your child's responses.

Avoid being judgmental. Avoid comparisons ("When I was your age . . ."). Be sensitive, loving, understanding. Set clear rules about drugs and alcohol, and explain why. Be clear where you stand on these issues. (For example, if you smoke marijuana, how do you feel about your child using drugs? If you drink when you get home from work, what do you want your kids to do about drinking?)

Keep your kids busy. Arrange for them to take music lessons, scouting, sports, and other activities after school. Get them started on hobbies at home. Do things with them as a family: bike rides, swimming, games. (See Part Five.)

Help teach your child to say no. When Shepherd's kids were teenagers, he told them that anytime they got into a situation where they did not want to go someplace with someone, drink, try drugs, or whatever, they were to blame their "no" response on him. That is, encourage your kids to use the excuse: "I can't do that. My Mom/Dad won't let me." If it has to be tougher, try: "I can't do that. My Mom/Dad will kill me if they find out." Let 'em know it's true, too!

I argue that the best way to handle alcohol and drug abuse is to set a good example as a parent. If you get sloshed after work, you are telling your kids a lot about handling stress, fatigue, anger, and frustration. They'll start getting sloshed after school. If you smoke marijuana or use cocaine or other drugs—including amphetamines (perhaps as diet pills), caffeine, or tranquilizers—your kids will see that solutions to their problems may be found in a joint or a pill too. Just as you should set an example in terms of improving your kids' fitness, so you should set an example in terms of improving their wellness.

Help. If you have a kid who drinks a lot or is using drugs, what should you do? Don't blame yourself. Don't nag your child. Try love and assurance and understanding—but also listen, be firm, clearly state the perceived problem and choices. Get outside, professional help. This is no time for amateur psychologists or scam therapies. Get yourself and your child into therapy, preferably not together.

In the case of drinking, be certain to teach your kids about the "designated driver" rule. As they reach drinking age—eighteen to twenty-one, depending on your state—they must be encouraged to have a designated driver at every party. This can be rotated among friends. But that person must not drink *any* alcohol (or use any drugs) at the party. It is his responsibility to get his friends home safely. This doesn't mean not having any fun; it means loving one's friends above all else. Alcohol is the largest single cause of death in traffic accidents—more than half of all deaths are caused by drinking.

As in the case of fitness, you and I as parents have a lot of work to do. We need to engage this wellness/abuse issue directly, fully, and permanently. Make it part of our lives, although it would be much easier to turn it over to someone else. Listen to this:

- In a national study of fourth- through sixth-graders conducted by *Weekly Reader,* 41 percent of those who had tried marijuana said they did so "to fit in" with other kids. Others said they did it "to feel older," "to have a good time," "to not feel bad."
- More than 40 percent said they felt that kids their age felt "some" or "a lot" of pressure to try cigarettes.
- About 34 percent said kids their age felt "some" or "a lot" of pressure to try wine coolers.
- Almost 25 percent said kids their age felt "some" or "a lot" of pressure to try cocaine or its variation, crack.

These are our ten-year-olds!

28

Stress Management

As Shepherd and I wrote in *The Runner's Handbook:*

> Stress is essential to life, but a cause of death. It sweetens victory, and
> defines defeat. It relieves boredom and helps us maintain life, resist
> aggression, and adapt to changing external influences. It may be pleasant
> or unpleasant, damaging or helpful. Its effect, especially its negative
> impact on our bodies, may be long-lasting, even occurring after the
> stressful event has passed.

What do we mean by stress? Clinically, stress is different from anxiety
or depression. Depression manifests itself in prolonged feelings of sadness,
hopelessness, guilt, and worthlessness; in a sense of doom, disturbed sleep,
or changes in your weight or appetite. In mild cases, psychotherapy is
helpful; drugs may be necessary in severe cases. Anxiety causes excessive
worry, irritability, anger, nervousness, panic disorders, palpitations, chest
pain, dizziness. It can be helped with psychotherapy and some drugs.

Stress is something we all face at one time or another. It may have some
of the symptoms above or irritability, rapid breathing and heart rate, tense
muscles, queasy stomach, vomiting, headaches, skin problems, chest pains,
sexual dysfunction, or drug, alcohol, or food abuse. It can usually be eased
with simple relaxation exercises and deep breathing, or by vigorous exercise.

WHAT CAUSES STRESS?

Living. It's the wear and tear on us caused by life. It may be at work,
school, play, or at home. There are various kinds of stress: emotional
(caused by a family argument, the death of a loved one); environmental

(caused by heat or cold); and physiological (caused by an outpouring from the adrenal glands, which control heartbeat, breathing, and muscle tension and are extremely sensitive indicators of stress). There may also be perceived stress. How we see an event may make it more stressful than it inherently is. Children, as we shall see, appear to be particularly vulnerable to this kind of stress.

Some stress is good for our lives. It can help us concentrate, perform, focus, and reach a peak level of efficiency. Many people, in fact, do their best work under the pressure of stress. Changes in our lives, whether good or bad, cause stress. And stress itself, whether good or bad, may impair the way we work, live, and feel.

What actually happens to us under stress? Imagine that you are facing a deadline. The boss or teacher comes in and tells you that what you've done so far is awful and that you'd better get the job finished, in good shape and on time. Your body reacts to this stress and prepares for action. The stress excites your hypothalamus (a brain region near the base of your skull), which produces a substance that stimulates the pituitary gland to discharge the hormone ACTH (adrenocorticotrophic hormone) into your blood. Signals begin rushing to all parts of your body. Adrenaline pours into your bloodstream. The adrenaline increases your heart rate. Your heart demands more oxygen and there is an increase in your respiration. Now your heart is pounding, your blood pressure is up, and your palms, armpits, stomach, or back may be sweating. You are ready to act. But too often in our society, instead of taking action or fleeing—the fight-or-flight reaction of our ancestors—we merely sit and seethe.

The repeated suppression of this natural sequence strains our bodies. Fewer than 5 percent of American workers have jobs that keep them active, and in the electronic and computer age, that figure is dropping. Our lives and our children's lives create stress. In truth, sometimes we create stress for our kids and they for us.

The impact of stress on us is measurable. Stress changes us physically and can cause a variety of medical illnesses, some imagined and some very real, painful, even lethal. Each period of stress, especially from frustrating, unsuccessful struggles, leaves some irreversible chemical scars, says Dr. Hans Selye, author of *Stress Without Distress*. When we become overburdened beyond our stress tolerance, we may become ill, develop emotional illnesses, or suffer physical breakdown. The list of disorders caused by negative stress is long: high blood pressure, mental depression, insomnia, impotence, viral infections, asthma attacks, ulcers, migraines, rashes, overeating, various heart diseases, and arrhythmias. "The relationship of stress and behavior to cardiovascular conditions is well documented," says Dr. David Jenkins, professor of preventive medicine and community health at the University of Texas in Galveston. "What is not widely known is that, through its ability to depress the body's immune system, stress probably also influences the development of cancer."

WHAT'S STRESSFUL?

How we handle stress can literally determine how well we are. One of the earliest studies on the effects of stress was done by Lawrence E. Hinkle, a reseacher in the 1950s, who determined that people do not become ill equally or randomly. His research of telephone company employees showed that 25 percent of the people had half of all the illnesses; another 25 percent had less than ten percent of all the illnesses. This was true regardless of how severe the illness. Hinkle also found that the illnesses occurred in "cluster years"—that is, one-third of the illnesses occurred in one-eighth of the time studied. Hinkle concluded that the way we react to the events in our lives plays a significant role in at least one-third of all our illnesses and their severity.

The employees Hinkle studied became ill when they saw their life situations as negative, unsatisfying, threatening, overdemanding, or unchangeable. Other researchers tell us that high levels of stress wear down the body by direct damage to tissues. Stress also suppresses the body's immune system. This makes you more susceptible to all kinds of infections, abnormalities (such as cardiac arrthymia), and even, as mentioned, cancer.

Dr. Roger Meyer, a noted pediatrician, studied a group of healthy children and recorded the incidence of strep throat over several years. His throat cultures discovered that 30 percent of all the well children had streptococcus bacteria present in their throats at any one time, but showed no symptoms of the disease. Dr. Meyer concluded that "peaceful coexistence [between the child and the bacteria] is the rule, disease is the exception." What, then, triggers disease?

Dr. Meyer found that 25 percent of the strep throat he and his researchers saw followed a family crisis. An ill child was four times as likely to have experienced a recent stressful episode as a well child. Stress, therefore, increased the probability of a child's getting a strep throat.

In *The Well Child Book*, Mike and Nancy Samuels report on Dr. Klaus J. Roghmann's study of stress as a cause of *all* illnesses in children. Dr. Roghmann found that a stressful episode doubled the probability of illness in both mothers and children. "The day *after* a stressful episode," the Samuels write, "the probability of a mother or child becoming ill was even higher—three times more likely than normal." The stressful episode was usually a family fight or job or school tensions.

STRESS AND ADULTS

Drs. Thomas H. Holmes and Richard H. Rahe, psychiatrists at the University of Washington Medical School, attempted to rank stressful events and their impacts on us. They interviewed 394 men and women and asked them to assign a relative number value—using marriage as the equivalent to fifty on their scale—to all kinds of life events. From this they devised a "social adjustment scale" of stressful events, which has proved to be a highly accurate tool in the statistical prediction of illness.

The Holmes-Rahe scale places death of a spouse as the most stressful event we experience. Corroborating this, the doctors discovered that widows and widowers are ten times more likely to die within the first year after the death of their husbands or wives than all other people in their age group. The Holmes-Rahe scale lists divorce as the next most stressful event. Here, too, they found that divorced men and women, in the year following their divorce, had an illness rate twelve times higher than married people.

These stressful events work on our adult bodies in obvious ways. In a well-known study about heart disease and behavior patterns, Drs. Meyer Friedman and Ray H. Rosenman of Mount Sinai Hospital in San Francisco examined some 3,500 men during a four-year span. They broadly divided the behavior patterns they found into two types: A and B. The Type A man, they reported, was aggressive, ambitious, and success oriented; he competed against everyone and himself. The Type B man was calmer, working at his own pace and under little self-imposed stress.

Not surprisingly, Drs. Friedman and Rosenman found that Type A men had two and a half times more heart attacks than Type B men. They also reported that emotional stress and tension played a relevant role in coronary heart disease. The Friedman-Rosenman study has been challenged several times since it was conducted in the early 1980s. But I still see a lot of Type A men—and now women—in my exercise classes.

Type A adult exercisers are easy to spot. They exericse with tight face muscles, tight and high shoulders, and a short, choppy running style. The Type A exerciser I see is a successful woman or man who works hard and believes that she or he has to exercise hard. They exercise, in part, as an escape from self-imposed pressures. They may be too busy to warm up, stretch, and then begin exercising slowly. They think cooling down is for other exercisers.

The Holmes/Rahe Social Readjustment Rating Scale

Life Event	Mean Value
Death of spouse	100
Divorce	73
Marital separation	65
Jail term	63
Death of close family member	63
Personal injury or illness	53
Marriage	50
Fired at work	47
Marital reconciliation	45
Retirement	45
Change in health of family member	44
Pregnancy	40
Sex difficulties	39
Gain of new family member	39
Business readjustment	39
Change in financial state	38
Death of close friend	37
Change to different line of work	36
Change of number of arguments with spouse	35
Mortgage over $10,000	31
Foreclosure of mortgage or loan	30
Change in responsibilities at work	29
Son or daughter leaving home	29
Trouble with in-laws	29
Outstanding personal achievement	28
Wife begins or stops work	26
Begin or end school	26
Change in living conditions	25
Revision of personal habits	24
Trouble with boss	23
Change in work hours or conditions	20
Change in residence	20
Change in schools	20
Change in recreation	19
Change in church activities	19
Change in social activities	18
Mortgage or loans less than $10,000	17
Change in sleeping habits	16
Change in number of family get-togethers	15
Change in eating habits	15
Vacation	13
Christmas	12
Minor violations of the law	11

STRESS AND CHILDREN

Not surprisingly, the Type A exerciser tends to create a Type A child. Researchers at Stanford University made a three-year study of seven hundred children in grades five, seven and nine. They found Type A kids—intense, competitive, impatient, angry—just like Type A adults. And like adults, Type A kids in this survey had more sleep disturbances than Type B kids. They also suffered more headaches, sore throats, colds, flus, and allergies than other children. Robert E. Kowalski, author of *Cholesterol and Children*, writes:

> Interestingly, often the high Type A youngsters—and their parents—would ignore the symptoms, perhaps because they occurred so frequently. In any case, the Type A's wouldn't miss school because of those symptoms; they would just go on. And, I suppose, they would grow up to "tough it out" by going to the office and perpetuating the problem.

Children under stress who are developing into Type A kids and adults show one characteristic behavior pattern: they are unhappy. They cannot enjoy accomplishments; they seldom please their parents; and they lose the ability to please themselves. Dr. Karen Matthews of the University of Pittsburgh has developed a questionnaire for teachers of children. You might ask yourself these questions about your own kids:

- Does your child like to argue and debate?
- Does your child work quickly and energetically rather than slowly and deliberately?
- Does your child become impatient waiting for others?
- Does your child generally do things in a hurry?
- When your child plays, is the play competitive?
- Does it take much to make your child angry?
- Does your child interrupt others more than usual for his or her age group?
- Is your child a leader in various activities?
- Does your child become easily irritated?
- Does your child perform better when competing against others?
- Is your child patient when playing with other children who are slower?
- Does your child get into fights?
- Does your child place a great deal of emphasis on winning rather than having fun at games or school?
- Whether working or playing, does your child try to do better than other children?
- Can your child sit still for extended periods?

Kowalski added other relevant questions to Dr. Matthews's list. Does your child flaunt victory over others? Does your child pause to reflect on achievements or immediately go off to another task or challenge? Does your child ever gain a sense of serenity and contentment over a task well done?

Competitive drive and impatience are also seen in adolescents. Here, too, anger, impatience, a sense of frustration, and competitiveness are characteristic traits. Kowalski suggests that they identify not only Type A kids and teenagers, but "those destined to develop a major risk factor for heart disease."

Some parents are pushing their kids too hard to succeed; they want to add "parent of superkid" to their résumés. These parents are reinforced by some school systems; they both want kindergartens with homework, foreign languages, and grades. They want "superpupils." As a result, our kids are paying a price.

These pushed kids are showing signs of early stress. Stanford researcher Carl Thoresen sees increasing evidence of Type A behavior—even in preschoolers. "These kids are over-scheduled," he says. "They are hurried, harried, competitive, quick to anger." They are showing early symptoms of stress, such as high blood pressure.

What sets off stress in children? Two researchers, building on the work of Holmes and Rahe, have devised special stress scales for children of different ages. Like Holmes-Rahe, these scales are proving to be accurate tools to understanding what events trigger stress reactions in our children. Children deal, however, with a different set of life events: rather than losing a spouse or divorce, for example, the children's scale ranks such things as beginning nursery school and discovery of being an adopted child.

The reseachers, R. Dean Coddington and J. Stephen Heisel, studied children in hospitals and outpatient clinics suffering from a wide range of illnesses. According to *The Well Child Book*, "They found that children who were sick were three times as likely to have experienced more frequent or serious life events in the year prior to the onset of their illnesses." Other reseachers have also found that children experiencing high stress had three times as many accidents as children in low-stress lives.

For a child, beginning any new stage of life—nursery school, first grade, high school, or a new school—creates the greatest stress. That is a time of great change and uncertainty, when parents should give their children strong support. It is also a time when parents may see some of the symptoms of stress mentioned above.

Many parents put pressure on their kids, from toddlers to adolescents. The results may be emotional illness—stomachaches, headaches, eating disorders, drugs or alcohol use, depression, or even suicide. "The degree

Stress Rating Scale for Children

LIFE EVENTS	PRE-SCHOOL AGE	ELEMENTARY AGE	JUNIOR HIGH AGE
Beginning nursery school, first grade, or high school	42	46	45
Change to a different school	33	46	52
Birth or adoption of a brother or sister	50	50	50
Brother or sister leaving home	39	36	33
Hospitalization of brother or sister	37	41	44
Death of brother or sister	59	68	71
Change of father's occupation requiring increased absence from home	36	45	42
Loss of job by a parent	23	38	48
Marital separation of parents	74	78	77
Divorce of parents	78	84	84
Hospitalization of parent (serious illness)	51	55	54
Death of a parent	89	91	94
Death of a grandparent	30	38	35
Marriage of parent to stepparent	62	65	63
Jail sentence of parent for 30 days or less	34	44	50
Jail sentence of parent for 1 year or more	67	67	76
Addition of third adult to family (e.g., grandparent)	39	41	34
Change in parents' financial status	21	29	40
Mother beginning to work	47	44	36
Decrease in number of arguments between parents	21	25	29
Increase in number of arguments between parents	44	51	48
Decrease in number of arguments with parents	22	27	29
Increase in number of arguments with parents	39	47	46
Discovery of being an adopted child	33	52	70
Acquiring a visible deformity	52	69	83
Having a visible congenital deformity	39	60	70
Hospitalization of yourself (child)	59	62	59
Change in acceptance of peers	38	51	68
Outstanding personal achievement	23	39	45
Death of a close friend (child's friend)	38	53	65
Failure of a grade in school		57	62
Suspension from school		46	54

LIFE EVENTS	PRE-SCHOOL AGE	ELEMENTARY AGE	JUNIOR HIGH AGE
Pregnancy in unwed teenage sister		36	60
Becoming involved with drugs or alcohol		61	70
Becoming a full-fledged member of a church/synagogue		25	28
Not making an extracurricular activity you wanted to be involved in (i.e., athletic team, band)			49
Breaking up with a boyfriend or girlfriend			47
Beginning to date			55
Fathering an unwed pregnancy			76
Unwed pregnancy			95

Used by permission from *Journal of Pediatrics* 83 (1973): 119.

to which parents are out of their children's lives is the degree to which children are vulnerable, " says Lee Salk, child psychologist. "The family must help children develop skills to meet life's problems and pressures."

Recognizing stress in older children can be harder than in younger ones. Eating disorders, withdrawal from school activities, or preoccupation with a video or computer game can go unnoticed.

Another study shows a different interesting pattern. Kaoru Yamamoto, a psychologist at the University of Colorado, has done extensive research on children's own perceptions of stress. There is an important difference here: usually, researchers report what *they* perceive to be stress-causing events in a child's life. Dr. Yamamoto is studying what children tell him is stressful to them.

And what do our kids rate as most stressful? The fear of being humiliated. Second, children say they fear incidents that would make them look "bad." Other troubling events, in a child's perception, are being kept back a grade, wetting his or her pants in class, and seeing their parents fight.

What do you notice about all of these stress-inducing fears? First, they are all in some way humiliating to the child. (If the child's parents fight in public, that's humiliating too.) Second, they underscore the prominence of school life and peer opinions in the child's world. School and peer life— together with family—play a significant role in shaping the child's perceptions of accomplishment and personal worth. All of these stresses are injuries to the child's sense of self-esteem.

This research is vital to us as parents. Events that we see as not being so bad—getting low grades, witnessing parents fight, wetting pants—are seen by our children as stressful and humiliating. This extends to sports.

Coaches who bench kids for making mistakes, chew them out in front of teammates or crowds, or embarrass kids in other ways are humiliating them. And, says Ann Epstein, a child psychiatrist at Harvard Medical School: "One of the most common triggers of suicide in children and teens is a humiliating experience."

Stress and humiliation may be important in understanding one of the saddest statistics we have discovered in researching this book: suicide among our children is rising sharply. Successful suicides by teenagers have tripled during the last thirty years. The adolescent suicide rate for boys increased almost 50 percent between 1970 and 1980. Suicide is now the second leading cause of death (automobile accidents is first) for children ages fifteen to twenty-four. I've even heard first-graders talk about killing themselves because they are unhappy.

According to the 1988 National Adolescent Student Health Survey, one out of every two girls and one out of every four boys say they have seriously thought about killing themselves. About 18 percent of our teenage girls and 11 percent of our teenage boys say they have tried to commit suicide.

As much as our kids are in physical fitness trouble, so they are also in emotional difficulty. Some 34 percent of our girls and 15 percent of our boys say they often feel sad and hopeless. About 18 percent of our girls and 9 percent of our boys claim they have nothing to look forward to.

DEALING WITH STRESS

Dr. Meyer Friedman, the researcher who did the initial Type A/Type B studies, has a challenging idea. Kids, adolescents, and heart attack patients who exhibited Type A behavior "lacked a 100-percent commitment of love from parents."

Dr. Friedman argues that Type A people—kids and adults—are striving to gain love from parents who have made that love conditional on performance. Kowalski, in discussing Friedman, writes:

> Thus a hug from a parent and a fervent statement of love for "no good reason" is more nurturing than a hug given for achievement of some task. Not that we shouldn't praise our children's accomplishments. Rather, let's all try to love our kids completely, even when they're not doing something brilliant.

> Dr. Friedman believes this is dramatically true for girls. When they don't receive that unconditional love from their fathers, they become overly competitive and driven to achieve goals which they believe, unconsciously, will please those parents and thus "earn" their love.

This alone may explain the unanswered question in the statistics on suicide. Twice as many girls as boys say they feel sad and hopeless most of the time and that they have nothing to look forward to. Twice as many girls as boys think of suicide and twice as many actually attempt to kill themselves. It's probably unfair to blame all this on fathers and hugs. But unconditional love of a parent for a child is clearly a factor in that child's self-esteem and happiness. And, as research mentioned above shows, self-esteem and happiness are central to our children's well-being.

How can we deal with stress in our lives?

Become a good role model. As in the case of exercise, how we behave teaches our kids how to behave. Do you teach your kids Type A behavior by yelling and swearing at small disturbances? How do you deal with major changes—positive or negative—in your life? What do you do when you are really overloaded by stress and faced with situations beyond your control? You might also ask yourself the following:

What do I do for fun and to relax?

Do I ever allow myself time to "play" as an adult?

Do I ever take quiet time for myself during the week?

Do my kids see me only when I'm working or upset?

Change and control the way you live. There are several things you can do here. First, eliminate the minor irritations in your life that cause chronic, negative stress. For example, join a car pool to avoid rush-hour traffic that makes you tense and angry.

Second, learn to meditate or simply sit calmly and let your mind float in any direction it wants.

Next, understand what makes you happy and gives you pleasure, and do these things. Allow yourself time to "smell the flowers."

Take a break when you know you are getting stressed.

Distance yourself from your problems. Take them one step at a time.

Nutrition. Eating properly is an important part of stress management. Junk foods and refined sugars are low in nutritional value and high in calories. Colas and other soft drinks have high levels of caffeine. Kids who eat chips and soda for meals are cheating themselves nutritionally, which puts stress on the body. Adults who have coffee and doughnuts are doing the same thing.

Plan your meals around the four basic food groups: proteins, dairy products, grains, and fresh fruits and vegetables. Limit your use of salt, caffeine, and alcohol to help promote good health and reduce stress. I'll say more on this in the next chapter.

Exercise. Physically fit people handle stress better than those who are unfit. Perhaps this is simply because fit people feel better about themselves. But there is also something to be said for getting out and running, swimming, biking, cross-country skiing, or walking when you feel tense and stressed. Why not be active and get fit? Whatever exercise you choose, the best one is the one you stick with on a regular basis.

As this book emphasizes, the best regular exercise program includes some form of aerobic activity. This helps your body use oxygen more effectively, strengthens your heart and lungs, and, along with the stretching before and after, helps relieve muscle tension and diminish stress. Engage in regular exercise in a gentle manner. This confers physical and psychological/emotional benefits.

What can we offer our kids?

Spend time with them. One of the themes of this book has been family togetherness. Take your kids out to play and exercise, and attend games and the theater. Do things together. If you don't, one day soon you'll look up and they will be on their own, far away from you physically and emotionally.

Make some quiet time for your family. Take time to read to your child. Show, by your example, the strength of quiet reading in your home. Kids who read are less likely to grow into frenzied adults constantly in search of a stimulus. If you have a hobby, share it. Build models with your kids.

Just reading to your kids can be wonderful. Whenever Christopher feels especially stressed, I pull out one of his favorite books: *Albert the Running Bear Gets the Jitters,* by Barbara Isenberg and Diane de Groat. In it, Albert gets very nervous about an upcoming race which is causing him stress and anxiety. Norman the zoo keeper writes out a program to help Albert relax. Here it is:

R—Recognize that you're upset. Talk things over with someone you trust (a parent, teacher, or friend). After Christopher talks about his fears and stresses, he feels much better. We often talk over problems while going for a walk.

E—Ease your mind. Tell yourself that you can calm down.

L—Loosen up. Take ten slow, deep breaths. As discussed in Chapter 11, belly breathe to promote relaxation.

A—Allow your imagination to help. Close your eyes and picture a place where you feel relaxed and happy. Albert likes to imagine his cozy bed with his special pillow and his teddy bear. Christopher feels better when he imagines lying in bed with his mom on one side and his dad on the other giving him "kisses on both sides." Sounds good to me!!

X—Marks the end, says Norman the zoo keeper. Open your eyes when you feel calm.

This simple relaxation device works for Albert every time! It may help your child deal with stress too.

Consider the role of spirituality in your family. Take the time, even if you do not consider yourself a religious person, to talk with your children about values, honesty, trust, and respect for others. These are long-term, basic truths; learning and discussing them help you and your children place short-term, everyday frustrations and stress in perspective.

Where should you begin? Outside of any formal religion, I suggest the Golden Rule. How do you and your children feel about "doing unto others what you would have them do unto you"? Type A people sometimes joke about "doing unto others before they have a chance to do unto you." There is fear and anger in this thought and you might want to discuss it with your children.

Next, you might want to talk about secular concepts such as those embodied in aphorisms or proverbs: "A penny saved is a penny earned"; "One for all, and all for one"; "Help the other fellow"; "Waste not, want not"; and so forth. Discussing Benjamin Franklin, Ralph Waldo Emerson, Abraham Lincoln, the Psalms, the Beatitudes—whatever you choose—is a good way to get you and your family thinking about more profound ideas than usual.

Listen to your kids. Find out what's happening in your children's lives and how you might help or be part of those lives. For a parent who wants to understand the troubled child, make a special effort to let the child be heard—have his or her say—without being judged. Simply listen and ask neutral questions: Did that bother you? How do you feel about that? Do not tell your child, "Do this," or "You did the right thing," and so forth. That's judgmental.

"Parents are too quick to impose what they think is going on in the child's mind, and make a snap decision about what's best for them," says Dr. Robert Coles, an eminent child psychiatrist at Harvard University. "You've only got to pause to hear what the child is really seeing and feeling."

Remember the study about humiliation mentioned above. What we adults see as causing stress in our children is not what they find stressful at all. Listen to them and listen hard for what they find troubling, not what you think may be troubling them. Hug and kiss your kids every time you can. And hug and kiss 'em in public, in private, in front of their friends and yours. When the urge hits, hug 'em!

Exercise and relaxation. When you're in shape—and even when you're just working on it—encourage your kids to get into an exercise program. Southern Methodist University researcher Jonathon Brown studied the role of exercise in counteracting stress in adolescents. He found that stress declined as physical exercise increased. "Exercise is good for people under both low and high levels of stress," he reported in the *Journal of Human Stress.* "It is not just aerobic fitness that enables one to handle stress;

adherence to a regimen provides a beneficial time out from the world." Perhaps most important, Brown found that "stress had a substantial debilitating effect on physical and emotional health among those who exercise infrequently, but not among those who exercised regularly."

When Brown and Judith Siegel, a behavioral scientist at the School of Public Health at the University of California, Los Angeles, did a follow-up study on teenage girls, the outcome was similar. Stress had a significant debilitating effect on the health of those teenage girls who exercised little. But stress had only a slight effect on the health of girls who exercised a lot. Brown concluded that exercise appears to be especially beneficial during periods of high stress. "Our data further suggest," he wrote, "that during periods of continued high stress those who exercise very little are much more likely to become ill. Exercise appears to be capable of protecting against the development of illness for as long as eight months."

Helping your kids get started on an exercise program is half the struggle. You should also help them to relax. Try *Albert the Running Bear Gets the Jitters*, for young kids. To help older children and teenagers cope with stress, Barbara Kuczen, author of *Childhood Stress: How to Raise a Healthier, Happier Child*, suggests teaching them deep breathing and muscle relaxing exercises. Laughter and positive thinking also help our kids to relax, she adds.

The notion of deep breathing as a form of relaxation is ancient. It has been practiced for hundreds of years by the Hindus through their yoga and breathing exercises. It is also the basis for all meditation programs. Shepherd has tried several different meditation programs, both before and during running, and still likes Dr. Herbert Benson's *The Relaxation Response*. Sometimes called the poor man's Transcendental Meditation or, more often, "a terrific aspirin," this popular meditative technique employs the traditional components of meditation coupled with some reassuring medical findings about reduced blood pressure and stress syndrome. You can do this alone, and then help your kids learn how to do it.

There are four traditional components to meditation:

1. Find a quiet environment that will help you concentrate.
2. Employ a mental device to help shift your mind from the external stress-filled world to an inner, peaceful world. Such a stimulus may be a word, sound, or phrase that's thought or spoken repeatedly.
3. Assume a passive attitude. This includes not worrying about your mind wandering or about how well you are performing.
4. Be comfortable. Some people sit in a cross-legged "lotus" position. Shift around. Dr. Benson warns, however, that "if you are lying down, there is a tendency to fall asleep."

Relaxation is simply quiet stillness, with a word or sound repeated. You are awake and in control. Start with meditation, stretching, and warm-up and then do your aerobic exercising; repeat your word or sound through the entire exercise process.

Dr. Benson and runners at Harvard's Thorndike Medical Laboratory developed a variation on the four meditative components.

- Sit quietly in a comfortable position, close your eyes, and deeply relax all your muscles.
- Breathe through your nose. You might try breathing in through one nostril and out through the other (block the first by pressing a finger against it). Continue gentle, rhythmic breathing for several minutes. Then, as you breathe out, say the word "one." Continue for fifteen to twenty minutes. You may open your eyes to check the time, but don't use an alarm. When you finish, sit quietly for a few minutes, first with your eyes closed, and then with your eyes open.
- Maintain a passive attitude. Permit relaxation to occur at its own pace. Try to dismiss all distracting thoughts. Continue repeating the word "one" (or any other soothing word). Do not worry about whether or not you achieve a deep level of relaxation.

With a bit of practice, you may come to enjoy these quiet, relaxing, meditative times. Your sessions should be regular, and then you may want to practice the relaxation response when you get tense or come under stress.

As you learn this method, teach it to your children. It can help them during stressful times at school and college. Kowalski suggests that you let your children become the "leaders" who "guide the family group through the breathing and guided imagery"—that is, imagining walking through a woods, watching a snowfall, sitting in front of a fire with the embers glowing. "You'll be surprised at how well even the smallest child can do the job," he writes. Moreover, you will be helping your kids deal with stress and enhance their overall wellness.

Nutrition

What we eat can make us sick as well as strong. The combination of eating too much and exercising too little can, in fact, kill us. Five of the ten leading causes of death in this country—heart disease, cancer, stroke, diabetes, and atherosclerosis—are conditions caused by poor diet. What you eat may also contribute to obesity, high blood pressure, osteoporosis, and dental disease. The *Journal of the American College of Nutrition* reports that one out of every three Americans will develop a cardiovascular complication before reaching age sixty—mostly caused by poor diet.

In a 1988 report Dr. C. Everett Koop, the U.S. Surgeon General, said: "If you are among the two out of three Americans who do not smoke or drink excessively, your choice of diet can influence your long-term health prospects more than any other action you might take."

To maintain a healthy, nutritious diet means understanding what to eat and the basic value of the four food groups: proteins, dairy products, grains/cereals, and fresh fruit and vegetables. All foods we eat contain some of these nutrients. They provide our bodies with heat and energy, and the materials for growth and the repair of body tissues. We need all the nutrients, but the amounts we need vary according to our age, sex, body size, environment, exercise level, and nutritional condition.

As the result of a four-year study, Dr. Koop reported in 1988 on the status of nutrition in the United States. He found that the top nutritional problem was eating too much fat at the expense of carbohydrates and fiber (nuts, grains). He called for reducing fats, cholesterol, sugar, salt, and alcohol in our diets while increasing the proportion of fiber and complex carbohydrates. These are whole grains, fruits, and vegetables. Some of the highlights of the Surgeon General's report include:

Fat. We should reduce the saturated fats in our diet. These are the red meats (beef and pork, for example) or vegetable fats that stay solid at room temperature, such as butter and palm oil. Instead, we should substitute vegetables, beans and peas, fish, poultry with the skin removed, lean meats, and low-fat dairy products.

Deep-fried chicken and fish are not low on fat. Hamburgers, hot dogs, French fries, high-fat ice creams, and other common foods account for the fact that dietary fat makes up at least 37 percent of the caloric intake of most Americans. The level recommended by the National Cancer Institute is less than 30 percent.

Salt. Our daily average intake of sodium (salt) is four to six grams, well above the National Research Council's recommended range of 1.1 to 3.3 grams.

All of us should reduce our salt intake. We should take the salt shaker off the dining-room table and decrease the use of salt in the preparation of food. We should stop eating junk foods like high-salt potato chips, salted popcorn, snack chips, and pretzels. We get enough salt in a balanced diet to meet our body's needs. Excessive salt increases our blood pressure and is a factor in some heart and kidney diseases.

Fiber/complex carbohydrates. These are the good guys. We should eat more of them: whole grain foods, bran cereals, beans and peas, vegetables, and fruits (especially the outer skin, which contains the most fiber). Researchers have found a link between diet and cancer, especially cancer of the colon, and recommend that we cut down sharply on red meat and increase sharply the amount of fiber we eat.

Alcohol. The Surgeon General's report suggests that we reduce alcohol consumption to two mixed drinks a day or less. Pregnant woman are advised to avoid alcohol altogether. Wine and beer should be consumed only in moderation.

Iron/calcium. Women of child-bearing age, children, and adolescent girls should eat more iron-rich foods such as fish, cereals, beans, and lean meat. This will help balance their diets and prevent anemia. They should also consume low-fat dairy products and vegetables. This will help build strong bones in growing children and prevent osteoporosis in women.

Vitamins. Some 40 percent of Americans spend about $1.5 *billion* a year on vitamins. That gives us the most expensive urine in the world, for few of us need additional vitamins added to our already elaborate and balanced diets. But if you eat a balanced diet you do not need vitamins.

The U.S. Department of Health set some goals for us in 1980, to be achieved by 1990. Here are three of the most important ones:

Weight. The report recommended that Americans lose weight. About one out of every four Americans needs to lose 20 percent of his or her weight, compared to the 1990 goal of 10 percent for men and 17 percent for women.

The report also recommended that half the overweight Americans get on a weight-loss program of diet and exercise. But surveys indicate that while half the nation's overweight adults are trying to lose weight, only 25 percent of them are using diet and exercise in combination. Thus, only 25 percent of the nation's overweight people have a good chance of losing weight and keeping it off.

Diet. The goal here is to drop the average American adult's serum cholesterol below 200. The national averages are 211 for women and 215 for men. The report called for all packaged food to list "useful calorie and nutrient information" and nutritional counseling in "all routine health contacts" between patients and health professionals. In 1985, nutritional counseling was done in only 30 percent of the contacts with patients, and in 1988 only 55 percent of packaged food was properly labeled.

Youth. The Department of Health wanted the American people to assure that no U.S. child's growth would be retarded. In 1986, some 20 million U.S. kids went to bed hungry. A second goal of this category was to establish nutritional education as a requirement in all school curricula in every state. In 1985, only twelve states had such a requirement.

THE FOUR BASIC FOOD GROUPS

I believe the old maxim "We are what we eat." The foods we select and consume become part of us, and add to our growth or hurt us. No single food or food group supplies all the nutrients we need. By eating wisely and well we will get a variety of the foods that are good for us. Each day, we should choose from each of these four basic food groups:

Grains/cereals. This category includes cereal, whole grain breads, muffins, rice, oats, corn meal, and pasta. Recommended amounts: four to six or more servings daily.

Dairy group. Milk, cheese, and yogurt. Especially healthful are low- or non-fat products such as skim milk, cottage cheese, or low-fat yogurt. Recommended amounts: two servings daily for adults, two to three for children, and three to four for adolescents.

High-protein foods. Meat, fish, eggs, poultry, legumes, and nuts. Recommended amounts: two servings a day, except eggs and red meat, which should be eaten a few times per week. Excellent meat substitutes are legumes and nuts.

Vegetables/fruits. Citrus fruits, fleshy fruits (apples, pears); green, yellow, and root vegetables. Recommended amounts: four servings daily, including citrus fruit or juice, a green or yellow vegetable, and some fresh, raw vegetables.

The National Cancer Institute reports that 40 percent of all Americans do not eat a single fruit on a typical day.

NUTRIENTS

There are six classes of nutrients: water, carbohydrates, fats, protein, minerals, vitamins.

Water. We could go for weeks without much food, but we would die quickly without water. Our bodies, which are mostly water, need replenishment every day. There is little danger in drinking too much water; any excess is flushed away as urine by the kidneys or released as sweat. Water is the main component of our cells, urine, sweat, and blood. When you get dehydrated, your cells become dehydrated and cannot function properly; you don't produce urine, and toxic waste products build up in your bloodstream. You need to replace those lost fluids quickly.

Cold water is your best bet. Your body requires about six glasses of water every day. Some comes from the food you eat. But most comes from what you drink. When you exercise, you need more fluid; you should drink at least two or three quarts of fluids, half of it water. You should drink water before, during, and after your aerobic exercise, especially on hot days. But don't forget to drink water before and after exercise in cold weather, too.

Some commercial drinks replace fluids, lost minerals, and other elements. Water is absorbed the fastest and is my preferred drink. Besides, water can do double duty: you can also pour it over your head and body on hot days to help you cool off. Don't try that with those sticky commercial drinks!

Carbohydrates. The Surgeon General's report recommends increasing the amount of complex carbohydrates in our diet. These are the energy foods that aid in muscle exertion, and assist in digestion and the assimilation of other foods.

Simple carbohydrates include candies, soft drinks, and other sugar foods. We should eat fewer of those. But complex carbohydrates—grains, cereals, vegetables, fruits, and pasta—offer a nutritious energy source of vitamins, minerals, proteins, and water.

Fats. The good news here is that fats are the most concentrated source of energy in our diet. They provide the body with a variety of essential nutrients. Fats include butter, oils for salads and cooking, cream, egg yolk, avocados, and whole milk. Fats are also in meats, cheeses, and other dairy products. The bad news is that fats also contribute to many health problems, as mentioned, including heart disease and cancer.

Broadly, there are two types of fats: saturated and unsaturated. The saturated—with the exception of coconut oil—come mostly from meats.

The unsaturated (the good guys) include polyunsaturated fats and come from vegetables, nuts or seeds, and olives. Whenever possible, substitute saturated fats with unsaturated fats in your diet. Bake or broil foods instead of frying. Replace red meat with chicken and fish, whole milk with skim milk. Make sure your salad dressing is made with unsaturated fats.

Proteins. These body builders help bone and tissue grow and repair. They are major builders of muscle, blood, skin, hair, nails, and the internal organs, including the heart and brain. They aid in the formation of hormones that control growth, sexual development, and the rate of metabolism. They control the balance of acids and alkalines in the blood and they regulate the body's water balance.

Unused protein is converted in the liver and stored as fat in body tissue. Too little protein consumption will cause health problems, especially in growing children. Too much will cause fat storage.

Most protein contains a high level of fats. Many doctors and researchers now urge us to replace red meat as our primary protein source with fish or poultry. Red meat contains fat and takes too long to pass through our digestive system. Vegetable protein can be as nutritious and less of a hazard to our health. Some of the best protein sources are nuts, beans, whole grains, cereals, milk, and cheese.

Minerals. These basic chemicals are found in the soil and picked up by plants. We get out minerals by eating plants or animals that have eaten plants. Minerals, therefore, exist in most foods and in our bodies. Seventeen minerals are essential to human mental and physical well-being.

These minerals are usually supplied in sufficient quantities in a balanced diet. They include iron, calcium, phosphorus, sodium, potassium, and magnesium. The Surgeon General's report emphasized the need for adequate iron and calcium for children.

Vitamins. Natural vitamins are found in plants and animals as organic food substances. Because our bodies cannot synthesize vitamins (with a few exceptions), we must supply them with our diet or with supplements.

Vitamins help regulate our bodies, convert fat and carbohydrates into energy, and form bones and tissues. There are about twenty active vitamins in human nutrition; the important ones for active exercisers are A, the B-complex, C, D, and E. A good, balanced diet will supply you with all of these vitamins. You and your children, if you are uncertain about the vitamins in your diet, may wish to take a vitamin supplement in the form of a standard daily multi-vitamin.

JUNK FOODS

On the other side of the dietary table are foods like hot dogs, candy, potato chips and other salty snack foods, and soda. These "foods" contain little besides calories, salt, and fat. Eating junk food increases your intake of sugar and salt, and raises your cholesterol level.

To get out of the junk food habit, try switching to fresh fruits, vegetables, and unsalted nuts for snacks. Raisins (alone or with unsalted nuts), apples, oranges, carrots, and celery all taste delicious, especially after exercising. Drink tap or bottled water, or unsweetened fruit juice diluted with ice or water or both.

Sugar. No other food has been as over-emphasized in our diets as sugar. But sugar contains little food value. White, refined sugar lacks any nutrient value at all and, in fact, requires vitamins (especially vitamin B) for its digestion. Since you supply the B vitamins from your system, sugar actually steals vitamins from you for its digestion.

One myth states that sugar increases your energy. But studies show the sugar actually decreases energy over several hours because it requires those vitamins from your body for its digestion. Pure sugar passes quickly through your intestinal walls into your bloodstream. The result is an immediate rise in our blood-sugar level, which some exercisers think gives them quick energy. But that rise is as quickly followed by a dramatic fall in blood-sugar levels below your body's norm; to counteract this, you must ingest more sugar, and thus the cycle continues. Excessive sugar also causes cavities in our teeth, some forms of heart disease, stomach and bowel disorders, and some forms of cancer.

Salt. A little salt adds a lot of flavor to foods. But most foods do not need added salt, and most recipes call for far too much salt. You can cut your salt intake by halving the amount called for in recipes, eliminating all salty junk foods (chips, nuts) and taking the salt shaker off your dining-room table. Taste food before you salt. Most foods do not need any added salt.

CHOLESTEROL AND TRIGLYCERIDES

Your blood contains two fats that are essential to life, but can also be killers: cholesterol and triglycerides.

Cholesterol. There are two sources of cholesterol: our bodies manufacture it and we consume it in foods of animal origin. Cholesterol is a natural part of your body; it is synthesized in the liver and almost every tissue and organ. It is an indispensable component of cellular structure. But there is a sharp difference between the cholesterol your body produces and that ingested from foods.

High cholesterol is often the result of diets high in fat, particularly saturated fats found in red meat and high-fat dairy products. Your inherited genetic character may also contribute to a high cholesterol count. Elevated cholesterol counts have been shown to increase your risk of heart disease and other related illnesses. High cholesterol in the blood increases the risk of deposits on the artery walls and the clogging of arteries. If arteries to the heart are blocked, a heart attack usually results. If an artery to the brain is blocked, a stroke may result.

Ideal cholesterol levels are about 170 milligrams per 100 milliliters of blood serum. We Americans average closer to 215 milligrams, down from 240 two decades ago.

Research suggests that the amount of serum cholesterol in your blood is not as important as the ratio of high-density lipoproteins (HDL, or "good" cholesterol) to low-density lipoproteins (LDL, or "bad" cholesterol). LDLs are considered "bad" because they carry cholesterol into our tissues, where it may clog our arteries. The HDLs, on the other hand, clear away cholesterol from our artery walls and prevent it from being deposited there. Thus, HDL protects against heart attack and stroke. The ratio of HDLs to LDLs in your blood determines your risk of heart attack or stroke. If HDL levels are high (60 or above) and the ratio of LDL cholesterol to HDL cholesterol is 4.0 or less, your risk of heart attack or stroke is low, even if your cholesterol levels are moderatly high.

Studies show that HDL cholesterol levels are improved by aerobic exercise, keeping a lean body weight, and by not smoking. LDL cholesterol— the "bad" guys"—can be lowered by reducing your intake of saturated fats, cholesterol in other animal and dairy form, and refined sugar.

Triglycerides. These are fatty molecules that thicken the blood. Our bodies manufacture them and we consume them in food. Triglycerides are formed in the breakdown of carbohydrates and may be as dangerous to your health as cholesterol. Refined sugar and alcohol are two examples of food and drinks converted to triglycerides.

Triglyceride levels under 175 are considered ideal. Above 200 milligrams is high and increases your risk. The amount of triglycerides in your blood can be reduced through regular aerobic exercise, by maintaining a lean body weight, and by reducing your intake of alcohol, refined sugar, and saturated fat.

FIBER

Fiber may not be a true nutrient, but is has important nutrition and health functions. High-fiber diets have been shown to prevent cancer. According to the American Health Foundation, 75 percent of cancer of the colon and 50 percent of cancer of the breast can be prevented by reducing fats and increasing fiber in our diet.

Fiber is a natural "internal broom" that sweeps through our intestines and moves food along quickly and easily. It softens, adds bulk, and attracts water to our stools. It thus prevents constipation, hemorrhoids, and colon and rectal cancers.

The National Cancer Institute suggests that Americans increase their fiber intake by 25 to 35 grams a day. Good sources of fiber are fruits and vegetables. But an easy way to get fiber in your diet is to start the day with whole grain or bran cereals.

GOOD EATING HABITS

Dr. Kenneth Cooper, in his book *The Aerobics Program for Total Well-Being,* states that we each need an individual, sensible, well-balanced eating pattern. Dr. Cooper designed such a program, which he called P.E.P. (for Positive Eating Plan). Here are some highlights:

- Eat a balanced diet, with a variety of foods at each meal that includes 50 percent carbohydrates, 20 percent proteins, and 30 percent fat.
- Establish consistent eating patterns, including three meals a day.
- Decrease calorie intake and increase calorie expenditure.
- Eat fewer foods high in fat.
- Eat less sugar.
- Eat more low-calorie, high-volume, high-fiber foods.
- Eat smaller meat portions.
- Eat more lean meats, poultry, and fish.
- Prepare foods in a way that minimizes the use of fat.
- Limit your consumption of alcohol.
- Eat low-calorie snacks.
- Drink six to eight glasses of fluids, preferably water, daily.
- Eat slowly and in a relaxed manner; chew your food well.
- Choose "crunchy" foods over "soft" foods.
- Pre-plan your meals to avoid impulse eating.
- Limit your sodium intake.
- Eliminate external food "cues." By that, Dr. Cooper means store food

out of sight; serve only the amount you want to eat rather than be tempted by excess food.

- Establish a regular exercise pattern; get more physical activity into your daily life.
- Find ways to deal with stress effectively, without food or alcohol.
- Establish lifelong eating and exercise habits for permanent weight control.

KIDS AND NUTRITION

Healthy diet and good health are constant companions. They are part of our kids' lives from birth. But the reverse is also true: poor diet and poor health go together and can be the scourge of our children. As Jane Brody wrote in her *New York Times* column:

> Coronary heart disease is rarely thought of as a youthful affliction, but this disease, which kills more Americans than any other, has its roots in the dietary and other habits—sedentary living and smoking among them—adopted during childhood and adolescence. By age four, the average American child has already reached a serum cholesterol level that is as high as it should be in adulthood if coronary arteries are to remain unclogged by fatty deposits. About 30 percent of the nation's youngsters have cholesterol levels that most experts consider abnormally high, levels likely to grow increasingly worse when the children become adults.

The good news here is that we can do something about this. Most of our children's health problems, in fact, are diet related. We and they can cut back on cheeseburgers, French fries, ice cream, sodas, and luncheon meats. Dr. Charles J. Glueck, a pediatrician at the University of Cincinnati School of Medicine, told the *New York Times:* "Modest and easily achievable dietary modifications can produce an average reduction of nearly 30 milligrams in the youngsters' cholesterol levels." The U.S. Department of Health states: "Adequate nutrition during adolescence is essential for normal development and may help to avert many chronic diseases."

The irony is that most of us know all this. Parents, children, and adolescents understand the need for wise nutrition and exercise. For example, in a national survey 73 percent of the adolescents said they knew that eating food high in saturated fat was related to heart problems; 79 percent said that eating too much salt was related to high blood pressure; 94 percent knew that diet is the key to curbing cholesterol intake.

Nonetheless, four out of every ten adolescents said that they eat fried foods four or more times a week. On average, students reported in one survey that they ate three snacks a day, and more than half of those snacks were food high in fat and/or sugar. A 1988 Gallup poll reported that most teenagers don't know that eggs and ice cream contain high quantities of cholesterol.

What's going on here? "First, there's not enough basic nutritional education," said Dr. Peter Kwiterovich, a professor at Johns Hopkins University. "Second, the schools are setting a very bad example with the lunches." If this were to change, it would have an immediate impact on our children's diet and health. According to a *USA Weekend* survey of 34,000 readers ages seven to sixteen, half changed what they ate when they learned about better nutrition. All we need to do is teach them.

Not all dietary changes are beneficial. A growing number of children under age two are victims of misguided parental ideas about a healthy diet. They put their kids on a stringent low-fat diet to prevent obesity and heart disease. A 1987 Beech-Nut study of 243 mothers of three-month to sixteen-month-old babies showed that 44 percent worry that their child will grow up to be overweight. Thirty-seven percent think a chubby three-year-old will be a fat adult, though odds of this being true are only one in four. The study showed that well-meaning parents were starving babies by feeding them low-fat, low-calorie diets such as they eat themselves. But, as Dr. Michael Pugliese, a pediatric endocrinologist at North Shore Hospital in Manhasset, New York, points out, such restrictive diets for kids that age account for 25 percent of the cases of babies failing to thrive at his hospital. These diets are more appropriate for adults than babies or children. Once the kids are back on an expanded diet, they recover quickly.

"Infants should decide how much they eat," nutritionist Jo Ann Hattner of the American Dietetic Association told *USA Today.* "Look for cues such as pulling away or closing the mouth. Stress nutrition, but don't be neurotic."

Another controversial topic here is testing kids for cholesterol. The American Academy of Pediatrics recommends a cholesterol test for all children age two and older who have a family history of high cholesterol (200 mg/ ml), or premature heart attacks. For other children, Dr. Glueck recommends a cholesterol test between ages seven and twelve.

You can prevent high cholesterol in you and your children by gradually changing your diets, reducing stress, and increasing your aerobic exercise. You can start, as I've said, by eliminating or drastically reducing junk food, switching from whole milk to 1 percent or skim milk, and from butter to soft margarine. Do this gradually and carefully.

NUTRITIONAL TIPS FOR CHILDREN

During the first six months of life, breast milk is the best source of nutrition. Many pediatricians also prescribe supplemental liquid vitamins for breast-fed infants, since breast milk lacks sufficient vitamins C and D. If breast-feeding is not possible, commercial formulas given under a doctor's direction may be adequate. Around six months of age, a baby should be eating some solid foods.

Pre-schoolers need large amounts of calcium in their diets to help build strong bones and teeth. Dairy products are good sources of calcium, but, as I've suggested, you should stick to low-fat milk, yogurt, and cheese. Pre-school kids need one to three cups of milk, at minimum, a day. They should also get four to five servings from the protein group—meat, fish, or poultry—a day, or one egg or half a cup of dried beans or peas. Include two servings of fruit and servings of bread and cereals—a bowl of cereal and a slice or two of bread, minimally.

There appears to be some justification for giving pre-school children vitamin supplements. Surveys of pre-school children indicate that the nutrient missing most often in their diets is iron, followed by vitamins A and C. These can be met with vitamin supplements.

To get kids interested in their diet, include them in the meal planning, shopping, food preparation, and table setting. Help them understand your efforts to give them a balanced diet, and to avoid foods and snacks that are unhealthy for them. "Make a variety of interesting and attractive foods available to your children," says Barbara Levine, director of the Nutrition Information Center at New York Hospital/Memorial Sloan-Kettering Cancer Center. "Don't keep foods around the house that you don't want your kids to eat."

Elementary school children need special watching; at this age their peers and school begin to dictate what they eat. They are also more susceptible to advertising, and may want foods because some athlete or rock star claims to eat them. Habits picked up now will carry into adolescence, so it is a good time to work with your kids on their diets.

The same principle of providing foods from the four food groups applies to these children. The elementary school child needs three daily servings of milk or other dairy product; a cup of yogurt or a glass of milk is a serving. He or she also needs two to three ounces of proteins a day—either meat, fish, poultry or substitutes like beans or peas. Peanut butter is all right, but two spoonfuls add about seventeen grams of fat to the diet. Two servings of both vegetables and fruits should be eaten daily by a child in this group. Breads and cereals round out the diet.

Teenagers have similar nutritional needs—only more of them. Calcium should be emphasized now to aid rapid growth. Calcium sources may include sardines and salmon with the bones, leafy green vegetables, or corn tortillas. Girls may want to take a calcium supplement to help prevent future development of osteoporosis. An iron supplement may also be added as girls begin their menstrual cycles.

The rest of the teenage diet is largely the same as it was in pre-school—proteins, fruits, vegetables, breads, and cereals—only more of it. Remember: Keep food around the house that you want your kids to eat. Make it available—fruit in a basket, for example—and they will munch, snack, and nibble throughout the day. But they will also be getting a good, balanced diet because of your care for them.

You should also plan snacks as carefully as you and your children plan meals together. Fruit, vegetables, yogurt, or bran or oatmeal cookies are good choices. Candy, potato chips, and other high-salt, high-fat, high-calorie foods are best left unpurchased. I suggest just leaving the food out, or easily available in the refrigerator.

If there are athletes in your home, remember that a low-fat, high-carbohydrate diet helps build up energy stores and improve performance. Pre-game meals are not magic: just have your kids eat a well-balanced meal that easily agrees with a nervous stomach three hours before the game. This eliminates all fried foods, chips, and junk snacks. Extra water and other fluids are essential for exercising athletes.

I have already discussed school lunches. Most of them are carbon copies of fast-food meals: cheeseburgers, French fries, and cheese pizzas. Encourage your kids to carry their lunches at least twice a week. This eliminates standing in lunch lines, gives them more time to eat, and lets them (and you) control the diet.

FAMILIES AND MEALS

I'm a big believer in three square meals a day and having all family members sit down together for dinner every evening. In any case, eating regular meals and eating breakfast regularly are two of the seven good health practices linked to living longer—not to mention living better.

Eating three meals every day prevents a wide change in your blood sugar, which in turn affects your appetite, energy level, and ability to handle stress. That is why people sometimes feel "on edge" when they skip a meal or have a meal out of schedule. If you have to skip a meal, skip lunch; never skip breakfast.

Breakfast

In my work as the national director of the Post Raisin Bran Family Fitness Program, I'm often called on to discuss the merits not only of family excercise, but also of the nutritional value of the family breakfast. That's a natural for me, since I start off almost every day with a healthy breakfast with Christopher.

Breakfast is considered the most important meal, primarily because it provides the fuel needed to get our engines running for the rest of the day. We should provide that engine with premium fuel: complex carbohydrates, bran, vitamin C, calcium, iron, and potassium. The National Cancer Institute reports that 80 percent of Americans eat no high-fiber cereals or whole-grain breads at all, let alone at breakfast. Start your day with a high-fiber cereal topped by fruit.

Why bother? Studies show that people who eat breakfast tend to be more alert, productive, and efficient than people who skip this meal. They are also more likely to perform well at sports. There are four major dietary ingredients to athletic success, says Nancy Clark, a Boston nutritionist and author of *The Athlete's Kitchen: A Nutrition Guide and Cookbook*. These are iron, calcium, carbohydrates—and breakfast. A good, balanced breakfast would solve all four needs. Clark wrote in *Runner's World:*

> A substantial breakfast sets the stage for a productive, high-energy day. And when you eat healthfully (a wholesome breakfast rather than the 10 o'clock sweets binge), you feel not only better, but also better about yourself. . . . If you skip breakfast, your ability to concentrate is likely to be diminished later in the morning, and you will work or study less efficiently. You may feel irritable and short-tempered. You may fall short of energy for your afternoon run. And, worst of all, you may gain rather than lose weight.

Clark notes that research subjects who ate 2,000 calories a day at one meal all lost weight when that meal was breakfast. When that meal was dinner, four of the six subjects gained weight. Shepherd practices the old English adage: eat breakfast like a king, lunch like a prince, and dinner like a pauper. That is, have your largest meal in the morning, your smallest (in terms of calories) in the evening.

Clark suggests eating a solid breakfast and then dieting during the rest of the day. "If you overeat at breakfast, simply eat less at lunch and dinner," she writes. "The calories that get you into weight trouble tend to be the ones you wolf down when you're ravenously hungry because you've skipped breakfast and trained hard."

Clark rates cereal at the top of her good breakfast list. So do I. Many cereals are rich in carbohydrates, the best source of energy for your muscles, and loaded with fiber and iron, but low in calories, fat, and cholesterol. Cereal can in fact form the center of a convenient, balanced breakfast that starts you on your full and active day. But I also recommend that you read the cereal nutrition labels on the sides of the cereal boxes. You will be surprised to find that many cereals are high in salt.

Breakfast should provide 25 percent of your daily calories, proteins, and essential vitamins and minerals. A cereal breakfast does that. I recommend: a bowl of bran cereal topped with sliced bananas, half a cup of low-fat milk, a glass of orange juice for vitamin C, an eight-ounce glass of low-fat milk, and a slice of bread or toast topped with margarine or jam. This should give you the fuel to handle an active day of work, or school and exercise.

You don't have to eat cereal every day. When you have the time, perhaps on weekends, you may want to cook eggs, pancakes, waffles, or other traditional breakfast foods. But breakfast should never be a cup of coffee and a doughnut on the way to your office or school.

Teenagers need special attention to make sure they eat a good breakfast. According to the 1988 National Adolescent Student Health Survey (NASHS), half of our teenage girls and one-third of our teenage boys reported eating breakfast on only two days or less during the previous week. They are missing out on two things: a nutritious start to the day and family time together. Ernesto Pollitt of the Department of Applied Behavioral Science at the University of California at Davis, told the *Reader's Digest:* "Kids are especially sensitive to the effects of skipping breakfast. Studies show this reduces their reflective and analytical abilities." Too often, these kids will skip lunch, too. This makes breakfast doubly important to them.

Lunch

Lunch is a time to re-charge, but always re-charge with nutritious foods, not junk. "Brown-bag" lunches will guarantee that you get a healthy and light meal. Adults either eat too much—the proverbial business lunch— or skip this meal. The "two-martini" lunch leaves you bloated, groggy, and soon overweight. You are better off skipping it.

According to the NASHS, about 25 percent of our teenage boys and 33 percent of our girls reported skipping lunch at least twice during the previous week. The Department of Agriculture's Food and Nutrition Service reports that half of today's high-school students don't eat lunches provided at school. It also noted that those other students who do eat the school lunch have a significantly higher energy level than those who skip lunch. Other studies link poor eating habits with weak academic performance.

But should our students eat the school lunch? A 1988 report by the

Public Voice for Food and Health Policy states that school lunches are healthier than a decade ago, but they are still too high in fat, sugar, and salt. Eileen Kugler of Public Voice told *USA Today:* "We'd like to see more schools serve healthfully modified lunches that are still attractive to school children, like spaghetti with meatballs or baked potato with chili. The idea that the school lunch has to mimic fast-food restaurants is something we don't buy." (See Chapter 8 for a model nutritious school lunch program.)

How does exercise fit with lunch? Exercise done at lunch time suppresses appetite. Instead, you can exercise and eat a light, nutritious lunch at your desk, such as yogurt or fruit. Shepherd, when working at the South-North News Service in Hanover, New Hampshire, often runs at noon and then brown-bags his lunch. He shocks co-workers, with yogurt, nuts, and an orange or apple: "That's not a lunch!" one of them told him.

Dinner

Traditionally, dinner is the main meal of the day for the American family. But it is also the largest meal, and that adds calories. You exercise little after dinner. A full stomach does little for a sound sleep. Dr. Cooper's research indicates that exercising vigorously about two hours before the evening meal is more likely to cause a loss of body fat than exercising at other times of the day. Dr. Cooper believes this is because the exercise depresses your appetite just before the heaviest meal of the day. Exercise after work may also increase your metabolism at the same time you exercise, thus doubling the body's burning of calories.

Do children skip this meal, too? Yes, but not as much, says the NASHS report. Many teenagers miss two dinners a week; 20 percent report eating dinner less than five times a week. Too often, kids eat in a hurry, if at all, because their parents aren't around to prepare a meal and eat with them.

THE FAMILY MEAL

Dinner is supposed to be a time when the family gathers at the end of the day and eats together. Sociologists report that the family dinner provides a sense of security and identity to family members. Research by Dr. Steven J. Wolin, a professor of psychiatry at the George Washington University Medical Center in Washington, D.C., indicates that families who maintain regular meals together, vacations, and bedtime routines protect their members from alcohol abuse, depression, and family violence.

"Healthy families spend time together on a regular, daily basis," Dr. Wolin told the *New York Times.* "Every family has a deep cultural need to do things together around food." Dr. John DeFrain, a psychologist and co-author of *Secrets of Strong Families,* finds that strong families believe that regular dinners together contribute to a sense of belonging, commitment, and ability to cope with stress. "To succeed as a family," he told the *Times*, "folks have got to spend time together. And dinner time is one of the best for throwing all the good things and bad things into the family melting pot."

But the sad fact is that fewer and fewer families exist in the traditional pattern—Mom, Dad, and Kids. And fewer of those families bother to take the time to eat together. The kids eat as they watch TV; their dinner is usually snacks. In 1976, according to a Roper Poll, 72 percent of U.S. families ate dinner together frequently. In 1986 that had dropped to 63 percent. The reasons: More women work and family members are scattered about, busy with activities.

Because families are busy in the evenings, breakfast is starting to replace dinner as the family meal. At least everyone comes home at some time to sleep. And when they wake up—often to get ready to go off to work or school again—breakfast is a good time to gather. My own family is an example of this. We eat breakfast together and then I walk Christopher to school. We often don't eat dinner together, since I often run after work and then teach fitness classes at least two nights a week. When I return, Christopher has already eaten, and most often with Virginia.

Set a family goal: eat together for breakfast or dinner—or perhaps a combination. Maybe breakfast on the weekdays and a family dinner on one weekend night. Whatever your pattern, make the gathering sacrosanct. Do not let television, phone calls, work, or anything distract you from this. Use the time to talk to each other about each person's life: What have you learned? What are you planning? Make contact with each member as though you had met him or her for the first time; in a sense, you have.

The Shepherds take the phone off the hook, clear the newspapers from sight, and sit at a special table. They make it a point at this one special dinner with their kids to join hands and pause for a moment of silence before eating. At first, the kids thought it was corny. Now, when they come home from college or jobs, sometimes with friends, it is the kids who pause, reach out with their hands, bow their heads, and seek the moment of peaceful quiet before the joyful hubbub of a family dinner.

30

Weight Management

You cannot lose weight without exercising. All those fancy and often expensive diets are fine; they may take pounds off of you. But to keep the weight off, and to tone flabby muscle and skin, you'll need to exercise. Vigorous exercise increases your metabolic rate, and that rate is sustained for more than fifteen hours, during which you are burning calories at a higher rate than if you did not exercise at all. So, I'm suggesting now that if you want to lose weight, combine diet with exercise.

Any aerobic exerciser will tell you that if you exercise vigorously and regularly you can ignore going on a diet. Your weight will stabilize. The food you eat will be burned up in exercise, and nutrients absorbed more readily. For example, a study by Dr. Peter Wood at the Stanford University Medical School indicates that people who run six or more miles a day eat about six hundred more calories daily than people who do not exercise at all—yet the exercisers weigh 20 percent less!

Studies with rats indicate the same pattern. Rats that exercise moderately actually eat less than rats that do not exercise at all. When rats exercise more than two hours a day, putting extra energy demands on their bodies, hunger is stimulated and food intake increases to match energy output. The same mechanism keeps the weight of humans who exercise regularly at a constant level.

Researchers at Cornell University have learned that if we exercise within two or three hours after eating we burn up more calories than identical exercise on an empty stomach. In addition, as mentioned, vigorous exercise tends to suppress hunger for hours.

"Diet and exercise go together," Dr. Clayton Myers writes in his *Official YMCA Physical Fitness Handbook*. "If you diet without exercising the result may be a thin weak person in place of a fat weak person. Muscle tissue that is not used will atrophy and proportionately become fatter even though the intake of calories has been reduced."

CALORIES

Our cells obtain and use food through the three-step process of digestion, absorption, metabolism. Basically, the foods we eat are broken down in the body to simpler forms, taken through the intestinal walls, and then transported by the blood to the cells. Food intake is measured in calories. A calorie is the amount of heat required to raise the temperature of one gram of water one degree of Centigrade. A pound of body weight averages 3,500 calories of energy. To gain a pound, you must eat and store that amount of energy; to lose that pound, you must get rid of it.

All carbohydrates, fats, and proteins contain calories; water, minerals, and vitamins do not. As we all know, it's easier to feed calories to the body than to burn them up.

This is another example of why we need more, not less, exercise as we grow older. Dr. Ralph Nelson of the Mayo Clinic has demonstrated that a 154-pound man at age thirty who maintains a constant level of exercise and food intake will weigh more than two hundred pounds by age sixty. To stay at the same weight while doing the same amount of exercise, this man must reduce his caloric intake by 11 percent.

Most of us gain weight when we stop exercising, usually within a decade or so after we leave school. Being a few pounds overweight isn't a serious health hazard. But it can lead to one. Remember, research indicates that overweight men and women can reduce their risk of heart attack by as much as 25 percent with a regular exercise program.

WEIGHT

Excessive weight is a well-known health problem. But so is being underweight. The National Institutes of Health estimate that 34 million Americans need to lose thirty-five pounds or more; one American in every four is twenty pounds overweight and thus is considered obese. The President's Council survey found one American child in every three overweight: perhaps as many as twenty million kids! Obese children are three times more likely to grow up to be obese adults.

On the other side of the scale, bulimia and anorexia nervosa are two psychiatric eating disorders that primarily affect women and girls. Bulimia is characterized by someone eating large amounts of food and then making herself vomit. Anorexia is the refusal to eat almost anything at all, even though the individual is hungry and obsessed with food. The anorexic wants to be extremely thin. Bulimia often leads to anorexia, or follows it once the anorexic begins eating again.

These disorders are most commonly found among adolescent girls from middle- and upper-income families. Dr. David Herzog of the Eating Disorders Clinic at the Massachusetts General Hospital in Boston estimates that one out of every five female college students has bulimia.

These diseases are different from other eating disorders, or even ordinary dieting. At any one time, according to a 1988 University of Michigan study, a third of all U.S. girls ages ten to twenty are on a diet; this rises to 42 percent for ages sixteen to twenty. Most of them are not fat, but are succumbing to social and cultural pressures to diet. Although only 15 percent of the girls were found to be overweight, half of the girls' mothers thought they were overweight, as did 38 percent of the girls themselves. Half of the girls in the study said that their mothers encouraged their dieting. The study also pointed out that most girls with serious dieting problems have mothers who diet constantly and yet are overweight.

Your bone structure and metabolism determine what is too much or too little weight for you. To determine your best weight consider the following points. Then consult the following charts to *estimate* the best weight for you. Check with your physician for the healthiest weight for you and your family.

What did you weigh at ages eighteen to twenty-five?

During those years, many of us are too active to get fat. (Others, who are already fat, tend to stay that way.) Theoretically, we stop growing in our early twenties. No one should gain weight as he or she ages. Life insurance charts that show people weighing more as they get older simply reflect what is happening, not what should happen. As we age, our metabolism slows. To counteract this, we should eat less and exercise more, and make sure that our weight levels off rather than continuing to increase. Your weight at age twenty-five, therefore, should be a goal.

How do you look and feel?

Here is the moment of truth, your time in the ring with the great bull. Dr. Cooper suggests that you stand nude in front of a full-length mirror. Don't even bother sucking it in. Look at yourself. If you are fat, admit it.

Still lying? Try running in place and look at the jiggles, especially your thighs and stomach. Go ahead, suck it in now; it's still gonna jump around. If you are like the majority of Americans, you will come away from this moment of truth with two convictions: diet and exercise, just like ol' Bob Glover said. While you exercise, stay out of the ring with the bull in it for about six months; then step back in front of the mirror and compare. You may be able to say "Olé!"

How do you compare to the popular weight formulas?

Using the formula in the Wellness Quiz in Chapter 27, you can estimate your ideal weight. Men take their height in inches, multiply it by four, and subtract 128. Women take their height in inches, multiply it by 3.5, and subtract 108. If you are large boned, you may add 10 percent.

How do you compare to the weight charts?

Check yourself against the charts below developed by the Metropolitan Life Insurance Company. Remember, these height-weight mortality charts are based on what people who have the lowest mortality rates actually weigh, not what they should weigh to increase longevity. They do serve as good guides for estimating desirable weight. Aim to stay below these recommended figures.

METROPOLITAN LIFE HEIGHT/WEIGHT TABLE

MEN					WOMEN			
Height		Small	Medium	Large	Height		Small	Medium	Large
Feet	Inches	Frame	Frame	Frame	Feet	Inches	Frame	Frame	Frame
5	2	128-134	131-141	138-150	4	10	102-111	109-121	118-131
5	3	130-136	133-143	140-153	4	11	103-113	111-123	120-134
5	4	132-138	135-145	142-156	5	0	104-115	113-126	122-137
5	5	134-140	137-148	144-160	5	1	106-118	115-129	125-140
5	6	136-142	139-151	146-164	5	2	108-121	118-132	128-143
5	7	138-145	142-154	149-168	5	3	111-124	121-135	131-147
5	8	140-148	145-157	152-172	5	4	114-127	124-138	134-151
5	9	142-151	148-160	155-176	5	5	117-130	127-141	137-155
5	10	144-154	151-163	158-180	5	6	120-133	130-144	140-159
5	11	146-157	154-166	161-184	5	7	123-136	133-147	143-163
6	0	149-160	157-170	164-188	5	8	126-139	136-150	146-167
6	1	152-164	160-174	168-192	5	9	129-142	139-153	149-170
6	2	155-168	164-178	172-197	5	10	132-145	142-156	152-173
6	3	158-172	167-182	176-202	5	11	135-148	145-159	155-176
6	4	162-176	171-187	181-207	6	0	138-151	148-162	158-179

Weights at Ages 25-59 Based on Lowest Mortality.
Weight in Pounds According to Frame (in indoor clothing weighing 5 lbs., shoes with 1″ heels).

Source of basic data: *1979 Build Study*, Society of Actuaries and Association of Life Insurance Medical Directors of America, 1980.

BODY COMPOSITION

Your body consists of two types of tissues, fat and lean, as well as bones, organs, and muscles. The amount of fat you carry is called your body fat percentage. It is determined by dividing your total body weight by the weight of your fat.

Body fat percentage is commonly estimated by using calipers to measure the fat under the skin (skinfolds), or by an underwater weighing technique. The latter is more accurate, but both are good estimates. You can usually have a skinfold estimate taken by your local fitness club or YMCA. Your child's physical education teacher should be able to measure his or her approximate body fat percentage.

Why should we want to know this? Body weight and body fat are closely linked. And body weight and body fat tell us about how fit and healthy we are. Dr. David Costill, director of the Human Performance Laboratory at Ball State University, has found that each pound of fat added or lost can result in an increase or decrease of body fat percentage by as much as half a point. Some people may weigh within the standard ranges but have a high percentage of body fat. They are underweight but overfat.

A desirable goal for adults is 10 to 15 percent of body fat for men, 14 to 22 percent for women. Men with 20 percent body fat and women with 28 percent or more are considered overweight.

LOSING WEIGHT

No other topic so obsesses the American people. We spend billions of dollars a year to lose weight. More than 60 percent of our adolescent girls diet (28 percent of the boys), and they try diet pills, vomiting, or laxatives. Adults try fad diets, diet books, resort diets, Mexican diets, even diets named after expensive suburban towns. Still we remain the world's most overweight people. We could save all that money by doing two simple things: eating less, exercising more.

If you want to lose weight, here are some suggestions for you and your family:

- The key, as I just said, is to exercise more, eat less; burn more calories, consume fewer calories.
- Keep track of what you eat. Even keep a log. If you are honest, it may shock you.
- Switch to lower-calorie items—water instead of soda; an apple instead of a candy bar.
- Learn to eat slowly and enjoy your food and meals. This will keep

you from eating too much. Also, do not read or watch television while you eat; you will tend to eat more and to create a stimulus-response reaction (every time you read or watch TV, you will want to eat).

• Eat smaller amounts, more often. This is a good idea for teenagers in your home. Sometimes they cannot eat a lot at one sitting, but need to keep calories coming. When he was a young adolescent, Shepherd's son Caleb ate about every two hours all day long. Research indicates that you gain more weight by eating one large meal than by eating three to six smaller ones.

• Cut out desserts and high-calorie snacks. Keep evening meals light.

• Be disciplined. Set a reasonable goal, such as five to ten pounds off within two or three months. As you get older, taking off weight gets harder. Remember, it took a long time to put it on; take time getting it off. Don't try to lose too much too soon, certainly not two to three pounds a week. Keep a weight diary to make you stick with your goal.

• Don't reduce your fluid intake. No one loses weight permanently from sweating. That's a myth. You just replace fluids lost by sweating.

• Forget spot-reducing gimmicks! The only thing that will lose weight is your bank account. Aerobic exercise combined with some weight training should take care of specific areas of your body you want to firm up. Spot reducing is a myth and a rip-off.

• Children who are overweight have a better chance of losing weight and keeping it off if the entire family diets and exercises with them. If only one child needs to diet, rearrange the family's meals to accommodate that child. Get the sodas and fatty (and salty) snacks out of the house; don't even buy them. Take the opportunity to redesign your family's eating habits and diet.

WEIGHT FOR CHILDREN

You should monitor, within reason, your child's weight and growth. This does not mean standing by the scale every week; parental obsession about a child's weight could lead to eating disorders or at least uncooperative eating behavior. But some monitoring should take place. The best way is simply to ask the child how he or she feels, and to look at the youngster when he or she is undressed or in a bathing suit or exercise outfit. Compare him or her to other children of about the same age and height when they are playing.

I do not want to overstate this. Kids grow at different speeds. They go through periods when they are a little chubby, or a little thin. If your child is physically active, generally happy, growing, and developing, you have nothing to worry about. The following formula and chart may be of some use in understanding the proper weight for your child.

Always check with your doctor if you are concerned about your child's weight. Never start your child on a restrictive diet unless your doctor prescribes it and monitors it.

By age two, most babies have grown to more than thirty inches and weigh between twenty-five and thirty-five pounds. But this, too, varies. Baby fat is not a concern. But using a low-fat diet to reduce a baby's weight or to get a headstart on preventing heart disease could interfere with the baby's normal growth. Pediatricians recommend that babies drink whole milk until age two; half the calories in breast milk—a highly recommended food source for babies!—come from fat.

The first three years are the quickest stage of growth. From ages three to nine, kids grow at a slower but steady rate. Then comes another growth spurt. Girls between nine and twelve and boys between eleven and fourteen grow quickly in height. They also gain a proportional amount of weight over a two- or three-year period. After about mid-adolescence, growth slows; by age sixteen or so for girls and age twenty or so for boys, growth rates have begun leveling off.

A Formula for Children's Body Weight

A simple estimated ideal body weight for children can be determined by using the following formula. But remember that this is an estimate and an ideal.

Children forty-two to forty-eight inches tall should weigh one pound for each inch of their height. Children forty-nine to sixty-four inches tall should add 4.5 pounds for each inch over 48 inches. (For example, a fifty-inch child should weigh 48 plus 9 [2×4.5], or 57 pounds.)

Height and Weight Charts for Children

Your family doctor can tell you if your child's height and weight are normal. Here is a chart to use as a guide. Take your child's height and weight without shoes.

Don't worry if your child does not fit the charts. Christopher doesn't either. He is small in height and weight for his age, but his weight is ideal for his height. About 10 percent of all U.S. children will be about 10 percent smaller or bigger in height and 10 percent lighter or heavier in weight for their age. For these kids, you may want to determine weight from their height on the chart, not their age. Also, a child may be 10 pounds heavier or lighter than the chart's averages and still be "normal." Remember, this chart is only a guide.

HEIGHT-WEIGHT CHARTS FOR CHILDREN

BOYS

Age	Weight (pounds)	Height (inches)
5	42	44
6	48	46
7	54	49
8	60	51
9	66	53
10	72	55
11	80	57
12	90	59
Teens	102	61
	112	63
	118	65
	126	67
	134	69
	142	71
	150	73

GIRLS

Age	Weight	Height
5	41	43
6	47	46
7	52	48
8	58	50
9	64	52
10	70	55
11	79	57
12	90	60
Teens	106	62
	113	64
	121	66
	129	68

SUMMARY

Let me underscore the two basic themes of this book. First, set an example as an adult and parent. You are being watched by your kids and other children. What you do is what they do, and will do. Become a good role model for all of our children. Exercise regularly. Exercise with them, if you can. Include them in your life in every way possible.

Second, include your children in your discussions about stress, nutrition, and weight management. Let them help in the planning and preparation of meals. Make wellness a part of your home, just as exercising is part of your lives.

These are among the lifelong gifts you give your children. They are things you control, you can do—and they pay off. Someday, when your kids are out cross-country skiing, running along a country road or city park, lost in the motion of a long swim, feeling the wind on a bike ride, they will think of you, and what you stood for and taught them and gave them. And they will thank you, once again, for your gifts.

Maybe this book will have played a role in those gifts. Christopher and I hope so.

APPENDIX

Appendix

The Post Raisin Bran Family Fitness Program

Bob Glover developed and serves as the National Director of this program, which consists of family fitness events—non-competitive runs for pre-schoolers, youth, and families—in cities across the U.S.A., and a public service brochure which provides guidelines for exercise and nutrition for the entire family. For more information, contact Robert H. Glover and Associates, Inc., 236 East 78th Street, Box #6, New York, New York 10021.

Fitness Organizations

American Alliance for Health, Physical Education, Recreation and Dance (AAHPERD)
1900 Association Drive
Reston, VA 22091
703-476-3400

A non-profit, membership organization of over 30,000 professional educators in physical education, health, fitness, sports and athletics, recreation, dance, and related diciplines. Founded in 1885. The purpose of the Alliance is to improve the health and fitness of Americans by improving our country's educational programs. The AAHPERD brings together teachers, administrators, researchers, coaches, students, and others with career interests in its specialized fields. The Alliance works to improve education programs in the schools and the community, and to encourage all Americans to make fitness and health a part of their daily lives.

The Alliance also relates to its members through its six national associations: National Association for Sport and Physical Education; National Association for Girls and Women in Sport; Association for the Advancement of Health Education; American Association for Leisure and Recreation; Association for Research, Administration and Professional Councils and Societies; and National Dance Association.

The Alliance publishes a newsletter, three professional periodicals, and a series of books and booklets (see publications). The Alliance supports research projects, conducts training sessions and seminars for members, lobbies Congress on legislative issues, develops programs for schools, conducts surveys, and provides information to the media.

Among the AAHPERD programs: the health-related fitness test and educational program for schoolchildren (Physical Best), the National Youth and Children Fitness Study, the Jump Rope for Heart program, and Shape of the Nation—a study of the status of physical education in each state.

Association for Fitness in Business (AFB)
310 N. Alabama Street, Suite A100
Indianapolis, IN 46204
317-636-6621

An organization for personnel associated with fitness in corporations, clubs, hospitals, and other businesses. Provides promotion, training, educational information, employment information, research briefs, etc. Provides support for assistance in the development of fitness and health promotion programs in business. Publishes a research summary and a membership newsletter.

The Institute for Aerobics Research (IAR)
13300 Preston Road
Dallas, TX 75230
214-239-7223

A non-profit research organization founded by Dr. Kenneth Cooper. The Institute studies the effects of exercise as a preventive tool. It also provides training and certification programs and consults with corporations, agencies, and schools. Its Fitnessgram program, available to schools at a low cost, is a computerized youth fitness reporting and motivation system for use in the school setting.

National Strength and Conditioning Association (NSCA)
300 Old City Hall Landmark
916 O Street
P. O. Box 81410
Lincoln, NE 68501
402-472-3000

An organization of strength coaches, exercise physiologists, and physicians that provides information, training, and certification to members and disseminates information to the public. Its goal is to facilitate a professional exchange of ideas in the area of strength and conditioning development as it relates to the improvement of athletic performance and fitness.

President's Council on Physical Fitness and Sports (PCPFS)
450 5th Street, N.W.
Suite 7103
Washington, DC 20001
202-272-3421

The principal federal organization for physical fitness and sports, it was established by an Executive Order to serve the President in promoting national physical fitness and sports programs. The Council's goal is to advance the physical fitness of children, youth, adults, and senior citizens by encouraging the development of community recreation, physical fitness, and sport participation programs. Among its services: public service advertising to inform and motivate the American people, preparation of articles and booklets (see publications: US Government Printing Office). Among its programs: The President's Challenge (youth fitness testing); Presidential Sports Award (a national sports participation and incentives program for persons aged fifteen and over; awards available in forty popular participant sports, from archery to weight training); and the PCPFS School Population Fitness Survey.

YMCA of the USA
101 N. Wacker Drive
Chicago, IL 60606
312-977-0031

Develops national programs and publishes books in adult and youth fitness and sports (see publications: Human Kinetics Publishers). Provides facilities and programs for infants to senior citizens in hundreds of branches across the USA. Programs include "The Y's Way to Physical Fitness," "The Y's Way to a Healthy Back." Directs programs and provides coaches manuals for several youth sports, including basketball, soccer, gymnastics, flag football, racquetball, softball, tennis, volleyball, wrestling, and swimming. Also provides programming to schools and corporations. Provides training and certification programs in physical fitness.

Lifetime Fitness Sports Organizations

Aerobics

Aerobics & Fitness Association of America (AFAA)
15250 Ventura Boulevard
Suite 802
Sherman Oaks, CA 91403
818-905-0040

Provides education, training, and certification to aerobic exercise instructors and serves their professional interests. Publishes a magazine, *Aerobics & Fitness*. Promotes "Superclass," an aerobics program for youth.

International Dance-Exercise Association (IDEA)
6190 Cornerstone Court East, Suite 204
San Diego, CA 92121
619-535-8979

A professional association for aerobics and fitness instructors; conducts training and certification programs for instructors; promotes aerobics dance exercise.

Biking

American Youth Hostels (AYH)
1332 I Street N.W., Suite 451
Washington, DC 20005

Contact for information about biking, biking equipment, and bike tours. Local associations across the country. Members include both young and old.

Bicycle Federation of America
1818 R Street
Washington, DC 20009

Promotes the safe use of bicycles for transportation and recreation. Offers brochures on bicycling skills, safety, and maintenance.

U.S. Cycling Federation (USCF)
1750 E. Boulder Street
Colorado Springs, CO 80909
303-578-4581

Governing body for cycling competition. Provides educational materials and information to grass-roots clubs and publishes newsletter, *Cycling U.S.A.*

Canoeing/Rowing

United States Canoe Association
4169 Middle Brook Drive
Dayton, OH 45440-3311

United States Rowing Association
251 N. Illinois St., Suite 980
Indianapolis, IN 46204
317-237-2769

Cross-country Skiing

United States Ski Association-Nordic
P. O. Box 727
Brattleboro, VT 05301

Running

American Running & Fitness Association (AR&FA)
9310 Old Georgetown Road
Bethesda, MD 20814
301-897-0197

A membership organization that promotes running and fitness. Publishes *Run-*

ning and FitNews, provides a speakers bureau, serves as a clearinghouse for information on running and other forms of aerobic fitness.

The Athletics Congress (TAC)
200 S. Capitol St.—Suite 140
Indianapolis, IN 46225
317-638-9155

Governing body for the sports of track and field, racewalking, and long-distance running. Conducts a Junior Olympics Track program for youth.

New York Road Runners Club (NYRRC)
9 East 89th Street
New York, NY 10128
212-860-4455

An organization of over 25,000 members, primarily in the New York City area. Programs include running classes (directed by Bob Glover for beginners through marathoners), stretching classes, over one hundred races per year, educational clinics and brochures, magazine, youth running sessions and events. Achilles Track Club program for disabled adults and youth. The Junior Road Runners Club for youth was developed by Bob Glover.

Road Runners Club of America (RRCA)
629 S. Washington Street
Alexandria, VA 22314
703-836-0558

An organization of hundreds of local chapters across the country. Local clubs promote running, racing, and educational programs—including youth running.

Swimming

American Red Cross
17th and D Streets, N.W.
Washington, DC 20006
202-639-3259

Offers training programs for swimming instructors, booklets for pre-schoolers, and youth swimming safety.

United States Swimming, Inc. (USS)
1750 E. Boulder St.
Colorado Springs, CO 80909
303-578-4578

Governing body for swimming competition.

Tennis

U.S. Tennis Association (USTA)
1212 Avenue of the Americas
New York, NY 10036
212-302-3322

National governing body for tennis. Sponsors recreational-development programs for youth through its Junior Tennis Program.

Walking

The Rockport Walking Institute
72 Howe Street
Marlboro, MA 01752

Free information and booklets from the Rockport walking shoe company.

Walking Clubs
P. O. Box 509
Gracie Station
New York, NY 10028

Information on walking and walking tours.

The Walkways Center
Suite 427, 733 15th Street, NW
Washington, DC 20005
202-737-9555

A national non-profit organization formed to promote walking, provide information on walking, represent the needs of walkers, and work with local communities to improve walking facilities. Membership includes access to a toll-free telephone information service, a newsletter, resource book on walking, and tip booklets.

Medical Organizations

American Academy of Pediatrics (AAP)
141 Northwest Point Boulevard
P. O. Box 927
Elk Grove Village, IL 60009
312-228-5005
800-433-9016

An organization of 32,000 pediatricians dedicated to the health, safety, and well-being of infants, children, and adolescents. One of its major goals is to educate the pediatrician and the public on exercise and fitness for children and on the care of the young athlete. Has published a position statement on "Physical Fitness and the Schools" and a brochure "Sports and Your Child," which are available to parents and teachers. Has worked with the AAHPERD to campaign for improved physical education in the schools.

American College of Sports Medicine (ACSM)
401 West Michigan Street
P.O. Box 1440
Indianapolis, IN 46202
317-637-9200

The College is engaged in the study of sports medicine. It conducts research, publishes educational material (see publications), sponsors seminars, conferences and workshops, and serves as a resource clearinghouse. The College consists of over 12,000 members representing many disciplines from the three main areas of medicine, basic and applied science, and education and allied health, such as physicians, educators, athletic trainers, nurses, biological scientists, exercise physiologists, behavioral scientists, and students. The College provides a continuing education program to its members, and provides certification programs for exercise/health program directors and instructors.

Sports Organizations

American Athletic Union (AAU)
AAU House
3400 West 86th Street
P. O. Box 68207
Indianapolis, IN 46268
317-872-2900

The AAU is the largest non-profit, volunteer organization in the United States dedicated solely to the promotion and development of amateur sports and physical fitness programs. The AAU provides for participation in a variety of sports. Among its programs: The Chrysler Fund/AAU Physical Fitness Program (fitness testing), the Junior Olympics, and AAU Senior Sports for adults. Junior Olympics (ages eight through eighteen) includes competition in baseball, basketball, field hockey, gymnastics, karate, soccer, swimming, and wrestling

American Coaching Effectiveness Program (ACEP)
Box 5076
Champaign, IL 61820
217-351-5076

A training and certification program for coaches, administrators, physicians, and others associated with youth sports programs developed by *American Coach* newsletter. ACEP teaches coaches to: focus on their athletes' well-being first and winning second, reduce the risk of injury to their players and provide better first aid when injuries occur, teach the skills for playing sports and living life more effectively. Leadership training seminars conducted around the country. Advanced courses available in sports physiology, sports psychology, sports injuries, teaching sports skills, sports law, and time management. Self-study courses available. Resources include the basic program text, *Coaching Young Athletes*, guidebooks for each course, and specific sports' coaching guides, including baseball, softball, swimming, soccer, and more. Program is utilized by high schools, colleges, national organizations (such as the YMCA), and other groups. The USA's most widely used coaching education program has educated over 50,000 coaches.

Little League Baseball
P. O. Box 3485
Williamsport, PA 17701
717-326-1921

Programs across the country for boys and girls ages six through eighteen. Produces written information and training videos.

National Youth Sports Coaches Association (NYSCA)
2611 Old Okeechobee Road
West Palm Beach, FL 33409
305-684-1141

Provides a variety of publications and educational materials, training and certification programs, and technical assistance for youth sport coaches. Publishes a membership newsletter and a series of sports coaching books.

North American Youth Sports Institute
4985 Oak Garden Drive, Suite C
Kernersville, NC 27284
919-784-4926

Provides technical assistance, educational materials, training, and instruction for coaches.

Office of Youth Sport
University of Illinois
Champaign, IL 61820
217-351-5076

Provides technical assistance, publications, training, and other services through Human Kinetics Publishers. Developed and administers the American Coaching Effectiveness Program for training and certification, and publishes the newsletter *American Coach* and a long list of fitness and sports books.

Youth Sports Institute (YSI)
IM Sports Circle
Michigan State University
East Lansing, MI 48824
517-353-6689

Conducts research on youth sports and disseminates information.

Girls' and Women's Organizations

Girls Clubs of America
441 West Michigan Street
Indianapolis, IN 46202
317-634-7546

A national organization serving over 250,000 girls and young women members annually through 240 affiliated Girls Club Centers. Promotes sports and fitness for girls, as well as other issues. Provides a Sports Resource Kit for information as part of its Sporting Chance program designed to assist youth serving agencies in the development of sports programs for girls age six through eighteen.

The Melpomene Institute
2125 East Hennepin Avenue
Minneapolis, MN 55413
612-378-0545

An organization devoted to research and education in the area of women's and girls' sports and fitness. Holds frequent seminars, distributes educational information, and publishes a newsletter, the *Melpomene Report*.

National Association for Girls and Women in Sport (NAGWS)
AAHPERD
1900 Association Drive
Reston, VA 22091
703-476-3450

A member of the AAHPERD; the only national professional organization for girls and women in sports-related disciplines and careers. Works to provide communication networks, leadership opportunities, political action, international exchange, student participation, job placement, and advancement of coaches. Publishes educational materials, including sports guides and rulebooks in a large variety of sports. Conducts nationwide sports training seminars for coaches.

Women's Sports Foundation (WSF)
342 Madison Avenue
Suite 728
New York, NY 10173
212-972-9170
800-227-3988

Dedicated to educating the public on the value of sports for all girls and women and to providing opportunity for their participation. Founded by tennis great Billie Jean King to create a unified body to encourage and support participation of women in sports; further opportunities, facilities, and training; and educate the public on the value of participating in sports and fitness activities. Serves as a national clearinghouse for fitness and sports information for women and girls, and as a referral network. It also lobbies Congress for legislation affecting women and sports. Produces several publications, including its *Annual Scholarship Guide and Camp Guide* and the booklet "Parent's Guide to Girls' Sports."

Young Women's Christian Association (YWCA)
726 Broadway
New York, NY 10003
212-614-2851

Provides fitness and sports facilities and programs through its branches across the USA for women, as well as children from pre-school to teenagers.

Organizations for the Physically Disabled

The Achilles Track Club
New York Road Runners Club
9 E. 89th Street
New York, NY 10128
212-967-9300

A running and fitness program for adults and youth with chapters around the world. For all types of physically disabled.

American Athletic Association for the Deaf
3916 Lantern Drive
Silver Spring, MD 20902
301-942-4042

National Association of Sports for Cerebral Palsied
P. O. Box 3874, Amity Station
New Haven, CT 06525
203-397-1402

National Handicapped Sports and Recreation Association
P. O. Box 18664, Capital Hills Station
Denver, CO 80218
303-232-4575

Information on a variety of sports programs for the physically disabled.

Special Olympics
1350 New York Avenue, N.W., Suite 500
Washington, DC 20005
202-628-3650

Programs for the mentally handicapped.

United States Association of Blind Athletes
55 W. California Avenue
Beach Haven, NJ 08008
609-492-1017

Wellness Organizations

General

American Heart Association
7320 Greenville Avenue
Dallas, TX 75231
214-750-5300

Provides educational information on fitness, nutrition, and health. In association with AAHPERD developed the Jump Rope for Heart program and a series of booklets (see publications).

Smoking

Action on Smoking and Health (ASH)
2013 H Street, NW
Washington, DC 20006
202-659-4310

American Cancer Society
4 W. 35th Street
New York, NY 10001
212-736-3030
(Check phone book for local affiliate.)

American Lung Association
1740 Broadway
New York, NY 10019
212-315-8700

SmokEnders
50 Washington Street
Norwalk, CT 06854
800-243-5614

Nutrition/Weight Control

American Dietetic Association (ADA)
208 S. LaSalle Street
Suite 1100
Chicago, IL 60604
312-899-0040

Weightwatchers International
800 Community Drive
Manhasset, NY 11030
516-627-9200

Stress

American Institute of Stress
124 Park Avenue
Yonkers, NY 10703
914-963-1200

Fitness/Wellness Programs Available to Schools and Organizations

Physical Best
AAHPERD
1900 Association Drive
Reston, VA 22091
703-476-3400

A comprehensive physical fitness education and assessment program designed for schools to motivate youths in grades K–12 to participate in physical acivity to develop their personal bests. Combines health-related fitness testing with practical classroom instructional materials that teach how and why to stay fit for a lifetime. Educational kit includes an introductory letter to parents, fitness lesson plans for classroom or P.E. teachers, student contracts for individual goal setting, and a report card to parents.

The Body Shop
Methodist Hospital
P. O. Box 650
Minneapolis, MN 55440
612-932-6008

A weight-control-through-wellness program for young people ages eight through eighteen. Primarily available through hospitals across the USA.

Every Child a Winner
Box 141
Ocilla, GA 31774
912-468-7098

An alternative physical education program utilizing dance, gymnastics, and creative games.

Feelin' Good
Fitness Finders, Inc.
133 Teft Road
Spring Arbor, MI 49283
517-750-1500

Combines classroom health awareness instruction with creative aerobic exercise classes for kindergarten through grade nine.

Fit Youth Today (FYT)
American Health and Fitness Foundation
6225 U.S. Highway 290 East
Suite 114
Austin, TX 78723
512-465-1080

A complete program of health fitness for kindergarten through grade twelve endorsed by the American College of Sports Medicine. Includes a health-related fitness test, fitness curriculum for teachers, a progressive conditioning protocol for students, and educational information by grade level in the areas of exercise, cardiovascular risk factors, diet and nutrition, tobacco, stress, cancer, family role in health and fitness, and allergies/asthma.

Jump Rope for Heart (AAHPERD)
1900 Association Drive
Reston, VA 22091
703-476-3400

A program developed by AAHPERD for youth and adults designed to promote jumping rope for fitness and to raise money for the American Heart Association

Know Your Body
American Health Foundation
320 E. 43 Street
New York, NY 10017
212-953-1900

A comprehensive health education program for kindergarten through grade eight, including classroom instruction, teachers' guides, workbooks, and student "health passports." Topics included: self-care and self-responsibility, health decision-making, accident prevention, lifestyle decisions, substance abuse prevention, heart disease and cancer prevention, nutrition, exercise and physical fitness, and dental health.

Walking Wellness
Creative Walking, Inc.
407-S White Clay Center
Newark, DE 19711
302-368-2222

A series of workshops combining walking and wellness instruction for kindergarten through grade six. Includes teachers' guides and students' workbooks.

Fitness Testing Programs Available to Schools and Organizations

Physical Best (AAHPERD)
1900 Association Drive
Reston, VA 22091
703-476-3400

The nation's original health-related fitness test revised. Tests for the five key fitness components described in Chapter 2 with the following assessments:

Cardio-respiratory endurance—one-mile walk/run
Body composition—skinfold
Flexibility—sit and reach
Muscular strength/endurance (abdominals)—modified sit-ups
Muscular strength/endurance (upper body)—pull-ups

Includes health fitness standards based on a single age and sex-adjusted goal for each test item for youths in grades K–12. Reaching this goal is necessary for minimal health fitness. Awards available for meeting fitness participation goals, for meeting personal fitness goals, and for meeting the health fitness standards on all test items. Includes a computerized report. An educational program is combined with the testing and awards program.

President's Challenge
President's Council on Physical Fitness and Sports
450 5th St., Suite 7103
Washington, DC 20001
202-272-3421

Students, ages six through seventeen, who meet the "President's Challenge," by scoring at or about the eighty-fifth percentile (top 15 percent of all students of the same age and sex) on all five test items are eligible to receive the Presidential Physical Fitness Award. Program honors the very fit and motivates youth to reach the highest fitness goals.

Fitness tests administered include:
Cardio-respiratory endurance—one-mile run/walk
Abdominal strength/endurance—curl-ups
Arm and shoulder strength/endurance—pull-ups
Flexibility—V-sit reach or sit and reach
Leg strength/power/agility—shuttle run

Fitnessgram
Institute of Aerobics Research
13300 Preston Rd.
Dallas, TX 75230
214-239-7223

This organization produces for parents a very nice-looking, practical computerized report card with a comprehensive fitness profile and recommended exercises to help improve fitness. Tests for all the key fitness components.

Fit Youth Today
American Health & Fitness Foundation
6225 U.S. Highway 290 East
Austin, TX 78723
512-465-1080

Uses criterion reference standards based upon desirable health fitness levels for children in kindergarten through grade twelve, combined with a complete health education program. Tests include:

Cardio-respiratory endurance—twelve- to twenty-minute steady state jog
Muscular strength and endurance—bent-knee curl-up
Flexibility—sit and reach
Body composition—height and weight/skinfolds

Computerized report cards available. Awards available to students who meet the health fitness standards, as well as to those who don't but who have improved their fitness levels.

Chrysler Fund–AAU Physical Fitness Program (AAU)
AAU House
3400 W. 86th St.
P. O. Box 68207
Indianapolis, IN 46268

Standards based on data from previous tests for ages six through seventeen. Certificates awarded for participation and passing standards. Patches awarded to youths who meet all the standards. Tests utilized:

Cardio-respiratory endurance—one-mile run/walk
Flexibility—sit and reach
Muscular strength and endurance (abdominals)—bent-knee sit-ups
Muscular strength and endurance (upper
    body)—pull-up/flexed-arm hang (girls)

Optional tests available: standing long jump, isometric push-up (boys), modified push-up (girls), isometric leg squat, shuttle run, sprints.

Youth Physical Fitness Program of the Marine Corps League
United States Marines Youth Foundation
P. O. Box 8280
Sylvania, OH 80909
419-882-0051

For boys and girls ages six through seventeen who wish to attempt to meet the Marine standards or to compete in local, regional, and national contests. The five competitive exercises are pull-ups, sit-ups, standing broad jump, push-ups, and the shuttle run.

Publishers

AAHPERD Publications
1900 Association Drive
Reston, VA 22091
703-476-3400

Publishes over a dozen books per year in sports, fitness, and health, as well as three professional periodicals for members:

Journal of Physical Education, Recreation and Dance
Health Education
Research Quarterly

American College of Sports Medicine Publications
PO Box 1440
Indianapolis, IN 46206
317-637-9200

Publishes its journal, *Medicine and Science in Sports and Exercise,* books (including *Guidelines for Exercise Testing and Prescription*), position stands on important issues, and a series of booklets for the lay person, including "Alcohol in Sports," "Anabolic Steroids and Athletes," "Fitness in Healthy Adults," and "Weight-Loss Programs."

Consumer Information Center Publications
U.S. General Services Administration
Washington, DC 20405
202-566-1794

Publications on a wide variety of topics, including fitness and health.

Human Kinetics Publications
P. O. Box 5076
Champaign, IL 61820
800-DIAL-HKP

Publishes nearly one hundred books per year on sports, health, and fitness, including professional textbooks and reference books for physical and health educators as well as books for the general public. Also publishes all the educational books and materials for the YMCA.

Publishes several periodicals, including:

Adapted Physical Activity Quarterly (physically disabled)
Journal of Sport and Exercise Psychology
Journal of Teaching in Physical Education
Journal of Philosophy in Sport
The Sport Psychologist

Publishes *American Coach,* the publication of the American Coaching Effectiveness Program, and the ACEP textbooks.

Rodale Press Publications
Emmaus, PA 18098
215-967-5171

Rodale Press publishes over forty new book titles a year on topics like health, fitness, gardening, diet, and nutrition. Rodale publishes several fitness newsletters, including *Executive Fitness*. Rodale's magazines include: *Backpacker, Bicycling, Children, Cross Country Skier, Prevention,* and *Runner's World*.

U.S. Government Printing Office Publications
Superintendent of Documents
Washington, DC 20402
202-783-3238

Publishes information on a variety of topics, including fitness. Publishes President's Council on Physical Fitness and Sports instructor guide and survey, youth fitness handbook—*Getting Fit*.

Magazines/Newsletters

General Health

American Health Magazine
80 Fifth Avenue
New York, NY 10011
212-242-2460

Health and fitness for the whole family.

Health Magazine
3 Park Avenue
New York, NY 10016

Specializes in health and fitness for women and girls.

Hippocrates
475 Gate Five Road, Suite 100
Sausalito, CA 94965

Health and fitness.

Prevention Magazine
Rodale Press
Rodale Press Publications
Emmaus, PA 18098
215-967-5171

Seven million subscribers for this health and fitness magazine.

Sports and Fitness

American Coach
Human Kinetics Publishers
Box 5076
Champaign, IL 61820

The official publication of the American Coaching Effectiveness Program. A newsletter full of good tips for youth coaches.

The Physician and Sportsmedicine
4530 W. 77th Street
Minneapolis, MN 55435
612-835-3222

Excellent source for latest research and guidelines for sports, fitness, health, and sports medicine.

Running & FitNews
American Running & Fitness Association
9310 Old Georgetown Road
Bethesda, MD 20814
301-897-0197

A monthly newsletter which includes brief nuggets of information on a variety of topics, including research findings in fitness, health, and sports medicine.

The Walking Magazine
711 Boylston Street
Boston, MA 02116

A general magazine on walking and fitness.

Women's Sports & Fitness
World Publications
809 S. Orlando Avenue, Suite H
Winter Park, FL 32789
305-628-4802

Founded by the Women's Sports Foundation. Provides a variety of information to women and girls concerning sports, fitness, and health.

Parents and Children

Child
477 Madison Avenue
New York, NY 10022

Children
Rodale Press
Rodale Press Publications
Emmaus, PA 18098
215-967-5171

Parenting
501 Second Street
San Francisco, CA 94107

Parents Magazine
685 Third Avenue
New York, NY 10017

Index

Abbott, Jim, 288, 293
abdominal curls, 152
abdominal muscles, testing minimum
    strength of, 60
Achilles Track Club, 283–87
    Youth Program, 285–87
activities, physical:
    after-school, 55–56
    appropriate, year-round, quality, 89–
        93
    coed, 272–75
    continuous vigorous, 70–71
    encouraging variety of, 53–56
    girls dropping out of, 270–71
    in model school physical education
        program, 105–13
    in physical education programs, 89–
        93, 97–98
    quality of, 106
activity sessions, 110–13
Adams, John Quincy, 133–34, 155
adaptability, 134–35
aerobic activities, 107
    for children, 195
    home run, 177
    kite flying, 177
    selection of, 186–87
    soccer, 176
    volleyball, 176
aerobic exercises, 154–65, 168–69
    for children, 155–56
    dance, 194–95
    kinds of, 156–58
aerobic families, 39–40
aerobic tests, 69–74
after-school activities, 55–56
Albertson, L. M., 262

alcohol, 365
    abuse of, 345–48
Allen-Stevenson School, 103–17
    activity sessions of, 110–13
    aerobic activities at, 107
    fitness and sports activities of, 105–13
    fitness class of, 107
    fitness testing at, 113
    four cornerstones of physical educa-
        tion and, 105
    parental involvement at, 116–17
    philosophy of, 104–5
    quality of activity at, 106
    running at, 108–10
    walking program of, 107–8
    wellness education at, 113–16
ankle:
    rolls, 144
    stretches, 231
arm curls, 152
arthritis, 290
asthma, 290–91
athletes, code of ethics for, 310–11

baby bear sit-ups, 167
back muscles, testing minimum strength
    of, 60–61
backstroke, 234
Barnes, Joan, 259
baseball:
    snow, 179–80
    sports clubs, 315–18
basketball:
    fast-break, 177
    sports clubs, 318–19
belly breathing, 142–43
bench presses, 152

bends, forward, 231
Benson, Herbert, 362–63
Berenson, Gerald, 6
Berryman, Jack, 91
Beverly Hills School District, 128
biking and bikes, 196–206
  for adults, 200
  for children, 197–200
  clothing and accessories for, 204–5
  for families, 203–4
  getting fit with, 201–2
  right way of, 201
  safety guidelines for, 197, 198–200
  stationary, 205–6
Black Elementary School, 123–4
body:
  caring for, 326–27
  composition, 21–22, 384
  slamming, 178
Bradley, Bill, 343
Brandon, L. Jerome, 90
Branta, Crystal, 276
breakfasts, 376–77
breaststroke, 234
breathing, 233–34
  belly, 142–43
Brody, Jane, 372
Brown, C. H., 156
Brown, Jonathan, 361–62
Brox, Andrea, 38
Bunker, Linda K., 310
Butcher, Mike, 90
butterfly stroke, 234
Byron, Beverly, 84

calcium, 365
calories, 381
cancer, 291
canoeing, 191–92
carbohydrates, 365, 367
cardiac rehabilitation, 291
cardio-respiratory system:
  cool-down for, 138
  endurance of, 20–21, 154–65
  warm-ups for, 167–68
cardiovascular system, warm-up for, 138
Castelli, William, 15
cat backs, 144, 167
cereals, 366
children, 149–50
  aerobic activities for, 195
  aerobic exercise for, 155–56
  bikes for, 197–98
  competition for, 223–25
  elementary school age, 211–12, 213

encouragement for, 50–56
formula for body weight of, 386
learning to play like, 41
listening to, 361
nutritional tips for, 374–75
nutrition and, 366, 372–75
places to play for, 51
restraining of, 51–52
running and, 207–14, 223–25
running-based fitness programs for, 225
running tests for, 73–74
safety for, 198–200
sixth-grade, 121–22
smoking and, 343–45
spending time with, 360
sports and, 294–313
stress and, 354–58
swimming for, 226–28
unfitness of, 8
walking for, 237–43
walking test for, 71
weight for, 385–86
children, pre-school, 210–11, 253–62
  ages one to two, 256
  ages three to five, 257–58
  birth to one year, 254–56
  exercise programs, 258–61
  records for, 261–62
  terrible twos, 257
children, teenage, 149–51, 212, 213, 263–68
  eating with, 267
  exercising with, 268
  paying attention to, 267
  watching, 266–67
  what we can do for, 265–68
cholesterol, 369–70
Christie, Dame Agatha, 44
Clark, Nancy, 376–77
coaches, 279–80
  code of ethics for, 312–13
Coddington, R. Dean, 355
codes of ethics, 310–13
cold injuries, 330–31
colds, 331
Cole, Desmond, 104, 117
Cole, Jody, 289
Coles, Robert, 361
community, unfitness and, 13–16
competing, 202
  for children, 223–25
  fun racing and, 222–23
  with parents, 214
  in swimming, 228

complex carbohydrates, 365
conditioning, physical, 323–24
cool-downs, 137, 138–39, 150, 169,
    231–32
Cooper, Kenneth, xviii, 4, 6, 21, 24, 39–
    40, 74, 160–61, 183, 187, 189, 335,
    378, 383
cops and robbers, 171
Corbin, Charles, 92
Costill, David, 384
Creath, Curtis, 344
cross-country skiing, 187–89
Cureton, Thomas, 154
curls, 147, 148
    abdominal, 152
    arm, 152

dairy products, 366
dancing, 193–95
    aerobic, 194–95
Davidson, Sandy, 284
DeFrain, John, 378–79
de Groat, Diane, 360
d'Elia, Toshika, 288–89
DeVarona, Donna, 228, 233
diabetes, 292
diet, 366
Dietz, William, 5, 10–11
dinners, 378–79
Disney, Walt, 261
dodgeball, 176
dog stretches, 167
Donna DeVarona's Hydro-Aerobics, 228
Dow, Patty, 261
Down, Linda, 285
drugs, 324
    abuse, 345–48
    education, 113–15
Dybdahl, Thomas, 341
Dyment, Paul, 26, 53–54, 253–54, 260,
    268

eating, 267
    habits, 371–72
    see also nutrition
education, 44–45
    drug, 113–15
    physical, see physical education pro-
        grams
    wellness, 95, 99, 113–16
Eisenhower, Dwight D., 7
Ekblom, B., 156
elephant trunk swings, 167
Elkind, David, 253–54, 259–60
Elkton Elementary School, 128

emergencies, 327–28
emotionally disturbed, exercise programs
    for, 293
encouragement:
    in after-school activities, 55–56
    for children, 50–56
    comparison vs., 52
    of variety of activities, 53–56
endurance:
    cardio-respiratory, 20–21, 154–65
    muscular, 23, 62–69, 145–53
Engh, Fred C., 28, 306
epilepsy, 292
Epstein, Ann, 358
equipment, 216, 234–35, 242–43, 261–
    262, 279
    protective, 324–25
Evans, Raynette, 90
Ewing, Martha, 295
exercise physiology, 113
exerciser's triangle, 37
exercises:
    aerobic, 154–65, 168–69, 194–95
    family, 40–44
    flexibility, 141–42
    principles of, 131–39
    relaxation, 115, 138, 142–43, 166
    strengthening, 138, 167
    stress and, 359–60, 361–62
    stretching, 138, 141, 143–45, 167,
        231–32
    with teenagers, 268
    variation in, 134
    water, 228
exertion, perceived, 165
exploring, 241–42

Fahey, Thomas D., 297
family:
    aerobic, 39–40
    biking for, 203–4
    exercise, 40–44
    fitness evaluation of, 57–78
    involvement of, 37–40
    making quiet time for, 360
    meals and, 375–79
    relaxation and stretching program for,
        142–45
    role of, 33–56
    role of spirituality in, 360–61
    sports days, 319
    strength training program for, 146–49
    walking for, 237–43
fast-break basketball, 177
fast-moving action games, 170–79

fats, 364–65, 367–68
fellowship, 40–41
fiber, 365, 371
field days, 112–13
field sports, 110–12
Figgers, Linda, 124–25
Fisher, Judith Gaston, 122–23
fitness, 40–41
    activities and sports for, 27–30, 105–13
    benefits of, 18–30
    circuit training, 175–76
fitness classes, 107
    freeze aerobics, 169
    for handicapped, 287
    health-related, 20–23
    holistic approach to, 335–48
    meaning of, 18–20
FIT training method, 131–32
flexibility, 22–23, 140–45
    testing of, 61–62
flexibility exercises, 141–42
flu, 331
flutter kick, 232–33
follow the leader, 172
food groups, 366–67
football, Frisbee, 177
forward bends, 231
Fox, Sandy, 284
Frederick, E. C., 245
Freedson, Patty, 16
Fremont, Jim, 199–200
Friedman, Meyer, 352, 358
Frisbee football, 177
fruits, 366–67
fun, 40–41, 222–23

Gabriel, Paul H., 36
Galton, Lawrence, 277–78
games:
    fast-moving action, 170–79
    imaginative, 170–80
    parachute, 173–74
    during walks, 238–41
    winter, 179–80
Garrick, James G., 320
Gillette, Joan V., 321
giraffe neck rolls, 166
girls and women, 269–80
    boys and men vs., 276–80
    exercising quit by, 270–71
    history of athletic programs for, 269–272
    obstacles to, 275–76
    after puberty, 273–74
    before puberty, 272–73

Glueck, Charles J., 372–73
goals, establishment of, 53
Gold, Robert, 3, 13
gorilla pull-ups, 167
Gortmaker, Steven, 5, 10–11
grains, 366
groin stretches, 144
Gugenheim, J. J., 298
gym classes, 110

Haefele, Suzanne, 259
half squats, 148
hamstring muscles, 61, 231
handball, 190–91
hard-easy method, 132–33
Harris, Dorothy, 269, 280
Harris, Louis, 341
Hattner, Jo Ann, 373
Haycock, Christine E., 321
Hayes, Jessie-Lea, 104
head:
    lifters, 148
    rolls, 143
    turns, 232
health, holistic approach to, 335–348
health-impaired, 281–93
    fitness for, 287
    hearing, 288–89
    mainstreaming, 282–83
    orthopedically, 287–88
    visually, 289–90
health-related fitness, 20–23
heart rates, 161–64
heat injuries, 329–30
height charts, 386
Heisel, J. Stephen, 355
Hellstedt, Jon C., 304
Henschen, Keith, 253
Herzog, David, 382
hide-and-seek, 171–72
high-protein foods, 366
hiking, 178, 248–49
Hinkle, Lawrence E., 351
hip flexor, testing minimum strength of, 60
hip stretchers, 144
Hoeft-Varisto, Diane, 123–24
Holmes, Thomas H., 352, 355
home run aerobics, 177
Horizon School, 127
Howell, Mary, 34

ice-skating, 189–90
injuries, 278–79

causes of, 322
    cold, 330–31
    heat, 329–30
    prevention of, 216, 320–31
    R.I.C.E. routine for, 327–28
    supervision and, 325–26
    treatment of, 320–31
    warning signals of, 328–29
innovative school programs, 118–28
iron, 365
Isenberg, Barbara, 210, 360

Jeffords, James, 84
Jenkins, David, 350–51
Johnson, Lyndon B., 7
Joyner-Kersee, Jackie, 291, 293
jumping:
    kangaroo, 173
    rope, 192–93
junk foods, 369

kangaroo jumping, 173
Katz, Jane, 232, 234
keep away, 172
Kennedy, John F., 7–8
Kennedy, Joseph, Jr., 288
Kerry, Robert, 288
Kiesling, Stephen, 245
Kiser, John, 128
kite flying, aerobic, 177
Knack, Danny, 127
kneeling stretches, 144
Koop, C. Everett, 243–45, 364
Kowalski, Robert E., 354–55, 358, 363
Kraus, Hans, viii–xxx, 4, 6–8, 23, 34–
    35, 46–47, 59
Kraus-Weber Tests, 59–61
Kuczen, Barbara, 362
Kugler, Eileen, 378
Kuntzleman, Charles, 5–6, 15, 17, 90,
    156
Kuscsik, Nina, 121, 274
Kwiterovich, Peter, 373

Lappin, Pat, 104–5, 108
lateral raises, 153
Leal Elementary School, 122–23
Lee, Amelia M., 22
leg:
    extensions, 152
    raises, 149
Leon, Jeffrey, 286, 288, 293
Levine, Barbara, 374
lifestyle, unfitness and, 9–11
lifters, head, 148

logrolling, 174
lower back, 61, 231
Lugar, Richard, 18
lunches, nutritious, 115–16, 377–78
lunchroom, wellness education in, 95,
    113–16

McCary, Carolyn, 128
Macdonald, Donald Ian, 267
McInally, Pat, 149
Madden, John, 28–29
making tracks, 179
marching, 169, 248
Marcus, Michael, 126–27
Marshall, John, 278
Martens, Rainer, 29–30, 273
Matthew, Monica, 115–16
Matthews, Karen, 354–55
meals, families and, 375–79
Melleby, Alexander, 59–60
mentally handicapped, exercise programs
    for, 293
menus, 116
Meyer, Roger, 351
Micheli, Lyle, 322
minerals, 368
MiniThons, 121–22
moderation, 135
modified sit-and-reach, 61
modified sit-ups, 64, 147
Murphy, George, 16
muscular strength and endurance, 23,
    145–53
    testing of, 60–61, 62–69
    upper body, 66–68
Myers, Clayton, 380–81

Neeves, Robert, 242
Nelson, Ralph, 381
New York Road Runners Club Run-Easy
    Program, 219–20
Nixon, Richard M., 7
nutrients, 367–68
nutrition, 45–46, 324, 359, 365–79
    in breakfasts, 376–77
    children and, 366, 372–75
    in dinners, 378–79
    families and, 375–79
    good eating habits for, 371–72
    in lunches, 115–16, 377–78
    in model schools, 115–16

obesity, 292–93
obstacle courses, 175
ocean wave running, 178–79

Offer, Daniel, 263
Ojala, Carl, 270
one-and-a-half-mile run-easy program,
    218–19
1-2-3 method, 136–37
ostrich stretches, 167
overhead stretches, 231–32
overload, 131–32
overuse syndrome, 326

Pachter, Harvey, 120–22, 124
Page, Irvine H., 196
Pannell, Marlene, 124
parachute game, 173–74
parents, 150–51, 271–72
    bikes for, 200
    children started early by, 46
    code of ethics for, 312
    competing with, 214
    in model school physical education
        program, 116–17
    physical education in schools and, 83–
        88, 96, 97–102, 116–17
    responsibilities of, 44–50
    as role models, 36–37, 359
    role of, 33–56
    running test for, 74
    sit-ups for, 65
    starting point for, 33–36
    stress and, 352
    unfitness of, 8, 11
    walking test for, 73
    youth sports role of, 309–10
parks, 54–55
Parmalee, Patty Lee, 285
Pate, Russell R., 20
Paterno, Joe, 295
patience, 135
Paty Company, 118–19
peak work, 136–37, 138
pectoral stretches, 144
perceived exertion, 165
physical activity, see activities, physical
physical education programs, 262
    in elementary schools, 87
    fitness testing and reporting in, 93–95,
        98–99, 113
    four cornerstones of, 89–96, 105
    innovative, 118–28
    parents and, 83–88, 96, 97–102, 116–
        117
    physical activities in, 89–93, 97–98
    school model for, 1, 103–17
    in schools, 81–117
    in secondary schools, 87

wellness education and, 95, 99, 113–
    116
physically disabled, exercise programs
    for, 281–93
physiology, exercise, 113
playgrounds, 54–55
Pollitt, Ernesto, 377
pools, 235
pre-exercise health evaluations, 322–23
presses, bench, 152
programs:
    New York Road Runners Club Run-
        Easy, 219–20
    one-and-a-half-mile run-easy, 218–
        219
    pre-school, 258–61
    relaxation and stretching, 142–45
    running-based, for children, 225
    sports, 105–13, 314–19
    strength training, 146–49
    swim-for-fitness, for beginners and in-
        termediates, 230–31
    twenty-minute run-easy, 218
progressive relaxation routines, 139
progressive stress, 132
protein, 366, 368
Prudden, Donald, 197
P.S. 20, 126–27, 118, 124–25
P.S. 118, 124–25
Puffer, James C., 322
Pugliese, Michael, 373
pull-downs, 152–53
pull-ups, 67–69, 148–49
    gorilla, 167
    for upper body strength and endur-
        ance, 67–68
push-ups, 146–47
    for upper body muscular strength and
        endurance, 66–67
    wall, 143–44

races:
    for fun and competition, 222–23
    relay, 174–75
    sled pulling, 179
racewalking, 169, 248
racquetball, 190–91
Rahe, Richard H., 352, 355
raises:
    lateral, 153
    leg, 149
    toe, 153
Reagan, Ronald, 285
recovery, 132–33
regularity, 133–34

relaxation, 362–63
   exercises, 115, 138, 142–43, 166
   routines, 139
   and stretching programs, 142–45
relay races, 174–75
reporting, fitness testing and, 93–95, 98–99
Requa, Ralph K., 320
rewards, establishment of, 53
rhino hip rolls, 167
R.I.C.E. (rest, ice, compression, elevation) routine, 327–28
rock and roll, 173
Roghmann, Klaus J., 351
roller-skating, 189–90
rolls:
   ankle, 144
   giraffe neck, 166
   head, 143
   rhino hip, 167
   shoulder, 232
Rorabacher, Wisty, 254
Rosenberg, Lynn, 345
Rosenman, Ray H., 351
Rotella, Robert J., 312
routines:
   progressive relaxation, 139
   weight training, 151–53
rowing, 191–92
running, 108–10, 207–25, 256
   beginner, 217–21
   children and, 207–14, 223–25
   getting fit with, 217
   intermediate, 221–22
   ocean wave, 178–79
   places for, 213–14
   right way for, 214–16
   shuttle, 178
   speed in, 214
   starting children on, 209–14
   testing of, 73–74

safari aerobics, 168
Sage, John, 90
Salk, Lee, 357
salt, 365, 369
Samuels, Mike, 24–25, 30, 351
Samuels, Nancy, 24, 30, 351
Schlanger, Lou, 125–26
Schlein, Mort, 290
schools:
   activities after, 55–56
   administrations of, 97
   with innovative physical education programs, 118–28

with model physical education programs, 103–17
   philosophies of, 104–5
   physical education in, 81–117
   unfitness and, 12–13
   wellness education in, 95, 113–16
Seaton, Fred, 7
Seefeldt, Vern, 295
Segal, Marilyn, 227
Selye, Hans, 350
Senn, Karen L., 39
Sergeant Slaughter's march, 169
Seward, John, Jr., 119–20
sharing experiences, 135–36
Sheehan, George, 81–82, 331
Shephard, Roy, 27
shortcuts, elimination of, 46–47
shoulder, 231
   rolls, 232
   shrugs, 143
shrugs:
   shoulder, 143
   turtle, 166
shuttle running, 178
sidestroke, 234
Siegel, Judith, 362
Simon says, 173
sit-and-reach modified, 61
sitting stretches, 144–45
sit-ups:
   for adults, 65
   baby bear, 167
   modified, 64, 147
skiing, cross-country, 187–89
sledding:
   races, 179
   uphill, 179
sleep, 324
smokeless tobacco, 343–44
smoking, 342–45
   children and, 343–45
   how to stop, 344–45
   passive, 344
snail slides, 167
snow:
   baseball, 179–80
   shoveling, 180
   tag, 179
soccer, aerobic, 176
Solis, Sharmagne, 125
South Bronx High School, 125–26
South Huntington School District, 120–122
Southside Elementary School, 118–20
specificity, 134

sports, 27–30
  adult coed, 274
  benefits of, 28–30
  dropouts from, 301–2
  field, 110–12
  getting out from, 302–3
  model programs for, 105–13, 314–19
  participation in, 296
  role of parents in, 309–10
  selection of, 298–300
  stress related to, 303–5
  team and lifetime, 56
  when to start playing, 296–98
  winning and losing in, 305–7
  youth and, 294–313
sports clubs, 314–19
  baseball, 315–18
  basketball, 318–19
  organization of, 314–15
sportsmanship, 307–8
Square Deal, 89–96
squash, 190–91
squats, half, 148
standing stretches, 143–44
Stanley, Earl, 156
stationary bikes, 205–6
Stevens, Ted, 84
strength:
  exercises for, 138, 167
  muscular, 23, 62–69, 145–53
  training programs, 146–49
stress:
  adults and, 352
  causes of, 349–51
  children and, 354–58
  dealing with, 358–63
  diseases caused by, 351
  management, 349–63
  progressive, 132
  sports-related, 303–5
stretching exercises, 138, 141, 143–45
  ankle, 231
  dog, 167
  groin, 144
  hip, 144
  kneeling, 144
  ostrich, 167
  overhead, 231–32
  pectoral, 144
  sitting, 144–45
  standing, 143–44
  static, 141
  thigh, 143
Strong, William, 15
sugar, 369

Sweetgall, Robert, 242
swim-for-fitness program, 230–31
swimming, 226–35
  for children, 226–28
  competitive, 228
  getting fit with, 230–31
  right way for, 232–34
  safety guidelines for, 229–30
Switzer, Kathrine, 274
swivels, 143

tag, 170–71, 179
talk test method, 164–65
television watching, 47–49
tennis, 190–91
testing:
  of family fitness, 57–58
  in model school physical education
    program, 113
  in physical education programs, 93–
    95, 98–99, 113
thigh stretches, 143
thinking long term, 49–50
Thomas, Jerry R., 22
Thomas, Katherine T., 22
Thoresen, Carl, 355
three Fs, 40–41
toe raises, 153
Tom Sawyer adventure walks, 178, 241–
  242
touring, 202–3, 248–49
toys, 55
training:
  aerobic, 158–65
  for elementary age and teenagers, 213
  FIT, 131–32
  fitness circuit, 175–76
  frequency in, 159–60
  hard-easy, 132–33
  intensity of, 161–65
  1-2-3, 136–37
  time in, 160–61
  weight, 149–53
Traister, Michael, 259
Traum, Dick, 283–88
triglycerides, 370
trunk flexion, 61–62
tug-of-war, 172–73
turtle shrugs, 166
twenty-minute run-easy program, 218

Ullyot, Joan, 278
unfitness, 3–17
  causes of, 9–16
  challenging, 16–17

history of, 6–8
of parents, 11
of parents vs. children, 8
results of, 4–6
uphill sledding, 179
upper back, testing minimum strength
of, 60
upper body, 231
pull-ups for, 67–68
push-ups for, 66–67

vacations, 248–49
van Aaken, Ernst, 52
Vaughn, Lynne, 14
vegetables, 366
videos, 261–62
vitamins, 365, 368
volleyball, aerobic, 176

walking, 107–8, 236–49, 256
for children and families, 237–43
correctly, 243–44
getting fit with, 244–45
in groups, 242
increasing challenge in, 247–48
places for, 247
special supplies for, 237–38
starting with, 217
testing of, 71–73
times of day for, 245–47
Tom Sawyer adventure, 178, 241–42
wall push-ups, 143–44
warm-ups, 136, 150, 166–68, 231–32
cardio-respiratory, 167–68
cardiovascular, 138
water, 367
aerobic exercise in, 228
Watson, Robert, 263

Weber, Sonja, 6
weight, 360–61
charts, 383, 386
for children, 385–86
formulas, 383
losing, 384–85
management, 380–88
weight training, 149–53
routines, 151–53
workouts, 150–51
wellness education:
in classroom and lunchroom, 95, 99,
113–16
in model school physical education
program, 113–16
see also nutrition
wellness quiz, 337–41
Wells, Christine L., 155–56
whale spouts, 166
Whitley, Jim, 90
Wiegand, Robert, 288, 293
Wilkins, Kaye, 156
Wilmore, Jack, 15
Wilson, Patty, 292
winter games, 179–80
Wolf, Susan, 210
Wolin, Steven J., 378
Wood, Peter, 380
Wooden, John, 306
workouts:
imaginative, 166–69
samples of, 138–39
weight training, 150–51

Yamamoto, Kaoru, 357
Yanker, Gary, 244

Zanga, Joseph, 9, 267

FOR THE BEST IN PAPERBACKS, LOOK FOR THE

In every corner of the world, on every subject under the sun, Penguin represents quality and variety—the very best in publishing today.

For complete information about books available from Penguin—including Pelicans, Puffins, Peregrines, and Penguin Classics—and how to order them, write to us at the appropriate address below. Please note that for copyright reasons the selection of books varies from country to country.

In the United Kingdom: For a complete list of books available from Penguin in the U.K., please write to *Dept E.P., Penguin Books Ltd, Harmondsworth, Middlesex, UB7 0DA.*

In the United States: For a complete list of books available from Penguin in the U.S., please write to *Dept BA, Penguin,* Box 120, Bergenfield, New Jersey 07621-0120.

In Canada: For a complete list of books available from Penguin in Canada, please write to *Penguin Books Ltd, 2801 John Street, Markham, Ontario L3R 1B4.*

In Australia: For a complete list of books available from Penguin in Australia, please write to the *Marketing Department, Penguin Books Ltd, P.O. Box 257, Ringwood, Victoria 3134.*

In New Zealand: For a complete list of books available from Penguin in New Zealand, please write to the *Marketing Department, Penguin Books (NZ) Ltd, Private Bag, Takapuna, Auckland 9.*

In India: For a complete list of books available from Penguin, please write to *Penguin Overseas Ltd, 706 Eros Apartments, 56 Nehru Place, New Delhi, 110019.*

In Holland: For a complete list of books available from Penguin in Holland, please write to *Penguin Books Nederland B.V., Postbus 195, NL-1380AD Weesp, Netherlands.*

In Germany: For a complete list of books available from Penguin, please write to *Penguin Books Ltd, Friedrichstrasse 10-12, D-6000 Frankfurt Main I, Federal Republic of Germany.*

In Spain: For a complete list of books available from Penguin in Spain, please write to *Longman, Penguin España, Calle San Nicolas 15, E-28013 Madrid, Spain.*

In Japan: For a complete list of books available from Penguin in Japan, please write to *Longman Penguin Japan Co Ltd, Yamaguchi Building, 2-12-9 Kanda Jimbocho, Chiyoda-Ku, Tokyo 101, Japan.*